Brown has wrestled with the daunting task of finding language to illuminate what is almost entirely invisible—the prevailing social conditions we are immersed in that promote and foster trauma and traumatization. Those of us in the trauma field are just as submerged in these frameworks as anyone else, blinding us and radically limiting our effectiveness. That Brown took on this challenge in the first place is nothing less than heroic. That she succeeds is awe-inspiring … and, for those who dare to listen to her, powerfully mind-expanding.

—**Steven N. Gold, PhD,** Professor Emeritus, Nova Southeastern University, Fort Lauderdale, FL; licensed clinical psychologist in independent practice, Plantation, FL; author of *Contextual Trauma Therapy* and *Not Trauma Alone*; Editor-in-Chief of the *APA Handbook of Trauma Psychology*; and coeditor of *Dissociation and the Dissociative Disorders*

Brilliant! This book is for everyone interested in healing trauma. Laura S. Brown delivers a powerhouse in decolonizing trauma therapy.

—**Lillian Comas-Díaz, PhD,** Clinical Professor, Department of Psychiatry and Behavioral Sciences, George Washington University, Washington, DC

Kudos to Dr. Laura Brown for her manifesto, *Decolonizing Trauma Healing: Toward a Humble, Culturally Responsive Practice*, in which she builds and expands upon her 40 years' worth of scholarship, clinical and forensic practice, activism, and lived experience in trauma psychology. This book integrates a vast amount of information. It is a call to approach healing interactions with suffering individuals in a more humble, person-centered, and culturally responsive way that centralizes the traumatizing impact of social pathologies associated with colonization. Although as Dr. Brown recognizes, not all will agree with her approach, her ideas deserve close attention as they have the potential to move the frontiers and establish new methods of trauma psychology.

—**Christine A. Courtois, PhD, ABPP,** Delaware Licensed Psychologist and Board-Certified Counseling Psychologist; author of *Healing the Incest Wound: Adult Survivors in Therapy*; coauthor of *Treatment of Complex Trauma: A Sequenced, Relationship-Based Approach*; and coeditor of *Treating Complex Traumatic Stress Disorders in Adults, Second Edition*

W0230594

In this gorgeously written book, Laura S. Brown first exposes the ways the practice of trauma therapy—despite good intentions—has so often colluded with the oppressive and colonizing forces inherent in the harm of trauma. Then she offers an alternative approach for healers, one that humbly and repeatedly examines the political, intersectional, existential, and neurobiological realities that are inextricably linked to trauma harm and trauma healing. Once you start reading you won't want to put it down, because *Decolonizing Trauma Healing* is deliciously eloquent, brilliant, wise, and teeming with authenticity and compassion.

—**Jennifer Joy Freyd, PhD,** Professor Emerit, Psychology, University of Oregon, Eugene

Decolonizing
Trauma Healing

Decolonizing Trauma Healing

Toward a Humble, Culturally Responsive Practice

Laura S. Brown

 AMERICAN PSYCHOLOGICAL ASSOCIATION

Published by
American Psychological Association
750 First Street, NE
Washington, DC 20002
https://www.apa.org

Order Department
https://www.apa.org/pubs/books
order@apa.org

Typeset in Charter and Interstate by Circle Graphics, Inc., Reisterstown, MD

Printer: Sheridan Books, Chelsea, MI
Cover Designer: Gwen J. Grafft, Minneapolis, MN

Library of Congress Cataloging-in-Publication Data

Names: Brown, Laura S., author. | American Psychological Association.
Title: Decolonizing trauma healing : toward a humble, culturally responsive
  practice / Laura S. Brown.
Description: Washington, DC : American Psychological Association, [2025] |
  Includes bibliographical references and index.
Identifiers: LCCN 2024009937 (print) | LCCN 2024009938 (ebook) |
  ISBN 9781433840630 (paperback) | ISBN 9781433840647 (ebook)
Subjects: LCSH: Psychotherapy. | Mental health.
Classification: LCC RC480 .B73 2025 (print) | LCC RC480 (ebook) |
  DDC 616.89--dc23/eng/20240613
LC record available at https://lccn.loc.gov/2024009937
LC ebook record available at https://lccn.loc.gov/2024009938

https://doi.org/10.1037/0000421-000

Printed in the United States of America

10 9 8 7 6 5 4 3 2 1

Contents

Acknowledgments

In all of my years as an author I have rarely had a book that felt so large, with ideas that seemed difficult to tame and organize. No surprise, because every time I stopped for a month to write, I had read something new or the world had blown up in another terrible way. If it were not for Krissy Jones, editor extraordinaire, this book would have remained incoherent and disorganized. Were it not for her encouragement, her humor, and her willingness to genuinely collaborate with me, I might have given up due to what felt like the sheer magnitude of editing my allegedly final draft of this book. I bow deeply in gratitude to her; every author should be so fortunate as to have an editor this excellent.

I am also thankful to Meghan Quinn and the entire team of copy editors at Circle Graphics for tightening up my language, tracking down obscure references, and in general making me sound like someone who can write sentences that are not, like this one, run-ons. Editors are the lifeblood of academic writing, and they rarely get top billing in the Acknowledgments section of books.

I am alive to write these words thanks to my oncology team: Kim Gittere Abson, MD, my outpatient dermatologist, who decided from the outset, when she first diagnosed that cancer in January 2019, that I would not be her first patient to die of melanoma and who, in 2021, proposed the innovative treatment plan that has so far saved my life; Ata Moshiri, MD, whose skilled hands administered the most painful and healing injections in the world and who is a true healer as a human; Heidi Gray, MD, a thoughtful gynecological oncologist whose hands did their best to scar my body the least; Shailender Bhatia, MD, my primary oncologist, whose calm in the face of my terror has allowed me to move through the past 4 years of utter ambiguity about life and death; and all of the nursing staff, medical assistants, and receptionists at the Fred Hutchinson Cancer Center who accompanied me on this terrible path. I wouldn't have been here to write this book were it not for these skilled, smart people.

Thanks to the prophets: Paula Caplan, of blessed memory; Judith Lewis Herman; Mary Harvey; and Hannah Lerman, who taught me theory and who is the real mother of feminist therapy. To my elders and mentors, Florence Denmark, Nancy Felipe Russo, Lenore Walker, and Adrienne Smith of blessed memory.

Thanks to my sisters and brothers who I have found and embraced along the way: Lillian Comas-Díaz, Christine Courtois, Constance Dalenberg, Steven Neal Gold, Beverly Greene, Doug Haldeman, Ellyn Kaschak, Kathryn Norsworthy, Maria P. P. Root, and Mavis Tsai. A special thanks to my wing-women, Jennifer Joy Freyd and Kat Quina, the email triad that's been with each other for 3 decades. All of you have had a part in holding me up, sustaining me, teaching me, and getting me through hard times.

Thanks to my sisters from my earliest years in this endeavor of subverting the dominant paradigm, Nechama Liss-Levinson and Cynthia Villis, members of the Women's Caucus at Southern Illinois University, who have returned to my life in recent years. May you both live long and healthy lives.

Thanks to Flora Ostrow and Bobbie Stewart-Larson, who kept me sane during my VA internship and have gone on to become some of my longest and truest friends. Bobbie, I particularly appreciate what you have taught me about the subversive possibilities inherent in appearing to be normal; wow, did you fool them!

Thanks to the poets: Audre Lorde of blessed memory, Adrienne Rich of blessed memory, Mary Oliver, Joni Mitchell, Leonard Cohen of blessed memory, the various writers of the psalms of my people's scriptures; may you all rest in power, and Joni Mitchell, may you go forward in power. All of your works have inspired me and taught me how to think about pain and joy and healing.

Thanks to my aikido practice, to Kimberly Richardson Sensei, who created a dojo in which I could be a clumsy 50-year-old woman and be welcomed, and find my grounding and my joy. Thanks to my aikido community for holding me up during some spectacularly challenging times in my life; in particular thanks to my training partners Dennis Johnson, Regina LaGalbo, Jessica Levin, Michelle Pleasant, Mary Childs, and the many, many more whose names I cannot think of to list right now. Deep gratitude to Mary Heiny Sensei, who is the grandmother of my aikido lineage, and from whom I have the pleasure of continuing to learn directly. Mary Sensei decolonized the male-dominated world of aikido in ways that will reverberate through generations of aikido practitioners.

Thanks to my students, in particular Tyson Bailey, Marta Miranda, Joanne Sparrow, Micheal Kane, Michal Goldring-Keidar, and Samantha Slaughter, for teaching me how to be the best possible decolonial feminist teacher and supervisor. Special appreciation to my growing number of students in the People's Republic of China who read my work, sought me out, and are making decolonial feminist therapy a growing movement there in the face of growing suppression of feminist thought. They are brave, and brilliant.

Thanks to the many people who allowed me to be their healer. I cannot name you. I can only bow humbly to you in gratitude.

I learned a lot about trauma and healing in my own life from my more than 2 decades with my former wife, Lynn Brem, and especially about the challenges of living with and relating to neurodiversity. Much of what I have mentioned about that topic would not be in this book were it not for her. For that education, I am grateful.

As I write these words, the U.S. is less than 24 hours post the 34 guilty verdicts in the trial of the 45th President. I never thought I would live to see the day. I am thankful to the universe for allowing me to be alive to see this act of courage and wisdom on the part of ordinary people, taking power into their hands and trusting their abilities to know truth, and speak it to power.

Some of the early groundwork for this book was laid during the research and writing of my chapter, "Contributions of Feminist and Critical Psychologies to Trauma Psychology," which was published in Gold's *APA Handbook of Trauma Psychology: Foundations in Knowledge* in 2017.

Decolonizing
Trauma Healing

INTRODUCTION

We Meet Again

My heart is moved by all I cannot save: so much has been destroyed. I have to cast my lot with those who age after age, perversely, with no extraordinary power, reconstitute the world.

—Adrienne Rich, "Natural Resources"[1]

Not everything that is faced can be changed, but nothing can be changed until it is faced.

—James Baldwin, "As Much Truth as One Can Bear," *New York Times,* January 14, 1962

There is a crack, a crack in everything / That's how the light gets in.

—Leonard Cohen, "Anthem"

---

[1]"Natural Resources", from THE DREAM OF A COMMON LANGUAGE: Poems 1974-1977 by Adrienne Rich. Copyright © 1978 by W. W. Norton & Company, Inc. Used by permission of W. W. Norton & Company, Inc.

https://doi.org/10.1037/0000421-001
Decolonizing Trauma Healing: Toward a Humble, Culturally Responsive Practice,
by L. S. Brown

What is this book about, and why am I writing it now? It's about my attempt to develop a new paradigm—or perhaps to resurrect and reshape a very old paradigm—for how psychologists and those in related fields work with people whose lives, psyches, and souls have been affected by exposure to trauma. We, by which I mean you and me both, have been trained to think of trauma in ways that I have, over many years, come to find unhelpful, in large part because they are grounded in what can be described as "colonizing" epistemologies—ways of thinking about trauma and its healing that derive from models that pathologize those who suffer and that in turn are founded on Eurocentric models of human distress.

Why now? This book, which grew from the soil of my last foray into this topic as well as from everything I have been learning and doing since, reflects the depth and growth of thinking in both liberation psychology and the understanding of trauma, and of much human experience. While in the past the notion that trauma was a biopsychosocial/existential phenomenon had come to be generally accepted by most people working with trauma, our understanding as a field of the first part of that adjective, more specifically, of the neurobiological aspects of our responses to trauma, has become elaborated and sophisticated in the past 2 decades. Simultaneously, our understanding of how people's lived experiences, the lenses created by the many social locations that each person occupies and the identities that arise from those intersecting locations, has also become deeper and more sophisticated. The psychosocial part of that description of trauma now includes, for me, a consideration of how experiences of being colonized in the broadest possible meaning of that term have informed human psychosocial realities, which then interact with neurobiological trauma responses in a continuous iterative fashion in each person—and for the purposes of this book, each person exposed to trauma.

How is this different from any other contemporary exploration of trauma? My hope is that I may invite you, dear readers, to take a critical look at the entire field of trauma therapy through the lens I am offering here, the stance of being decolonial. This word gets tossed around a lot in the early years of this decade, so let me be clear about my use of the term. To be decolonial in the work of trauma healing does not mean that we are looking only at trauma in people who were colonized, within the past half millennium, by European powers, although the work done by decolonial scholars forms an epistemic foundation for how I have come to think about changing trauma practice. Rather, what I mean by this term is that we who work with traumatized people re-center our narratives, our authorities, and our paradigms for healing wounded souls outside of the matrices of systemic forms of marginalization and subjugation, interrogating the Eurocentrism that has plagued all of psychology and expanding our perspectives on what we mean by trauma and its healing.

I will invite you to learn how to detect the many ways in which our work of healing trauma has been intellectually colonized, because to become aware of this is central to understanding how to work differently. It is my contention that both our understanding of what constitutes trauma and our paradigms for how to assist suffering persons have been insidiously invaded and deformed by the norms of a dominant, Eurocentric culture, one that is so pervasive that it has been difficult, until very recently, even for those of us at its margins, to appreciate how fully it has permeated our work. This Eurocentric standpoint is defined by structural and systemic forms of oppression, hierarchies of devaluation that are so built into the culture as to be nearly invisible to those who sit at its center, although they are painfully palpable to anyone on the margins. This hegemonic Eurocentric epistemic framework functions to exclude and stigmatize other worldviews and to overtly or subtly dehumanize colonized and marginalized persons, a group that includes suffering, trauma-exposed people.

I refer to this culture as a Eurocentric one in that it derives from the values and practices of the Christian Europeans who physically colonized the Western Hemisphere and much of the Global South from 1492 through the present time. It is a worldview whose descendants constitute a shrinking numerical majority of people living in the United States at the present, as well as an also shrinking majority of people working in the field of trauma healing.

There is nothing wrong per se with the Christian Eurocentric perspective when we identify it as simply one among many ways of knowing, no better nor worse than others. The problem for trauma healing is that it has been imposed upon the rest of the world as a universal norm. In the field of trauma healing, it is intellectually and epistemically hegemonic. Because trauma truly is a universal human experience occurring in all places, to people of the entire range of worldviews and not only those organized around Christian Eurocentric epistemics, this colonized paradigm for responding to trauma introduces problematic dynamics of domination and subjugation arising from actual colonization that are inimical to a healing process.

To decolonize trauma healing is to uncover the presence of intellectual colonization and remove its influences, like the toxic shards of structural oppression that they are, from the ways in which we see and understand what constitutes trauma, doing what Bhatia (2021) refers to as "epistemic disobedience." It requires removing the Christian Eurocentric epistemic lenses that distort how we encounter and describe trauma-exposed suffering humans, as well as how we name and frame the roles that we play in the healing process.

Ultimately, this book is about overthrowing the intellectual overlords who have ruled our understanding of human distress, thanking them for their service, as this rule has been well-intended and at least served to put trauma into the lexicon of modern mental health. This book argues that we are ready to replace "trauma therapy as usual" with something that I hope will be different.

That different thing is what I am calling a decolonized, humble, culturally responsive set of healing epistemologies and methods, the decolonial, humble, culturally responsive (DHCR) model of trauma healing practice. This is a construct I will address in detail in Chapter 1. While I am proposing a name for the purposes of my discussion, I want to be clear that I am not inventing or discovering something here. It is simply a name that I find useful to describe this kind of practice which has emerged from my own continuing process of decolonization.

IT COULD HAVE BEEN OTHERWISE

I would not be writing this book if some of the earlier visionaries of trauma healing had been the ones whose voices were loudest as the field developed. I want to single out three people occupying the mainstream of the world of emotional healing, colleagues whose work, in my opinion, pointed toward the nonpathologizing constructs that I discuss in this volume. They are not the only ones; they are simply the ones whose work informs me that our field might have gone in a different direction.

W. H. R. Rivers

One might suppose that identifying a man who appeared on the surface to be the epitome of the colonizer mentality as a visionary figure in a decolonial analysis of trauma healing would mean that I had missed something important. And it is true that his intersectional identities were about as rooted in colonizer culture as one might find: a British army officer who had done anthropological work in the Global South during a period when the colonial view of "primitive" people prevailed in that discipline. He worked in a hospital for officers debilitated by shell shock in the First World War.

This makes him an excellent example of how not to be distracted by what we initially see. Both Judith Herman, more than 30 years ago, and Kay Redfield Jameson (2023), in her most recent work, have identified Rivers as a potentially revolutionary voice in working with trauma-exposed people. But had I not encountered him in the early pages of Herman's *Trauma and Recovery* (1992), I would never have heard of him because his vision died with him in 1922, to be supplanted by the problematic psychoanalytic constructions of trauma that I will explore later in this volume.

What made Rivers an ancestor of decolonial trauma healing? Several things. First, he adamantly opposed labeling the traumatized men he worked with as having something wrong with them. He was clear—the problem was that they had been witnesses to horrors, to the explosions of the bodies of their comrades, to the utter unpredictability and persistent life-threatening nature of a war that was interspersed with periods of boredom that gave illusions of safety. He saw these men as wounded, traumatized, but not as having something about themselves that was pathological.

This viewpoint was deeply countercultural in his time, given that most similarly traumatized soldiers were socially constructed as malingerers or cowards, if they were fortunate not to be executed by their superior officers for their inability to continue to fight. Rivers located the problem in the social pathology of war, although he did not frame war in those terms. He simply could see that being exposed to combat was the problem that his patients faced. Ironically, because he was a military physician, his job was to get his patients to the point where they could return to the battlefield, a painful paradox that has persisted for those assigned the task of patching up traumatized warriors through the present time.

The second facet of Rivers's role as an ancestor of decolonial trauma healing was how he approached the work. His approach with his patients was to be their witness, to listen to them. He did not see his job as interpreting dreams or delving into childhood experiences that might be symbolized by the trauma of exposure to this war. He valued the importance of exploring the moral wounds and apparently insoluble existential and spiritual dilemmas that were a component of his patients' suffering (Rivers, 1918).

Because Rivers's best-known patient was the British poet Siegfried Sassoon, we also know a great deal about the lived experience of being Rivers's patient. While various aspects of cultural privilege created the space for Sassoon's voice to be heard, not the least of which was his membership in the upper classes of British society and his prewar reputation as a poet of merit, his accounts of Rivers are decolonial because they center the voice and lived experience of the suffering person, Sassoon himself.

Consequently, we can know that Rivers did not simply preach the ideas of nonpathologizing a trauma response, nor those of listening carefully to the meaning of the trauma in the life of the suffering person. We can follow Sassoon's process through his work with Rivers and notice how true to those values this healer remained, despite the enormous pressures on him to conform himself and his work to the needs of the military establishment of which he was a part.

More than half a century later the trauma healers working with those harmed by the coups and dirty wars in Chile and Argentina would write about the use of testimonio, a construct I will explore in depth later in this book. *Testimonio* is the simple bearing of witness, listening to the traumatized person as long as needed for them to tell their story. Rivers (1918) appears to have done just that—or at least he did so with Sassoon and wrote about the importance of so doing.

Rivers, who had dealt with health problems of his own for most of his life, did not live long enough to advance his vision for what trauma healing might be, dying of a strangulated hernia in 1922. His methods, which came to be known as humane ways of responding to those traumatized by war, continued to be used by those he had taught and to be written of by those he had worked with. But the entire topic of trauma, and Rivers's predecolonial paradigm for understanding it and working as a healer, vanished from the narrative of the growing field of psychotherapy.

Jameson (2023) has written a full account of Rivers's life and his work with Sassoon, which, even more than Herman's (1992) briefer dive, describes his role as a progenitor of the modern field of trauma healing. This chapter of her book, which aligns with my own standpoint that humans have been seeking healing for suffering souls long before that work was colonized, is worth exploring for today's psychotherapists attempting to transform ourselves into DHCR trauma healers. Reading about Rivers's struggles to become the predecolonial healer he was has also been a source of grief for me about what might have been.

Judith Lewis Herman

Judith Herman's work has always been, at its core, decolonial. Her courage in exposing the realities of incest and her visionary description, as early as 1992, of the phenomenon she called "complex trauma," emerged from a clear and unstinting analysis of the politics of how people were traumatized and how traumatized people were marginalized among sufferers. *Trauma and Recovery* (Herman, 1992) was a shining beacon, a volume both scholarly and yet founded in her witness to the lived experiences of suffering, trauma-exposed people. While trained in psychiatry, she brooked its conventions; her feminist and other social justice commitments have always been primary in her writings and her work.

Herman (1992) has consistently defined trauma as a problem of what I call social pathologies, the effects of exposure to systemic and structural forms of oppression experienced at the individual level. And this was not a popular viewpoint. Biological psychiatry was emerging as the winner in the intellectual conversation about human experience, neuroscience was supplanting psychology, the notion being that the best understanding of human experience would emerge from brain science, with little to no reference to the larger political context in which that brain was living.

Herman was also sidelined from the discourse by her own physical trauma. Her friends and colleagues knew what she disclosed in detail in an interview published in the *New York Times* in April 2023 (Barry, 2023)—that since 1994, not long after *Trauma and Recovery* had been published, she has been struggling with chronic pain caused by an accident suffered during a speaking engagement. In the era before the internet and videoconferencing, at a time when to become more powerful in one's field entailed giving keynotes, in person, at conferences all around the world, she became unable to be present. Pain is also no friend to creativity, to writing, to engaging with the realm of ideas.

I have a vivid recollection of one of the last times I spent with her in person, in the period between the publication of her book and her injury. We, with several other feminist trauma workers, were sitting in a café in Amsterdam, where an international trauma conference was taking place. I was, of course, quite in awe of her and soaked up the discussion that she was spearheading about the debate as to how to name, and if to pathologize, the ways in which people who had survived repeated, usually developmentally early, trauma exposures suffered and functioned in the world.

At that same conference I was witness to an extraordinary debate about what precisely constituted trauma, a debate that exemplified, in retrospect, the tensions between a Eurocentric colonizer model and a decolonial, politically conscious one. At the time, trauma was officially defined as being outside the realm of usual human experience, frightening or threatening to almost anyone (American Psychiatric Association, 1987). One after another, the feminists, including Herman, and the Latin Americans in the room, rose to challenge this notion, to speak to the fact that trauma was not "outside the realm" but rather ubiquitous. A voice speaking to retain the official definition was that of one of the founders of the scientific society, a white-skinned European from a nation that had been colonized by its neighbors and occupied by the Nazi invaders during his youth; in other words, a person who was a survivor of the trauma of that brutal occupation and perhaps the generations of trauma of being a subjugated people.

Yet his message was that he could not bear to imagine living in a world in which trauma was not outside the realm of usual human experience. His impassioned plea to keep trauma defined as something not systemic, as something to which most humans would respond in the same manner, exemplifies the intellectual hegemony of the colonized narrative that has gone on to pervade the field of trauma studies despite tweaks to the official definition of a "real trauma," a debate I revisit throughout the volume.

Herman's work (1992), in which she lays out the essentially political and universal nature of trauma and traces that idea from Rivers to the time of her own writing, was profoundly decolonial well before anyone was using that term. She, like Rivers before her, drew upon the lived experiences of the people with whom she worked, mostly women and girls who had been sexually abused or assaulted, as her most important source of information about what a person in the role of trauma healer could do to alleviate suffering or to worsen it. The three-phase model of trauma healing, which she developed together with her colleague at the Victims of Violence program, feminist psychologist Mary Harvey (1996), a paradigm that has come to be the standard of care in this work, is an example of how what she wrote channeled the voices of the people she worked with. She was clear about patriarchy's role in the enormity of the problem of the sexual violation of women's and girls' bodies.

Having her body's suffering pull her off the stage just at the point where the field was defining itself created a vacuum into which others came, bearing biological psychiatry and exposure therapies for the alleged anxiety disorder that was called posttraumatic stress disorder. I hope that what follows in this book honors her vision, because it has always informed my own thinking. What would the field of trauma healing look like today had she not had to leave center stage? I imagine it would not need very many of the ideas in this book.

Yael Danieli and Intergenerational Trauma

The last marginalized visionary of modern-day trauma work who I want to discuss is Yael Danieli, who studied people like herself, children of survivors of the Shoah, better known as the Holocaust. While her work was lauded and visible in the very early years of the rediscovery of trauma, the importance of her uncovering the ways in which trauma need not be directly experienced but can become part of the relational and attachment experiences of those born to traumatized people (Danieli, 1980) has been curiously sidelined. Even the decolonial trauma healing literature, which refers explicitly to this construct that she first described and named, and to which she devoted her life's work, does not reference her as among the first voices on this matter, or even reference her at all as far as I have been able to find (cf. Comas-Diaz, Adames, & Chavez-Dueñas, 2024).

I have wondered if perhaps this occurred in part because most of the people she was writing about, herself included, had pale skin and both lived and died in Europe. Although the Jews of whom she wrote were not European colonizers but rather chronically oppressed and subjected to genocidal terror in

Europe for almost 2,000 years, it may be possible that the location of their exile from their Indigenous homeland excluded them from the decolonial discussions of intergenerational trauma that have followed.

Because her work preceded that of the earliest non-Western Indigenous decolonial authors in the field of trauma, whose work she promoted and included in volumes she edited (e.g., Danieli, 1998) and which work is often cited by current authors in the field of decolonial healing (e.g., Duran et al., 1998), her present-day near-invisibility, combined with what I experience as the marginalization of decolonial and non-Western Indigenous voices in the trauma healing field, has led to failures in understanding that trauma takes many forms, not all of which involve direct exposure to terrifying experiences. While Danieli did not formally conceptualize her work in this way, she in fact documented the effects on attachment systems that grew between children born to Shoah survivors and their parents (Danieli, 1980), a prescient vision of the phenomenon of attachment trauma that is now more widely accepted as part of the larger phenomenon of complex trauma.

Again, the question—what would the field of trauma healing look like if, rather than exoticizing Danieli's work as specific to one small group of people, Jews who had against all odds survived the death camps and then gone on to become parents, and the children born to those parents, applauding her, and moving elsewhere, this experience of intergenerational trauma, which is how systemic and structural social pathologies manifest everywhere, had become central to how trauma was understood?

This is not to say that there have not been many other visionaries in the world of trauma healing whose insights align with a DHCR paradigm and who yet were marginalized in some way by the mainstream of the trauma treatment world. These three, in particular Herman and Danieli, have greatly inspired my thinking. The question of "what if" leads inevitably to the next question: How is a decolonial trauma healing paradigm not just a fancy new name this author has made up?

My belief is that what I am going to spend the rest of this book talking about with you, dear readers, is not simply a fancy new name. As I notice my own struggles over the several years it has taken me to write this book, my own encounters with constructs that I then must interrogate and reconsider, I've had the experience of finding myself thrust into profoundly different ways of thinking about the suffering people I have been encountering in my work as I have been writing. When I talk about trauma with colleagues who are my friends, I notice myself chafing at typical ways of talking about people's distress, and, I hope, politely becoming a trauma world version of the person who says "may" instead of "can" (which I already am, thanks to my beloved eighth and ninth grade English teacher), substituting "distress" for "diagnosis" as we speak, then noticing what happens when I persistently do this, to me, to the interaction, with my colleagues.

TRAUMA IS AND IS NOT THE SAME

I started my last book on trauma work by stating that "trauma is, at the core, simply trauma" (Brown, 2008, p. 3). That was a naïve statement, one reflecting a colonized mindset in myself of which I was not yet aware. Even as I attempted to demonstrate in that book that intersectional identities, culture, context, history, and the relationship of the source of the trauma to the traumatized person matter deeply to how therapists ought to respond to that traumatized person, I was still trapped in what I now think was an archaic way of understanding the complexities of such psychic wounds. The last decade and a half have decolonized me a bit.

My ability to deeply appreciate the effects of the pathological social context was limited by the ways in which medical models leading to the professionalization of healing, making it the sole province of licensed mental health professionals, had colonized and limited my own capacities to think sufficiently radically about trauma healing. I thought one could become "competent," which stance reflected my own positionalities as a light-skinned, upper-middle-class, licensed, doctoral professional, as well as the ways in which my profession, psychology, spoke of responding more compassionately to marginalized people. The American Psychological Association has, after all, developed guideline after guideline for competent practice with an ever larger set of marginalized groups of humans (American Psychological Association, 2017b). As a psychologist emerging from that tradition, I even thought that we could use the *Diagnostic and Statistical Manual of Mental Disorders* and the framework of trauma response as pathology to respond to traumatized people in a competent manner. I was wrong about both of those assumptions. That's fine; one cannot know what one could not yet know, or could not yet allow oneself to know.

What was I right about? Quite a bit, and that carries over into this volume. I was right that intersectional identities are the intrapsychic and interpersonal lenses through which our bodies' responses to trauma are experienced, a construct foundational to DHCR practices. I was right that intersectionalities inform the ways in which a person experiences an event as traumatic, frames how they express themselves and their pain in the interpersonal field. As I wrote then, "trauma and its psychic aftereffects have a texture. The experience conveys meanings that derive from personal histories, cultural heritages, and the social, political, and spiritual contexts in which the painful event happens" (Brown, 2008, p. 3). I was right about the fact that everyone working with traumatized people needed to pay attention to those textures. I was right that every human has a neurobiology that responds in particular ways to particular kinds of trauma and that our neurobiological responses are simply human. I was right that trauma is a biopsychosocial/existential-spiritual phenomenon and that it is also a political phenomenon.

I didn't know enough then about the depth and breadth of that neurobiology to understand the degree to which the nature of response to trauma is all about that very human set of nerves at work. I failed to comprehend the magnitude of the problem I was attempting to address when I took on the problem of being culturally competent, nor even the problematic nature of referring to the possibility of a trauma healer (psychotherapist) achieving competence as a final and fixed state of affairs. I probably still don't quite get how big it all is. Humility, accountability, and repair are the types of competence that have become my guiding principles as I attempt to unpack colonizing forces.

I am grateful to the events in the world that have happened in the 17 years since I sat in my living room with a now long-dead therapy dog and wrote that book, to the thinkers and writers, to the activists and truth-tellers, to the colleagues and wounded people, who have expanded my outlook in the intervening years. I am even grateful to the tyrants, the strongmen, the fascists, the insurrectionists, the rogue law enforcement officers, to those whose sometimes all-too-public infliction of trauma on both the individual and cultural levels have taught me about how badly injured most of those people are too.

In this volume, which is not so much a revision as it is a successor to *Cultural Competence in Trauma Therapy* (Brown, 2008), I am attempting to propose a radical reconceptualization of the work of healing psychic trauma. I am also proposing a radical reconceptualization of what trauma is and how its wounds manifest. I am inviting you, my readers, to consider adopting a profound shift in the paradigm by which I and many others working with wounded souls have been guided until recently.

I am not the only person steeped in the world of trauma who is having this transformation of viewpoint. I apologize in advance if what I have to say here appears too closely to echo other work emerging at this potentially revolutionary moment for our species and the work of healing trauma. Many of us working with traumatized persons are having these insights simultaneously, reading each other's work (or not), and coming to very similar conclusions.

This paradigm shift in my own understanding of how healers, who like all humans are likely to be wounded by trauma themselves (Coale, 1998; Rippere & Williams, 1987), can develop genuinely healing relationships with other suffering humans mirrors other tectonic plate movements occurring in the social domains of the planet, as well as in the climatological realities that surround us in every moment we are alive. Without those enormous changes around me, I might never have had the words to describe what I hope is a decolonial, humble, culturally responsive—DHCR—model for how trauma might be healed.

How do we heal trauma even as its causes remain ubiquitous and persistent, even as the presence of trauma is continuous, even as most trauma is not behind us but with us as our constant companion? I don't think I can answer this question. I do believe that working from a decolonial standpoint might at least move the needle forward a bit toward an answer.

A New Way of Thinking About Competence

This book is not about becoming culturally competent because that notion of being able to achieve competence is, as noted in the first chapter, simply a shield behind which I and our field have protected ourselves from looking at our own collaboration with social pathologies. If we name ourselves competent, as if that is a finished state of being in which we can put ourselves forward into the world as expert, we can avoid knowing how many current models of responding to traumatized people collude with the fiction that trauma is a rare event and that the pathology is in the distressed person, not in the systemic and structural forms of oppression that do harm.

The construct of competence as it is commonly utilized, which I once embraced and wrote of, has, I now believe, been a way to bow to the existence of external phenomena that affect how humans experience things as traumatic while continuing to promote treatment modalities that in no way take those external realities fully into account nor do anything to overthrow those structural and systemic forms of oppression—although, to be fair, so many of us are direct targets of those systems that we often don't have enough energy to do our healing work, raise the next generation, care for elders, and in our alleged free time foment revolution. Cultural competence has been a hand waving at the ethics codes that say that therapists should be competent. But competent at what? And competency demonstrated how? This term is a terrifically misleading one; I want healers working with traumatized humans to be deeply steeped in knowledge about what trauma can be and how its wounds can manifest. I want those healers to have a humble, decolonial, culturally responsive practice, not to have taken a course and received a certificate and, based on that, declared themselves competent

Competence is consequently a moving target because intersectionality changes all colonized assumptions about separateness of group identities and experiences, allowing understanding of trauma to deepen and the way in which its wounds manifest to become ever more sophisticated. Competence as a finished product is thus unachievable because the very construct of competence as a finished product of a certain kind of education or training arises from a particular cultural model of who can be a healer, that is, someone who has studied the right things, jumped through the right hoops, and demonstrated an ability to say that they knew certain things, gotten the letters after their name or the certificate from a trauma guru on their way. This is not how I define competence, which would be demonstrated by the humble ability to sit in silent compassion, deeply honored, while a person in pain sobs for hours.

The woman who wrote *Cultural Competence in Trauma Therapy* and taught people how to practice in a culturally competent way now stands humbly before you to say: No. I allowed myself to be misled by the notion of competence as it is typically defined. I was seduced by my desire to simultaneously fit into my field while attempting to reform it from within. "Reform" is the problematic word; we did not then nor do we now need reform. We need to dissolve the old structures, with thanks and appreciation to what we could know and a filter that removes the toxins from the residue, so that we can build something from different materials entirely. Trauma healers must be competent; our competence requires something other than the ability to answer the questions to get credit for an online continuing education class.

Evidence? Whose Evidence?

In *Cultural Competence in Trauma Therapy* I was still giving some time and energy to a discussion of evidence-based treatments. It's not that I won't do that at all this time around, because there is evidence of a particular type that some of these healing modalities are helpful to some people who've experienced some kinds of things that I include within the broader rubric of trauma. I'm going to put my discussion of these interventions into some very different contexts than I did before. I will ask if a particular intervention supports a DHCR and relationally grounded trauma healing model that empowers sufferers to understand how they are not the problem and to see the presence of the social pathologies that have harmed them. I will allow you, my readers, to use your own critical thinking capacities to make decisions about what to incorporate into your work. I will be proposing some criteria of my own for whether or not your favorite trauma healing practice could be DHCR to aid you in making that assessment or in figuring out how to modify your practice to become closer to a DHCR paradigm.

In the interim since I first attempted to place trauma into the context of what is now called intersectional identities, the movement to decolonize the entire practice of healing of wounded souls (psychotherapy) rose out of its small corner in the universe of the discourses of the critical psychologies, among which my planet of intersectional liberatory feminist psychology has long rotated, and began to take what I consider to be its rightful and more central place in the discussion about what we're doing in our therapy offices. Decolonial psychology is the child of liberation and liberatory psychologies (Comas-Díaz & Torres Rivera, 2020), which are in turn the steps past the paradigm of cultural competence in psychotherapy, something that the person who coined that phrase now refers to as "cultural complexities" (Hays, 2022). As noted earlier, I have discarded "competence" in order to focus on humble, culturally responsive work with trauma as it emerges through people's intersectional identities. The intersectional identities generated by trauma are definitely complexities and not simply cultural ones.

YOUR AUTHOR'S INTERSECTIONAL IDENTITIES

So, who is writing this book? I believe it is useful to know an author's standpoints and biases. It is impossible for a human to be free of bias because we have a limbic system that adds spice and flavor and bias and meaning to the facts trickling through our so-much-slower frontal cortex. As I noted too many times to count in everything I've written in the last 4 decades, and will likely say again for as many years as I am given the opportunities to do so, neutrality and objectivity do not exist. They are the names given to the standpoints and biases of people who identify with dominant social pathologies, in my opinion, and who thus pretend to have no bias because their own blends into the background of the dominant culture.

I've left quite a bit of information about me along the way in everything I've written before. I still want to see if I can get the picture as fully drawn as possible in this book before you keep on reading. I can write this with ease, at last, because by the time this book is published I will no longer be practicing forensic psychology and thus no longer have to deal with accusations of bias from attorneys who are in denial about everyone having biases, just so long as they have a brain (no attorney jokes here, please, some of my best friends, as they say).

So, what are the component parts of Laura? I am a secular Jew of Eastern European origin, for whom the continued existence of Israel is existentially necessary and the rights of the Palestinian people to their own free and democratic state is also existentially necessary. I am a natal woman with a somewhat feminine of center gender presentation of the academic/old hippie, no makeup or high heels variety. I am not typically able in my body in several ways: I have spent most of my time in retirement from clinical practice dealing with a cancer that is so rare that there is no standard protocol for treating it; cancer, unlike response to trauma, is a pathology. As I write this in early 2024 I have been in remission for a year and hope to remain so well past this book's publication. As I edit this book, I am once again experiencing spasmodic dysphonia, a dysfunction of the nerve to my vocal chords that makes speaking difficult, an ironic affliction for a person who talks for her living.

I am a lesbian who came out in the early 1970s. I was raised in, and have always lived in close proximity to, the financial comfort that I now enjoy (being a poor student in grad school does not count because I had access to all of the social capital of having been raised in one of the top 10 public school systems in the country). I am damned lucky to be old enough to be on Medicare while receiving very expensive immune therapies for the above-mentioned cancer. My politics, if you hadn't already noticed, veer to the left in a democratic socialist, liberatory decolonial intersectional feminist sort of way.

I am a feminist who welcomes trans and nonbinary people into my life in the genders they know themselves to be, and I see that as part of my feminist commitment to undermining patriarchy and my DHCR commitment to honoring people's lived experiences, empowering them to say who they are rather than imposing my categories on them. I am also someone who understands that the experiences of natal women and those who are trans and nonbinary and were born with a uterus are different from those of natal men and nonbinary people or trans women who do not have a uterus. It is now more than 2 years since the *Dobbs* decision robbing women of the right to safe and legal abortion and reproductive health care in many parts of the United States, a day that was traumatizing and retraumatizing to many and has had immediate consequences for anyone who can become pregnant by accident or by force, which means anyone who has a uterus—thus, this biological aspect of some people's biopsychosocial realities matters in ways it hadn't in the half century of *Roe v. Wade*. Women are dying now because of this change.

I was born toward the end of the United States' un-war in Korea (we never declared it a war, it was a "conflict," like the American war on Vietnam wasn't officially a war either). I'm not sure I believe in divine beings, but I don't hold negative judgments of people who do, so long as they are not using their beliefs to uphold a social pathology or do harm to others. The divine being I'm not sure I believe in at the moment, which is a kind of vague spirit emerging from the universe and all in it, is a compassionate and inclusive one.

I am legally married and legally separated, both rights given to people in same-sex pairs in the entire United States only since 2015 and in my home state of Washington since 2012. I have lived by myself since late 2022. I am childless by choice. So far as I know I have never been pregnant nor have I ever aspired to be, even during my brief attempt at conforming to heteronormativity in my late teens. I am a survivor of childhood attachment trauma because I am the offspring of two people who themselves had complex trauma and am the descendant of people who were targets of anti-Semitic violence every day of their lives and who fled, carrying that intergenerational trauma, to what they believed was a safer place—which is becoming less safe every year. It would break my grandparents' hearts to see the upsurge in fatal anti-Semitic violence that has been happening in the United States in the last decade. They were very proud naturalized citizens of this country in which they did not have to hide in the basement several times to save their own lives.

Here's a rough one, but important to finally feel free to put in writing. I believe that I was sexually abused, briefly, by a nonparent family member when I was almost three, although all I have are vague memories, followed in time by the behaviors of a sexually abused child and then adolescent and adult. So I'm not sure and never will be more certain than I am today. I can simply back-engineer the behaviors that emerged after a particular point in time, behaviors that, had they been described to me-the-therapist, would have led me to say, "Hmm, sexual abuse?"

I have spent my entire adult life in Seattle, with gratitude to the Duwamish and other Coast Salish people on whose stolen lands I have had the privilege to live, people to whom I pay rent monthly for that privilege. To my great surprise as a former perpetually failed student of physical education, I hold the rank of second-degree black belt in aikido, and as I write this sentence I am slowly moving toward the next level, something I find both hilarious and profound. I love dogs, cats not so much. My favorite physical spaces are filled with books and art. My favorite spaces on the planet that are not here in the Pacific Northwest have sand: deserts, beaches.

I also do not work as a direct trauma healer any longer. I stopped doing that in December 2018 (just in time for the cancer diagnosis, which was not a thrilling surprise; retire day 1, day one plus a month getting surgery instead of flying to Israel to teach) because I knew that I didn't have enough left in me emotionally to keep on doing that work well, and I worried that I could start to do harm if I kept it up.

So what I still do: I consult with other trauma healers and people who train and supervise them. I teach, before the pandemic, around the world, since the pandemic, on the screen and around the world. I do forensic trauma work, although by the time this book is published I hope to be well and truly done with that.

Any clinical examples I give in this book from the lives of suffering people represent an amalgam of at least three people's lives and stories, unless I have at some time received direct written permission to utilize a disguised version of one individual's life story and have noted it separately. If you think you recognize yourself, it's not because it's you; it's because it's you-adjacent, as are so many stories of so many suffering people, and so many trauma healers.

The last time I wrote a book like this one I tried to use *Star Trek* ethnic groups for my examples when I could so as to avoid offending people. I am giving that strategy up; while such examples are useful when I'm teaching a brief workshop on trauma healing so that everyone in the room can keep their danger arousal systems deactivated, I've decided that the stories of the harm done by social pathologies ring truer when the story of the suffering person's intersectional identities can show where the wounds of the social pathology landed.

I will consequently offend some of you, my readers, some of the time, because I will get something wrong about you, about something in your intersectional identities that is dear to you, central to your communities, something that is tender and raw. I will anger some of my feminist friends because of my perspective on trans people. I will anger some of my trans friends because of my perspective on trans people. I have decided that if I am not pissing people off, I'm not writing truth as I see it. And being in my eighth decade of life, I don't care quite as much about not pissing people off as I do care about writing what I think might help people to heal.

That's where humility tries to come in. I humbly, and in advance, offer my sincere wish to have been able to repair that rupture by not having committed it. But because the last time I looked I was human, I will tear the fabric of human connection by what I write, without intending to, just as on the aikido mat I have stepped on a lot of bare toes without having the intent to do harm. Those toes hurt, nonetheless. I know, with deepening humility, that I am not the expert. I am simply one witness to suffering—older, still ignorant, more humble every day—who hopes that by writing about the suffering that follows upon wounds to the soul, the spirit, the body, our communities, the thing called trauma, and by inviting us all to decolonize this healing process, I can create some repairs. *Tikkun olam*, repair and healing of the world, is central to my values as a secular Jew. This book is an offering toward that end.

WHAT HAS MADE COLONIZATION TRAUMA INVISIBLE TO THE TRAUMA TREATMENT WORLD?

One of the hypotheses that I will be exploring in this book, in response to my own wondering about that question, has to do with how difficult it is for trauma healers to observe the colonizers and oppressors who are our literal or intellectual ancestors and whose ways of seeing people in pain constitute some of the challenging components of our own intersectional identities. A thing commonly called "privilege," which is frequently and unfortunately a source of shame rather than a door into deepened understanding of one's own place in the matrix of domination and subjugation, is one of the topics I will explore in this volume as it pertains to how we decolonize trauma healing.

The paradigm I am proposing is one that asks healers to turn inward as well as outward, to embrace and heal those monsters that live in our cultures, our families, our own life stories, so that we can be sources of healing for humans in pain without being tripped up by our own unexplored guilt or shame. We must embrace the monsters of our privilege in order to turn them into protective energies for alliance.

To change how trauma healers work with subjugated peoples is not the only step we need to take. The Indigenous peoples of the Western Hemisphere and the Global South who were colonized by Europeans between 1492 and the present are not the only colonized persons whose lives have been harmed in profound and painful ways. Thus, I am offering an expanded paradigm of what has constituted colonization in human history as it pertains to trauma that is passed on culturally and intergenerationally.

I am attempting not to appropriate the idea of decolonization, which is always the risk when people of the dominant culture take the work of the oppressed as our starting point. I hope instead to be inspired by and give full credit to the insights of the colonized, in order to think in what may be new ways about what it means to be colonized. My desire is to expand the reach of this paradigm, to construct of it an overarching metatheory of what has been, in my opinion, problematic in the field of trauma treatment, so that a decolonial standpoint cannot ever be dismissed as something peripheral to the core work of healing traumatized humans. This is not a book about special populations or adapting a method, both inherently colonial ways of responding to the reality of human intersectionalities. This book is about the intersection of trauma with all of the strands of which each of us are constituted.

AN INCLUSIVE CONSTRUCT OF COLONIZATION: TERRITORY, MIND, BODY, SPIRIT, THEORY

My project in this book is an ambitious one—perhaps overly ambitious. My broad vision arises from my own intersectional identities, which include both colonizer and colonized. I hope my vision is not an arrogant one. That risk is inherent in some of the strands of my intersectionalities. I intend on extending the construct of colonization beyond that of the physical colonization of Indigenous peoples, a continuing source of trauma to all of the descendants of those so colonized, to the interpersonal, intrapsychic, and spiritual/existential markers of ownership in traumatized humans without a recent history of colonization but instead, colonization by a toxic Eurocentric dominant culture. As Judith Herman wrote decades ago, "the systematic study of psychological trauma therefore depends on the support of a political movement" (1992, p. 9). The emerging politic of decolonial work is the movement that supports my systemic exploration of where our field has been distracted from the core.

1 INTRODUCING THE DECOLONIAL, HUMBLE, CULTURALLY RESPONSIVE MODEL

why some people be mad at me sometimes
they ask me to remember
but they want me to remember
their memories
and i keep on remembering
mine.

—Lucille Clifton[1]

TO UNCOVER, NOT DISCOVER: IT'S ALL IN HOW YOU TELL THE STORY

Think for a moment of the difference in the meaning of these two sentences:

In 1492, Columbus discovered the Western Hemisphere.

In 1492, Columbus initiated the European invasion of the Western Hemisphere and the decimation of its cultures and peoples through the introduction of new

---

[1]Lucille Clifton, "why some people be mad at me sometimes" from *How to Carry Water: Selected Poems*. Copyright © 1987 by Lucille Clifton. Reprinted with the permission of The Permissions Company, LLC on behalf of BOA Editions Ltd., boaeditions.org.

https://doi.org/10.1037/0000421-002
Decolonizing Trauma Healing: Toward a Humble, Culturally Responsive Practice,
by L. S. Brown

diseases, the use of advanced military technologies, the exploitation of the assumptions of good intentions of strangers in the cultures of the Western Hemisphere, and consequently to the inception of colonization and slavery.

The first sentence is the colonial story I was taught in the public schools of my upper-middle-class suburb in the 1950s, a story taught in almost every school everywhere in the United States, a story that, in 2024, some states are attempting to reassert as the only story that children may learn in school. The second sentence represents the facts, the memories of the ghosts who whisper their stories through the noise made by the colonizers. Nonetheless, if a child being given a standard test of cognitive capacity answers with the facts instead of the colonizing mythology, those factual answers have been, until recently, scored as incorrect because the colonial story was considered the only right answer. Whose memories become history? Whose memories are the "truth," whose a "mythology," whose "false"? Whose memories are we asked to remember? The memories of the colonizer? Or the colonized?

THE DECOLONIAL MOVEMENT IN MENTAL HEALTH

In the early 21st century a movement has arisen in the mental health fields that refers to "decolonizing mental health" (Comas-Díaz et al., 2024; Zapata, 2020). Almost everything that I have been studying on this topic has referred specifically to removing Global North/Christian-European models for healing distress from healing work with various groups of Indigenous, formerly enslaved, or otherwise subjugated people in the Western Hemisphere (Bhatia, 2021).

The people who are both the authors and the topics of this scholarship are most frequently those who were colonized by Europeans simply because the invaders had more advanced weapons technology. This brutal period of violent domination has lasted in some form or another from the 15th century until the present time. Decolonizing as understood in this particular discourse has been conceptualized as replacing Western models for treating trauma with healing modalities derived from the heritage of those Indigenous people (Comas-Díaz & Jacobsen, 2024; Comas-Díaz et al., 2024; Zapata, 2020).

The decolonizing movement in the field of emotional healing has focused its scholarship and activism on identifying those healing practices that would be more appropriate for work with colonized Indigenous peoples in distress than those used by Western medicine and mental health practices (Comas-Díaz & Jacobsen, 2024). This reclamation of Indigenous healing methods and viewpoints has been a necessary and important step toward challenging the hegemony of the Western medical model of trauma and its healing. It is a challenge I am hoping, humbly, to take on without prescribing the blanket adoption for non-Indigenous colonized persons in distress of these

Indigenous practices as an antidote to the Eurocentrism of our current models. The Indigenous epistemics, however, do offer a potential antidote, and it is to them I have looked for inspiration in writing this book.

The important work of decolonizing mental health opened many people's eyes to the narrowness of Christian-Eurocentric paradigms for responding to many forms of distress, not the least of which was the distress arising from exposure to trauma, of which colonization is one form. The decolonial discourse has, however, generally focused on the effects of colonization imposed by Christian Europeans on the Indigenous peoples of the Western Hemisphere, Australia, and New Zealand, on those living in the Global South, and on the enslaved persons hauled in bondage to the Western Hemisphere from Africa, much of which was also brutally colonized by European powers. This scholarship has been about the depredations and systemic forms of oppression brought to the Global South by the Christian colonizers of England, Spain, Portugal, France, Germany, the Netherlands, Denmark, Belgium—any European nation that could muster the ships and the weapons, driven by greed for what the rest of the world possessed, colonized. Then their descendants living on colonized lands extended colonization from the coasts to the interiors of continents; now there exists little to no uncolonized Indigenous land in the Western Hemisphere.

The epoch of Christian European colonization, from 1492 until now, involved the imposition of Christian Eurocentric rules, norms, languages, religions (all varieties of Christian, although few in agreement with one another), healing practices, and values on subjugated peoples. Colonization was not simply appropriation of land. It entailed mass and continuous trauma, the systematic destruction of cultures, languages, and spiritual and healing traditions, the processes of which were often intertwined. Colonization enabled, sometimes even blessed as a divinely given mission, the taking of lives that were defined as less than human: melanized lives, non-Christian lives. Colonization disrupted people's long-standing constructions of the legitimacy of relationships and identities, upending systems of meaning. Colonization has destroyed and continues to destroy millions of lives. For persons concerned with healing trauma, it seems impossible to proceed to work with anyone from a colonized community without understanding this terrible history or the ways in which healers might ourselves have become complicit in its continuing effects and aftermaths. Aligning trauma healing with the larger decolonial movement in mental health seems necessary.

In their wake, the colonizers left enormous burdens of every possible kind of trauma for the subjugated. This not-yet-postcolonial trauma is striking. It provokes me, and I hope you too, to wonder how so many well-meaning trauma healers looked past colonization as trauma for so long. Even if it was not named in any diagnostic manual, it was certainly being observed and recorded in the forms of higher rates of every possible somatic and psychic pain in the communities most deeply affected by colonization.

To overthrow a colonizer's rule over a physical space or nation does not eradicate the long-lasting internal colonization of the minds, hearts, and epistemic frameworks of the colonized, and of the colonizers as well. This "coloniality," as Maldonado-Torres (2007) has named it, represents the persistent dynamics of power the effects of which exist in the structures of psychotherapy, in the creation and authorization of knowledge, and in the ways in which both the larger culture and that of trauma therapy has responded to people who are suffering. Coloniality has made some traumas legitimate while casting others, the specific effects of colonization, as other than.

While, in the past decades, some pioneering critical theorists of trauma healing have been diligently rooting out coloniality with regards to how it has affected specific Indigenous or enslaved persons (e.g., Comas-Díaz et al., 2019; Martín-Baró, 1994; Morrow & Hawxhurst, 2013; Norsworthy et al., 2013), this book endeavors to move that work further, not to universalize, but to focus on the colonization that has not yet been written about or spoken of in the decolonial literature. I am gratefully borrowing this paradigm of decolonizing to propose a reconstruction of how trauma healers understand every facet of our work. Just as colonization dehumanized the colonized, so people suffering from their exposures to trauma have been stigmatized and treated as lesser forms of human by a Eurocentric culture that values stoicism. The parallels are powerful enough that this epistemic lens provides an opening into new ways of working with people in pain.

INTRODUCING THE DECOLONIAL, HUMBLE, CULTURALLY RESPONSIVE MODEL OF TRAUMA HEALING PRACTICE

Throughout this volume I will be leaning on a model that I have synthesized from the various trauma and decolonial healing practices and thinkers that I have studied. I call this the decolonial, humble, culturally responsive (DHCR) model of trauma healing practice. I do not claim originality of ideas here; this is simply how I have brought together what I have learned and what I now think about how to engage in trauma healing. Let me explicate next.

Decolonial

Decolonial practices grow from an epistemic base in which the influences of Eurocentric cultures are stripped out of every aspect of the trauma healing process. This requires interrogating how distress is understood and questioning the names we give to our roles as healers. Ultimately it necessitates a repositioning of authority about the trauma healing process from people with advanced degrees to suffering people themselves. Decolonizing our work means allowing ourselves to develop decolonial criteria by which a DHCR healer may assess whether a healing practice will be liberatory, emancipatory, and empowering to the suffering person seeking their care. DHCR work is technically integrative, but what a healer actually does in their work with a suffering, trauma-exposed person must be able to pass through the doors of such criteria in order to be DHCR trauma practice. It matters less what a healer does. It matters more how they frame it within a decolonial paradigm.

Decolonizing trauma healing involves demolition of the typical structures of power in the healing relationship. Such dismantling is required because the enterprise of what we now call psychotherapy has been colonized by various social pathologies over time, whether trauma is the topic or not. Decolonial trauma healing requires exploration of the interstices of all such practice. This radical paradigm seeks out the roots of the corruption, of domination and subordination, that are so normative within the cultures from which this discipline emerged that their presence, and their toxins, were invisible.

DHCR practice challenges a trauma healer to put their healing methods through the filter of a decolonial, liberatory lens so the juice of healing that pours through the filter is purified of toxicity. To decolonize psychotherapy and turn it instead into decolonial healing requires all of this and more. It's a complete reset that not only rejects Eurocentric practices, rather it de-centers them, reconsiders their value, and puts them into their place in the larger family of healing practices.

Feminist and liberatory healers have been engaging in this challenge to the power dynamics of emotional healing for half a century now, yet therapy as usual—indeed trauma therapy as usual—has yet to integrate the notion that abuses of power and experiences of disempowerment are unlikely to be healed in a setting where there is a clear hierarchy of power in which the healer/therapist is on top. DHCR trauma practice, like feminist, womanist, *mujerista*, and liberatory psychotherapies, is distinctive from other trauma healing practice in that the dynamics of power in the relationship are always interrogated, and that interrogation always integrated into what the healer does.

Humble

Humility is perhaps the hardest part of this entire paradigm for anyone who has trained as a psychotherapist/healer because it is a release of ego in ways that are, at times, painful, particularly as we gaze into the mirror of our own unwillingness to see and know and feel the pain of systemic trauma of which we have ourselves been a part or targets, or both. Humility emerges from a mindset of curiosity, open heartedness, a softening from the position of authority as it has been insinuated into the role of the healer in the Global North. It is a stance of knowing that we do not know, knowing what we cannot know, and searching to maintain a calm tentativeness about what we believe we do know. This is not a mindset conveyed in almost any postbaccalaureate training in the emotional healing arts; quite the contrary, the mental health fields have their own hierarchy, psychiatrists over psychologists, psychologists over social workers, everyone over master's level counselors, and no one with less than that degree admitted into anything other than the despised work of case management. DHCR trauma healing practice is much less concerned with the letters after a healer's name and much more interested in their ability to hold the space for the distressed person from a position of humility and compassionate curiosity.

Humility should grow naturally from understanding that the longer we practice, the greater we grow in our awareness of our ignorance; the longer we practice the more we treasure our capacity to be centered and engaged from a place of not needing to (pretend to) know what will happen next in a healing encounter. As in my martial art, where the achievement of a black belt means that a person is now truly a beginner, so humility in trauma healing work is not mistaking experience for wisdom, not allowing emotional muscle memory to substitute for being attuned, compassionately curious, and open-mindedly uncertain in the present moment.

Humility is an emotional, even spiritual, position where the healer seeks not simply a liberatory relationship with a suffering person in which the dynamics of power as dominance and hierarchy are structurally eradicated. It is also one where the suffering person's ways of knowing, their clarities, their growing sense of an embrace of their healing self are central to defining the process and outcome of the healing work, rather than a healer's ideas of what should work or what a good outcome would be.

Humility means that while the healer may read a manual, they will never make that manual more important than the suffering person's voice. Unlike trauma therapy as usually practiced, humble practice means that the voices of the suffering will be at least equal to those of our professions and professors. Humility changes power relationships.

Culturally Responsive

As I discussed in the introduction, let us cease to speak of cultural competence or diversity and inclusion. Notice who and what are centered in these terms: not subjugated or marginalized people but the dominant culture and its notions of what it takes to do decolonial work. Members of marginalized and subjugated groups are experts in understanding the cultures of the dominant groups because, after all, one must study the ways of the colonizer in order to survive them. All of us need, rather, to be culturally responsive, attuned to the many facets of each suffering person's intersectional identities and to the coloniality that surrounds the healer–sufferer pair and our work together. Cultural responsivity sees people in the contexts of their intersectional identities and social locations but does not subsume their experience into the healer's preconceived beliefs about what those identities and experiences might be. Instead, the healer listens, senses, responds.

Cultural responsivity leads to compassionate curiosity about how even the smallest or least easy to detect facets of a person's intersectional identities may be sources of trauma or may be affected by trauma. Responsivity also points to how these facets of identities may be wells of strength and resources for the healing process, wellsprings of capacities that can be specific to some or all of the trauma-affected person's healing experience. This is not, as I once thought, about understanding trauma through some specific component of a person's intersectionalities, disaggregating that component from the others. Cultural responsivity is the willingness to humbly and curiously invite the dyad of the suffering person and the healer to uncover the layers of experience that are manifesting as the biopsychosocial and existential markers of trauma exposure.

There are nearly infinite possible strands of the gorgeous braid that is a person's intersectional identity. Staying with this expansive vision gives a trauma healer the most powerful lens through which to detect the subtle, apparently small components of a person's intersectionalities that may emerge as most central to both the story of trauma and the path to healing. Trauma healers who have been on the path to decolonial work have tried, in the past, to find the complete list of possible strands (Hays, 2022), which has pointed us to the territory we are now exploring. Decolonial healing allows us to see that those strands we thought we knew about—and by "we," I include myself—were only the ones that a colonized taxonomy of humanity allowed us to include.

This differs enormously from all kinds of therapy as usual, whose response to intersectionality has been the construct of adapting the treatment to the person's group membership. Several problems are clear here from a decolonial standpoint. First, the person is reduced to their group. Second, the notion is that a methodology need not be interrogated for its possible colonial or oppressive dynamics but simply adapted, given the equivalent of cosmetic surgery rather than a radical restructuring. Culturally responsive trauma healing is not adaptation. It is transformation, with the liberatory lens of returning power to those who have been disempowered at its center.

SOME POSSIBLE STRANDS OF INTERSECTIONALITY: A COMPLETELY NONEXHAUSTIVE DISCUSSION

Consider for a moment some of the possible varieties of intersectionalities. All humans have various expressions of phenotype. We inhabit bodies with certain characteristics that are by and of themselves neutral yet are assigned meaning by the culture into which that body emerges and lives. Humans have experiences of scarcity or plenty or both. We have relationships to the languages spoken around us, mother tongue or not. We have lived in places on the planet, some of which are home, some of which we have fled to, some of which we have chosen, some of which ones to which we and our families were displaced. We all have lived to the age we are in the time of our world. We all have some kind of spiritual or existential meaning-making systems. We have talents and capacities, tasks with which we struggle or soar; experiences of being able or not in the world, born into disability or acquiring it as we go along, of being well or ill for shorter or longer times; of parenting or not, biologically, otherwise, by choice or not; of being partnered or not or both during a lifetime; experiences of where we are on the spectrums of kinds of intelligence, neurotypes, patterns of sexual and romantic relating, and much more. All of these strands of intersectionality may be locations where trauma resides or not.

Each person has a heritage, which may contain its own strands of trauma. Each person has experiences of attachment to other humans in which trauma may have occurred. And when a suffering person who has been exposed to something they experienced as traumatic seeks trauma healing, that trauma itself becomes another strand of intersectional identity.

Each of these strands of identity braid and rebraid repeatedly, sometimes across the course of a day, certainly during a lifetime, so that one strand more or less predominates, depending on the place and time in a person's life, on the social and political context, on what it means to be sitting with a healer—each of these strands of intersectionality marks the place where a decolonial healer brings their cultural responsiveness.

And we do not simply bring cultural responsiveness to the people seeking our care. Cultural responsiveness includes the healer's own in-depth exploration of their own intersectional identities, so that we might have a good set of working hypotheses about what we might represent to the trauma-exposed people who come to them. This self-examination also offers working hypotheses about what may, in turn, be activated in us by who walks in our doors. We become culturally responsive to ourselves as well as to those with whom we sit.

Cultural responsiveness as a construct defines culture as broadly as possible—for example, someone whose culture is, like that of one of my niblings, competitive speed-cubing with Rubik's Cubes, or, as is true for a friend, participating in canine agility, or as is the case for both those who are famous and those simply creating for pleasure, being a musician or artist or dancer or theatrical performer; each of these are components of intersectional identities and thus cultures. "Culture" in the culturally responsive framework is consequently construed as any set of important organizing principles in a person's intersectional sense of self, those that have been the places where marginalization and subordination have occurred as well those that have been locations of joy and power and play. In this model, a culture is a set of shared experiences, some of them internally generated, some of them externally defined, around which a person organizes some aspects of their sense of who they are which are important to them.

Sounds simple, doesn't it? Not really, because in order to get ourselves to this place from which to develop trauma healing, we must unpack a century and a half of what trauma healing has been until now, a half century of the mental health professions jousting with the concepts of diversity and inclusion, cultural competence and mnemonics for taxonomies of difference. Most of those experiences have not been DHCR in nature, although they have been shuffling in the right direction. They have been the first steps of the humble intellectual and emotional strivings stumbling in a DHCR direction for the last few decades.

Because this book emerged from those strivings, an enterprise of which I was a participant, it's helpful to clarify what DHCR is not. It is not the current realities of the intellectually colonized project of healing traumatized humans. That project was set in place by a politics of authority. Those structures authorized only professionals with advanced degrees to claim the territory of healing trauma. This required delegitimizing other kinds of healers whose methods were frequently discovered, that is, appropriated and given a new name, by the authorized people with the extra letters after our names. Indigenous healers and their practices were sent to the intellectual reservation called "culture-specific practices" to be performed only with those already living on those reservations. This is not what DHCR cultural responsivity is about.

BIOLOGY IS NOT DESTINY: IT SIMPLY HELPS US TO BE COMPASSIONATE REVOLUTIONARIES

Simply because something in the interpersonal and political realms arises from the typical workings of the human brain makes it neither immutable nor correct. Our default neurobiology is an artifact of human evolution that was necessary for our survival when we were a prey species 300,000 years ago. It, like many of the brain structures that allowed our species to persist, seems to have ceased to evolve in response to changes in our position in the natural order of the world, as we moved from prey to predator to super-predators on our own species. Understanding the colonized nature of how trauma is understood and responded to by the healing professions requires healers to push past this evolutionary structure and recognize that we are the predators now, not the prey, and that this shift in our place in the hierarchy of life requires us to move differently in the world. We can afford to be uncomfortable, to embrace ambiguity, to be humble—all of which is the foundation of emotional healing, no matter what we call it.

Consequently, starting to understand social pathologies as complex, elaborated extensions of this way that brains work within a given set of social and political realities might allow us to ask how we might use those same brain networks to decolonize our own thinking as healers. Deciding that evolution did not need to stop when we became *Homo sapiens* and were still prey, that the evolution of our capacities must continue into who we as a species and as trauma healers are today, can also revolutionize our understanding of what constitutes trauma and what makes for trauma healing. So let's take a deeper look at what our defaults have wrought, the social pathologies that I posit are at the core of almost all of what is traumatizing to humans.

SOCIAL PATHOLOGIES

In order to accomplish a move to a DHCR epistemology we need to explore what I conceive of as the large-scale emotional colonization of humans by what I describe in this volume as social pathologies. A social pathology is any form of structural and systemic oppression that exists in any given social and cultural context, whose effect is the domination, subordination, subjugation, and devaluation of identified specific humans, cultures, and/or ways of being. I know that in using this terminology I am using a pathology model; in this case, where I am referring to structural cultural forms of oppression, I have struggled to find a better term. I have stayed with *social pathology* because these things make humans ill in body, mind, and spirit.

I consequently will be internally inconsistent and refer to these social and political structural hierarchies of oppression as pathological because oppression is a social sickness, a large-scale set of structural toxins that poisons cultures and people and the planet. What follows assumes that most human experience of trauma is either created and sustained by social pathologies or aggravated by those social and political dynamics when they are not the specific source of what traumatizes.

Social Pathologies: An Explication of the Construct

The disorder is in the culture, not in the people in distress. What Kaschak (2021) has identified as the continuous presence of terror in the lives of many people is among the pernicious effects of the intersections of a number of powerful systemic forms of oppression, the many and varied social pathologies, which include, but do not end with, the two overarching phenotype supremacies of skin and sex: White supremacy in the Europeanized world and patriarchy everywhere, as well their toxic offspring,: systemic misogyny, xenophobia, anti-Semitism, ableism, classism, and of course colonialism, to name only a few. Social pathologies are the many heads of the monster of actual and psychic colonization, and they are poisonous. I know that to refer to something as a pathology means that my epistemic framework remains wedged against the ones I am attempting to leave behind. I nonetheless believe that this wording invites you, my readers, to consider where the problems are, even if the distress is residing in the person seeking healing.

Just as we know that a person bitten by a viper has been poisoned by its bite and has nothing otherwise wrong with them except that a horrible toxin has been introduced into their system, so the person bitten by the vipers of social pathologies is in distress, poisoned, but the distress engendered by the toxin is not the central problem, although it is something that a healer must attend to and often make primary.

But consider that the intended effects of these poisonous social pathologies are to create chronic, unremitting terror and feelings of alienation, disconnection, helplessness, and hopelessness, manifesting in various expressions of distress—in other words, to have people meet the diagnostic criteria for having been made disordered by being trauma-exposed or disordered in some way not directly associated, by narrow definitions of trauma responses, to being trauma-exposed. The trajectory of trauma to use of a substance to being unhoused to prison is, for me, the epitome of how trauma is the long arm of oppression. If trauma led to use of substance to soothe, then led to compassionate care— a rare storyline—the relationship of trauma to oppression would be much less simple to elucidate.

None of what is happening to people is posttraumatic when the vipers are still biting. The distress from a car accident might just be posttraumatic, if one leaves out the secondary trauma of pain, dealing with the car insurance companies, having to get back behind the wheel and spend half an hour every day driving to and from a job to which no form of public transportation goes, and so on. Or the tertiary trauma of not being able to get legally medicated for the pain, leading to ventures into the world of high-risk painkillers available on the street, leading to becoming unhoused or dying, all because there is a so-called war on drugs and physicians are terrified of prescribing enough pain medication for long enough for people whose pain from that accident is chronic but could be controlled with the prescription medication.

I worked with someone who had this story—terrible neurogenic pain from a car accident. This person happened to have, for most of the 20 years after that accident, a primary care physician who was trauma-informed, who trusted her patients, and who prescribed enough morphine for this person to go to graduate school, get a good job, and support a family. Then that physician retired. The new physician abruptly cut off the medicine. The person went through the pangs of withdrawal, becoming suicidal for weeks on end. I remonstrated with the physician, noting that this person had never taken any more than was prescribed and did not get high, which meant tolerance, not addiction. The physician, who knew nothing about trauma, was insistent that the suffering person was an addict, as evidenced by the withdrawal symptoms, and refused my entreaties.

The person, ironically, was fortunate to become terminally ill with cancer not long afterward and, through their oncologist, once again had access to sufficient opioid medication to quell the pain of both the car accident and the stage 4 disease. The person, in the brief interim, almost lost their home, did lose a job, and was in such torment that death seemed like a relief. The trauma of the car accident itself was something that had remitted long ago. The trauma of having medicine withdrawn abruptly and being marginalized as an addict followed this person to their grave as the horror of that first month away from medicine and the memories of the excruciating pain in which this person was forced to live for another year before they became terminally ill, not to speak of the trauma of the intensity of their suicidality, were all the story of how a trauma that is socially neutral turns into very socially constructed trauma. The disorder—the attitude of the medical professional toward this person's use of prescribed opioid medicine—was something that both of us were almost helpless to deal with. Thus, in general the disorder, the poison, is in the fangs of the social pathologies and not in those suffering from being bitten by these structural forms of oppression.

Phenotype-Based Social Pathologies

I posit that social pathologies referring to phenotype as a central construct are those which define aspects of a body as inherently better or worse. These are the most pernicious of the social pathologies, the metapathologies, the overarching conceptual frameworks for a given society that exist in almost every culture in some form and from which grow other more context-specific social pathologies. These phenotype pathologies, such as patriarchy or White supremacy, are so powerful that, as Kaschak (2015) learned in her in-depth study of blind people, even those who cannot see a person's phenotype express attitudes and values in line with the toxicities of social pathologies of their culture of reference.

Phenotype pathologies begin with patriarchy (G. Lerner 1986), which is about weaponizing the phenotype of the perceived sex of the body, something that each human is born into the world with, so as to create hierarchies of power and dominance. I have placed patriarchy at the top of the food chain of social pathologies not simply because intersectional feminist theory has guided my thinking, and thus pointed me at all things sex and gender for half a century, but more realistically because it exists in all cultures, given that all bodies are born with genitals. Not all bodies' genitals fit into a binary. Not all bodies' genitals are consistent with that body's reproductive organs or the so-called sex chromosomes. But the thing everyone can see is the thing that assigns humans at the moment of birth (or, in the technological world, during pregnancy via a sonogram) to being female or male, and with that assignment a place in a structural hierarchy of oppression based entirely on this phenotype. The horror stories of intersex children whose genitals were operated on, in what was for all intents and purposes the medical genital mutilation of late 20th-century Western patriarchy, surgeries performed so that the child's genitals would appear more "normal," that is, conforming to nonintersex genitals, are quite recent tales. The ideology that propelled them (Money & Ehrhardt, 1972) as squarely in line with patriarchy. If a baby girl's clitoris was too large, it should be amputated. If a baby boy's penis was too small, ditto, and that child raised as a girl.

Melanin-based body supremacy, which in European and Euro-colonized cultures expresses as White supremacy, although it takes other forms in other cultural contexts, is what I consider to be the next meta–social pathology. All humans are born with physical characteristics that are expressions of their genetics and that affect melanin in the skin, shape of eyes and nose, ways in which very early ancestors adapted to the specific climatological and geological aspects of their environments, and other aspects of bodily habitus. These two, patriarchy and melanin-based body supremacy, because they are attached to physical realities of phenotype that are then interpreted so as to create imbalances of power, are what I consider to be the two core social pathologies, the two social pathologies "to rule them all," to borrow a metaphor from J. R. R. Tolkien.

I conceptualize the phenotype pathologies as primary and central because it is my observation that most, if not all, other social pathologies—such as homophobia, xenophobia, classism, ableism, persecution due to gender expression or ways of enacting belief in a divine—tend to be somewhat more context-specific and to have roots in the two metapathologies of phenotype supremacy; they thus likely would not flourish as systemic forms of oppression in the absence of the two metapathologies.

All humans have phenotypes because those are a particular body's expression of its genetics for things like shape of genitals, presence of internal reproductive organs, degree of melanin in the skin, eye colors and shapes, hair textures and colors, average heights and weights. Thus all humans have characteristics that can be culturally constructed as being of value or worthy of maltreatment. The phenotype social pathologies create the vulnerable points at which trauma may be aimed or from which resilience may grow.

For instance, White supremacy, which is present in Christian Europeanized cultures, has historically been the source of anti-Semitism and anti-Roma and anti-Sinti bias. As Christian Europe colonized the Western Hemisphere and Global South this pathology began to be expressed as racism against Black, Indigenous, and people of color (BIPOC) people, both Indigenous and enslaved. Colorism, which is often seen in places that were colonized by Christian Europeans, is a subtype of White supremacy in which members of colonized BIPOC groups internalize White supremacy and oppress one for appearing darker-skinned.

Not all phenotype supremacy is White supremacy. Racism against Ainu people is a specifically Japanese phenotype supremacy, as is anti-gaijin (foreigner) racism. Phenotype supremacy culturally defines a phenotypic other as inferior or even subhuman. Anti-Semitism, conversely, did not exist in Japan until it was imported there during the Second World War by the Nazi allies of the Japanese empire. It is still a weak social pathology in that culture, as in almost all parts of East and Southeast Asia, where there have been very few Jews aside from tiny and no longer existing communities in Harbin, China, and Mumbai, India, or the group of German Jewish refugees who briefly found shelter in Shanghai after fleeing Nazi Germany. Instead, otherizing Uighur and Tibetan peoples is currently a phenotype supremacy practiced by the majority Han Chinese government of the People's Republic of China; persons of these groups are persecuted and oppressed, their lands and languages colonized by the Han majority.

As this illustrates, iterations of social pathologies in their expressions can be very specific to their era and geographic location. Yet all are variations of the overarching phenotype supremacy–based social pathologies that rely on real aspects of human physiology in order to claim superiority, dominance, and the right to colonize and subjugate for those with a particular typical phenotypic expression. All social pathologies, no matter their specifics, are structural forms of social hierarchies that are traumatizing both to their targets and, in different ways, to those who enact and appear to benefit from them.

A decolonized trauma healing perspective takes that last component of social pathologies into account in understanding trauma. That is, the default epistemics of a DHCR healing practice do not exclude the oppressor from being among those harmed by the social pathologies that have colonized their psyches and souls and the moral injuries incurred by participation in those systems of oppression.

CAN A HUMAN BE DISORDERED? SOMETIMES

I propose that we reserve the term *disordered* for those humans who have demonstrated that they lack the capacity to empathize with the suffering they inflict on others and seem to take joy in that suffering—sociopaths, in other words, be they performing their predations on humans at a large scale, like dictators and autocrats, or on a smaller yet equally destructive scale, like serial sexual predators and torturers. As the psychologist and social commentator Mary Trump (2020) has helped us to see in her excoriating and intimate descriptions of her uncle, the 45th president of the United States, this type of sociopathy and disorder also has its roots in trauma. As she described it, that man grew up in an atmosphere in which shame and humiliation and threats to attachment were omnipresent.

However, sociopaths' responses to trauma, to the degree that they have been available for observation, seem to be distinct from those of most human beings. For reasons not yet entirely clear to science, their response is not to suffer, or at least not to allow themselves to experience their psychic pain, but rather to identify with the source of the pain and seek to become a source of pain to others, to wallow in systemic and structural forms of oppression. There may be differences in their neurobiology, although this theory has not been adequately tested for me to subscribe to it, given the range of expressions of sociopathy. Apparently sociopaths either feel no emotional pain or avoid feeling pain by passing it along to others, what Anna Freud called the identification with the aggressor (1936/1966) or what decolonial thinkers would call the identification with and internalization of the systemic oppressor. This book is not about healing that particular dangerous manifestation of trauma, although I will address healing the traumas of those who have been entranced and betrayed by the sociopaths.

People can also have neurotypes that cause deep suffering and difficulties functioning in the interpersonal realm; autism, bipolar mania and depression, obsessive-compulsiveness, attentional difficulties, hearing voices and seeing that which is not there—each of these has its roots in a brain neurotype for which modern Western cultures are poorly adapted. I do not consider these neurotypes disorders, as their existence has been documented for millennia; in some places and times, the suffering emerging from these neurotypes has been responded to more or less compassionately than in the modern world. Persons with these neurotypes are often exposed to trauma because the expressions of these neurotypes in the interpersonal space create marginalization and often lead to cruel treatment at the hands of others, both individually and institutionally.

IT'S ALL IN OUR HEADS (PERHAPS)

Social pathologies may be as much a product of the human brain and nervous system as are the human responses to trauma, a product that goes wrong, becomes reified and associated with the cultural dominant. Similar to neurobiological responses in the various trauma response systems of the body that are expressed as distress in a trauma-exposed person, so it is very likely the case that the social pathologies that now seem entirely socially constructed represent expressions of other neurobiological realities, expressions that have become reified, given names, and then taken up as the ideologies of those in positions of power. Social pathologies are possibly a product of the brain's default mode network—in other words, of the neurobiology of how things "ought to be."

This default mode network, the DMN (Ma & Zhang, 2021), is a neural network that appears to operate to manage many other brain networks. It is hypothesized to run in the background of human brains like some kind of deep program for assessing what is normal and what is not in the life of that person. When not otherwise occupied by surprises and deviations from the default (such as, for instance, the bestowal of equal rights to previously disenfranchised groups, or the occupation of a position of power by a member of a group that was previously excluded, in other words, social change), the DMN seems to keep the human in question experiencing order in their cognition through the use of cognitive shortcuts. These shortcuts, which neuroscientists tend to describe as ways for the brain to be more efficient, contain the materials of social pathologies: stereotypes, rigid thinking, and reified beliefs about the alleged characteristics of people. This may start with our sense of self, our "me" being represented neurologically as a real and somewhat fixed thing. Think of how many times you've said, "I'm not a person who would do *x* thing." This is possibly your DMN in operation. Or, "This is what we do when working with a traumatized person." There's our field's default mode, which is a component of the faux competence we'll discuss throughout this book.

Imagine that the me in this case is a person whose characteristics have been sanctified by a social hierarchy, one emerging from structural and systemic forms of oppression, as divinely ordained. Perhaps this hypothetical me is endowed by some social pathology or another with the right to define other members of the human species, even to define them as not human or as property or as not worthy of equal access or treatment. Is this an expression of the neurobiology of social pathologies, a default mode that becomes systemic and part of dangerous hierarchies of value? Might the shaking up of social realities account for the fear that some people feel if the world around them becomes a truly more level playing field? Or if something happens to those allegedly invulnerable people, a something that is a trauma, that is not "supposed" to happen to "people like us" will it be perceived as so ferocious because it is disturbing a default neurobiology of a social pathology?

Because such a way of thinking about oneself and others could be a manifestation of a neurobiological default system, this hidden epistemic framework for life seems, when challenged, immutable, and the proposed changes to constructs of reality dangerous, to be stamped out, and quickly, so that the neurobiology of "how life ought to be" can keep humming along, making the person feel "normal" and safe.

The concept of a neurobiology of the social default also creates a sense of separateness between one human and another, and between humans and nature. This perceived separateness manifests as the depredations of social pathologies onto the environment and expresses, as well, as maltreatment of members of our species who are experienced, through the constructs of the nonconscious schemata of those in power, as most separate, different, not human creatures.

One hypothesis suggests that for many people, this default grows more influential in our ways of being in the world, or perhaps one might more accurately say, less plastic neurologically, as we grow older—thus the cliché about not being able to teach an old dog new tricks. The neurobiological default, which is still a very new construct, is perhaps organized differently in some cultural settings than others, especially those that value the notion of nonduality between beings. This last idea is entirely speculative on my part, relying on the observations that in some cultural contexts there is less of a separate me and more of a collective "I am because we are" way of experiencing the self. There are also some cultural contexts in which the default understanding of the world entails much less of a separation between me and all living creatures than in the collective defaults of European-influenced cultures, whose behaviors have led to the extinction of many species, including groups of humans excluded from the category of human, in the lands they colonized.

Children—whose neurobiology and thus their defaults is in a very active state of development, first with explosions, then pruning of neurons in the first years of life—don't participate very well in social pathologies at first. In the words of a song from the musical *South Pacific*, "You've got to be taught to hate and fear, you've got to be taught from year to year" (Hammerstein & Rodgers, 1949).

Rodgers and Hammerstein were on to something about how culture shapes the neurobiology of hatred and dangerous stereotyping, and thus of systemic and structural forms of oppression. The brain systems supporting those damages to the psyche through the processes of deforming the default neurobiology of young humans were only observable almost a century after this song was written, when neuroimaging technology has emerged that allows us to watch this process happening. Leaving the neurobiological aside, and turning back to the interpersonal and psychosocial, we can observe that children do not come into the world participating in social pathologies. They notice difference of all kinds. They require being instructed in the social meanings of difference for those to encode themselves into the default as the child grows older.

But in the Western societies in which most of you, dear readers, and in which I also have spent my 7+ decades on the planet, duality, separateness, and tight regulation of input from our senses and distance from the realm of what is often referred to as the mystical are rewarded and protected, and those who deviate from those values are persecuted in various ways. Nature and the other living creatures of the planet are "not me" for many humans in Europeanized cultures; those resisting such dualities are mocked and labeled "tree-huggers," a contempt which exposes the fear that a collective default might be required to move into new defaults.

The default of human neurobiology as currently understood appears to function as a filter, letting in the least possible information needed to allow the brain to keep humming along like a well-oiled machine. For the default, change, which includes the disruption and subversion of structural and systemic forms of oppression, is not experienced as a good thing because it is the opposite of the default. Our neurobiology of what is normal functions to reduce uncertainty. Certainty, or something masquerading as such, is soothing. This in turn supports the development of false certainties, for example, "the Jews control the money and the media," or "gay people are pedophiles," and enables the use of assumptions, which can also be soothing and in some instances lead a person to experience themselves as wise or powerful.

I hypothesize that social pathologies—the structural and systemic forms of oppression that are the sources of much human trauma—are the psychosocial, interpersonal, and political manifestations of this drive for epistemic homeostasis and emotional comfort. They are false certainties about the nature of other humans based on inadequate information, with the added element of being the predigested cognitions and overcertain belief systems that have been adopted by dominant groups and ruling elites in order to maintain social homeostasis. These rules are then imposed upon those with less social power. They keep colonized realities humming along until someone, rising up against oppression, throws a monkey wrench into oppression's well-oiled machines. The dominant fights back; it does not give up without a struggle. All decolonial practice in healing requires the throwing of many monkey wrenches into the default of the dominant, whether it is ensconced through internalized oppression within the self of a suffering person, in the social realities in which they live, in the dynamics of the healing relationship, or all of the above.

Decolonization of trauma healing is a challenge: as I throw monkey wrenches into trauma psychology, while I won't be burned at the stake, I will evoke discomfort in many of you who value what you do. I have certainly caused discomfort for myself as I review, in retrospect, my life as a trauma therapist. What you do, as a trauma therapist, is a good thing, even sometimes an astonishingly good thing. If you are willing to tolerate and even embrace the discomfort inherent in diving into a decolonial mindset, you could have more. Throwing off the colonization of your intellectual and professional identities will feel strange, and it will be consistent with the values that brought you into this field.

2 AN EXPANSIVE DECOLONIAL PARADIGM FOR TRAUMA

Trauma is the Greek word for wound. Wounds can be enormous and gaping, leaving permanent damage and horrific visible scars. Wounds can also be enormous and invisible. They can be cumulative. Trauma is a creature of many faces. The colonization of the field of trauma healing says, "No, there is only one face, the thing we call Criterion A." Decolonial, humble, culturally responsive (DHCR) trauma healing sees and names the many faces, the variety of wounds and kinds of trauma. Colonized trauma models create a hierarchy of what is "real" trauma and what is not, which means that many trauma-exposed humans find their suffering ignored or misconstrued. DHCR trauma healing has no such hierarchy or notion of what is real trauma. Instead, it uses the framework of colonization as an uber-trauma in order to understand the many ways in which a human can experience events or social realities as traumatizing.

Trauma is a reminder that we are mortal and that life might not have meaning after all. It is a wound to the psyche, sometimes accompanied by wounds to the body, sometimes by wounds to those around us, to our homes, our cultures, our languages. Colonized models of trauma follow the myths of colonizers:

https://doi.org/10.1037/0000421-003
Decolonizing Trauma Healing: Toward a Humble, Culturally Responsive Practice,
by L. S. Brown

thus, if your culture is wounded, well, that was because it deserved it, because its resources, human and natural, were needed by the colonizer or your culture spurned the colonizing cultures. In these instances, the wound to your culture that is colonization cannot be considered an official trauma.

The DHCR framework provides an expansive paradigm for what traumatizes humans, in contrast to the ever-tightening construct of what is traumatic as allowed in today's mental health disciplines. I have been complicit in building up that which I now plan to dismantle. Fifty years ago, I liked the idea that we could at last give a diagnosis to the effects of trauma and that there was a definition of what a trauma was. Fifty years ago, and 40, and 30, handing the latest iteration of the *Diagnostic and Statistical Manual of Mental Disorders* (*DSM*) to someone suffering from posttrauma symptoms and watching the relief on their face when they realized that there was a name for their suffering made that otherwise problematic book seem of some value.

As I said in a legal case in early 2023, which settled the day before I plunged into another period of working intensively on this book, it's possible to tell that something was a trauma because the neurobiology of trauma has been activated, and we can detect that activation in the distress a person is having, whether they can recall what the experience was or not. As van der Kolk (1994) said 30 years ago, our bodies keep the score, and also, I would add, call out the plays as they happen. This is true—and to decolonize trauma healing we cannot simply lean upon biological reductionism. The ways in which the neurobiology of the woman in the legal case was set on fire had to do with betrayal and violation, with being put in mortal danger by one of the longest-documented traumas of patriarchy: sexual assault by a person known to the violated woman. This woman's body responded the same way that of Dinah, the daughter of Jacob, is said to have responded after she was raped, one of the earliest stories in Hebrew scripture in which this weapon of patriarchy is so vividly described.

When the field of trauma is insidiously and not so insidiously colonized by the "six sessions and you're done" medicalized model of working with human distress, the body's unfortunate tendency to keep on knowing there is psychic pain for years and decades requires a DHCR healing practice, a recognition that in our intersectional identities we carry our own experiences, our cultures' experiences, the intergenerational pain living in our genetics, all mixing together in this moment in response to something today. We must not, however, succumb to the urge to make all of this pain about the body's response, because the body's response is simply the neurobiological underpinning of the biopsychosocial/existential phenomenon that is trauma. Ironically, the better the neurobiology of trauma has come to be understood, the farther away from its roots in social pathologies the field of trauma healing seems to have strayed. To do DHCR trauma healing work we must understand the body in the social and political realities in which that body lives and thinks and feels.

TRAUMA—THE CREATURE WITH MANY FACES

A rape. A terrible motor vehicle accident. Watching one's best buddy blown into pieces by the improvised explosive device that you drove over without being blown up only a second earlier. "It could have been me, but instead it was you" (Near, 1974). These are all among the kinds of emotionally enormous and gaping wounds that are recognized by the *DSM* and the *International Classification of Diseases* (ICD) as meeting Criterion A, the official formal colonized definition of a real trauma. Experiences such as these are sharply drawn encounters with the fragility of the human body and with how easily and quickly life, or bodily integrity, or the fantasy of safety, can leave us. Events such as these are less difficult for the cultures imbued with social pathologies to acknowledge, today in this third decade of the 21st century, as forms of trauma.

But it was not always thus. It may be hard for my younger readers to believe that in 1976, when I started my doctoral internship at a Veterans Administration (VA) hospital full of young men traumatized in Vietnam and old men traumatized in Korea or in the POW camps of World War II, the mental health staff were forbidden to use the concept of trauma with those men. We were taught that they had personality disorders, which I had difficulty crediting, having already worked with survivors of sexual assault and intimate partner violence and thus recognizing the similarities of distress between these people. It is no surprise that the movement to create a formal posttraumatic stress disorder (PTSD) diagnosis in psychiatry's diagnostic manual came simultaneously from the rape crisis movement and the VA in tandem.

Despite the grudging and hard-fought-for acceptance of the notion that yes, these are traumas, the culture of the Global North, particularly that of the United States, remains rife with persistent narratives that a person long affected by such enormous wounds is "malingering" or "wallowing," refusing to get on with life or has a preexisting condition that made them uniquely vulnerable. In other words, trauma should be rare. People should get over it, and quickly.

In fact, persons who have experienced these kinds of events are now confronted inescapably with the paradox of having to live while knowing that death or violation are inescapable. This is a kind of knowledge requiring a degree of courage that most people cannot easily manifest because few people learn it before they must call upon that courage. Most people exposed to trauma are not Elie Weisel or Christine Blasey Ford, Anita Hill or Nelson Mandela. They are ordinary people, not gifted with some kind of extraordinary internal resources.

Some of the ways in which people try to assist themselves in soothing their neurobiological responses to these experiences of trauma without exposing themselves to the gaze of professionals are themselves problematized by the dominant culture as pathological. Trauma can lead to use of substances that numb or de-numb, leading to dependence on the substance, for which one gets the label of substance abuser and subsequently experiences all kinds of disruptions in all spheres of life. The sheer number of stories in the popular press about military members returning from their 10th combat tour replete with the distress engendered by this kind of trauma exposure, then being discharged dishonorably from that same military shortly upon their return to the United States, largely because they were trying to assist themselves in coping with their pain with a substance, staggers the mind. The colonized narratives of masculinity and the warrior who absorbs trauma without a ripple leads these people to be discarded, denied even the rationed care that our veteran's health system can offer, spat out into the world as defectives.

The parallel stories about some of the same people who are now inhabiting the prison system because they acted criminally due to their use of a substance with which they were attempting to calm their neurobiology in a world that made their pain invisible or shameful is also evidence of how easy it is for a culture to transform a person from hero to zero. Trauma marginalization leading to incarceration is not an unusual pathway for people in a culture where to struggle with being trauma-exposed is to be labeled weak. Too many trauma-exposed people will go to great lengths to find a substance that will quiet the biology of their trauma while the psychosocial and existential pain are required to be hidden in order to uphold structural and systemic forms of oppression.

This downgrading the value of the person struggling with regulating their traumatized neurobiology in a manner that humans have done since trauma's distress was recorded in writing—that is, with a substance—is one piece of evidence of colonized thinking about trauma. The United States is a deeply puritanical society, quite literally infused with the precepts of Calvinist colonizers teaching that those who struggle, who lose faith, who cannot shut down what is happening within them, are sinners; that those in need of help from their communities are sinners, weak, and not worthy, not among the elect of the divine; such was, after all, the Calvinist theology of the particular group of Christian colonizers called pilgrims in U.S. mytho-history.

When these deeply psychically wounded people struggle with the messages of the social pathologies of toxic masculinity that proclaim that a real man—or, for women, a real warrior—does not have posttraumatic distress but instead drinks himself into a stupor, what was once praised as their valor and gave a sense of meaning to the pain and loss becomes invisible, hidden by the ways in which they are unable to hide their pain. Their drunkenness, their emotional extremity, their apparent nihilism, the behaviors and words that emerge from them and make them seem as if no longer themselves, all of this takes over the narrative of who this person was. "Whoever came back after those deployments is not the person we knew," say so many of their families and friends.

These stories about what is defined as real trauma and what, in real life, happens to many of those who experience its effects in ways that disrupt narratives about war and heroism are the tip of the iceberg of the colonization, by our dominant social pathologies, of the world of trauma healing. The official narratives have placed artificial limits on how healers of psyches and souls have understood trauma and understood the tasks in front of us. To engage in DHCR trauma healing practice requires us not only to respond compassionately and fully to those who have encountered the official traumas but also to expand our understanding of what constitutes trauma for humans, what creates the interplay between the interpersonal, the political, the contextual, and the neurobiological in such a manner that a person experiences themselves as not safe in the world.

LIMITING THE DEFINITION OF TRAUMA IS EPISTEMIC COLONIZATION

Artificial limits on how trauma and its healing have been understood and defined—limits that have grown ever more narrow in my half century of immersion in this work—now exclude much of what is experienced as traumatic by humans and much of the findings of scientific research into the broader reach of what is felt as trauma. This exclusion from the canon, aka the *DSM*, is a problem in numerous ways. Those limits ignore or define as "not real trauma" all kinds of things to which our neurobiology responds as traumatic or things that are disruptive to our relationships and meaning-making systems even when they do not lead to nightmares or flashbacks and about which decades of well-designed research can tell us are phenomenologically traumatizing. These artificial boundaries between "real trauma" and "something else maybe traumatic" create difficulties in the trenches as well. In the case of a person who was sexually harassed at work in ways that don't fit into the parameters of Criterion A, yet who has all the rest of the kinds of distress that inhabit the construct of PTSD, how does a healer practicing in, say, the forensic world name that distress? This is not a hypothetical difficulty but one faced daily by any practitioner, decolonial or not, who dives into the realities of trauma.

These human experiences of trauma excluded from the canon are often those that do not arise from a long-standing Eurocentric construct of trauma as an individual's intense fear experience, a construct that has prevailed through various theoretical models since Winter (2006) proposed that shell shock was a response to intense fear, persisting through Kardiner & Spiegel's construct of "war neurosis" (Kardiner & Spiegel, 1947). Trauma as fear also features in the work of more recent feminist students of sexual assault and intimate partner violence such as Herman (1992) and L. E. A. Walker (1979). Fear-induced trauma is trauma.

It is, however, but one kind, as Herman (1992), Freyd (1996), Gold (2020), and others have increasingly pointed out. Other kinds of trauma with which I am familiar include intergenerational trauma, complex developmental trauma, relational/betrayal trauma, postcolonial trauma, nonpost/continuing trauma, as well as the traumas of lifelong exposure to one of the social pathologies, such as racism, misogyny, or toxic masculinity, without any specific event marking the trauma of these social toxicities.

I could write entire chapters on the traumas engendered by these experiences and social pathologies. That's my old model, and I'm not using it in this book. No more writing about trauma through the lens of *x* type of intersectional identity because that paradigm reinforces colonial categories of humanity as being about one and only one strand of intersectionality, and by so doing undervalues how interactions of forms of oppression and positionalities in social hierarchies potentiate the experience of trauma. No more speaking of real trauma versus the other traumas. Rather, the epistemic framework that is core to a DHCR trauma healing practice is the range and scope of intersectional identities and the varieties of experiences that are traumatizing to people. One of the ways that Eurocentric, colonized intellectual realities have attempted to minimize the enormity of the scale of trauma, both directly and indirectly colonial, is to advance the claim that trauma is a modern invention and thus not a real thing.

But hark, the classics of the Western canon! In the *Iliad*, Achilles goes mad after the trauma of the battlefield death of his beloved Patroclus. Ezekiel, a Hebrew prophet has posttraumatic dreams and intrusive images—visions— after being taken captive by colonizing conquerors and thrust into exile.

All of this record of posttrauma distress comes to us from well before the Common Era, in Ezekiel's case, 586 years before year 1 of the Gregorian calendar by which we mark our time, which was the year of the sack of the First Temple in Jerusalem where Ezekiel served as a priest. Earlier societies, to the extent that we have their written records, were more able to include the traumatized among their midst, perhaps because the ubiquity of all kinds of trauma could not be hidden, mocked, or minimized as it has become in the 21st century. Oops. Trauma is not a new thing. It is, as Herman (1992, 2023) has pointed out, a thing that, despite all attempts to obscure, hide, and marginalize it, continues to assert its presence, defying colonial narratives that normalize structural forms of oppression and subjugation.

TRAUMA: A MORE COMPLETE PICTURE

When I wrote *Cultural Competence in Trauma Therapy* 15 years ago the science of trauma as a fear response and its related neurobiology was just starting to emerge. The science of trauma response had some, but not all, of the picture of trauma's neurobiology, with a primary focus on the fear model as its guide. Thus my earlier volume explored what was then known about the fear response system, the amygdala and the hypothalamic–pituitary–adrenal (HPA) axis, the fear and stress response systems that inform the activation of the sympathetic and parasympathetic nervous systems. The polyvagal model of the dissociative components of trauma response and the role of disruptions in the attachment system as forms of trauma were not as well understood by me or by most students of trauma at that time; data are now available, which I will discuss in many of the subsequent chapters, as I address integrating mind, body, and spirit.

At the same time as a more expansive understanding of the biological substrates of trauma was emerging, trauma healers whose social justice standpoints overlapped with my own were beginning to more deeply appreciate the ways in which the official definitions of trauma, primarily those in diagnostic manuals, were inadequate to explain what was emotionally wounding to humans and why that was so. People like me whose work focused broadly on the range of experiences of trauma had an inkling about that bigger picture, and my initial book reflected that inkling of just how much trauma was in our emotional atmosphere. But the depths and layers of trauma and the complex manners in which humans go about not knowing about trauma in our daily lives were only starting to be knowable to those of us who wanted to see and hear these things.

TRAUMA FOR EVERYONE?

The topic of psychic trauma has become common in the parlance of the first 2 decades of the 21st century because of how many of the official traumas have occurred in the lives and in view of members of the dominant culture. It's become mildly acceptable to speak of having PTSD because of the terror attacks of September 11, 2001, because of the rash of mass shootings that seem to happen daily, because of the wars that the United States waged in the Middle East for nearly the entirety of these 2 decades, because of the #MeToo movement, because of the bravery of the many girls and women in gymnastics digitally raped by the team physician, of the boys, grown into men by a coach at an Ivy League university, of the wrestlers sexually assaulted by their coach at a Big 10 university (while a man who now sits in the U.S. Congress, Jim Jordan, who knew about those abuses and attempted to shut the young men down, is today shouting and waving his hands around about imagined crimes committed when the government attempts to investigate corruption but remains silent on the abuse he enabled)—because all of these brave people are silent no longer.

Trauma has become harder to frame as something happening to someone who is already the other when it's happening to so many people next door, in our families, to people who were not on the margins. Nor are most of these public traumas among those that can be blamed on some action or inaction of those traumatized—although some commentators do, and have, blamed those people. The discourse about trauma has thus shifted subtly, in some places.

This near normalization of the discourse about certain kinds of trauma can be both enlightening and dangerous. Some of the change in the public trauma narrative is due to increased awareness of the actual ubiquity and the endemic nature of certain kinds of trauma. Veils have been pulled back, sometimes stripped away, from some of the more prominent forms of systemic social pathologies and thus from the wounds they inflict on the bodies, minds, souls, and cultures of people.

A 24-hour news cycle, the easy availability of social media, and the fact that many people carry recording devices on their persons at all times has revealed how frequently people are exposed to the worst sorts of traumatizing experiences. It flies in the face of reality for anyone to assert today that trauma is unusual. Yet some still do, and the exclusionary boundaries around Criterion A and the notion that it alone defines a trauma are a manifestation of that stance.

Unsurprisingly, some authors have critiqued this expanding awareness of trauma and describe the trauma narrative as "wearing thin" (Sehgal,

2022). Yes, being confronted with the ubiquity of traumatizing experiences that occur in and often uphold the social structures of social pathologies of the dominant culture is wearing on the dissociative strategies of anyone who is still working hard to pretend that the trauma narrative is being exaggerated or made overly inclusive. The colonizing epistemology that is the intellectual substrate of this weariness is one that I hope to expose here.

Because, dear readers, there is nothing new about the desire of the official voices of any culture that is upheld by social pathologies to be weary of the stories of the wounds that are inherently inflicted there. As Herman (1992) noted early in the struggle to unmask trauma's ubiquity and its role in maintaining the hegemony of social pathologies, the story of the reality of trauma in the lives of our species is one that is briefly allowed into the public view and then becomes hidden again. The truth is many times pushed out of cultural narratives with the same scorn, ridicule, and disbelief that then meets trauma survivors themselves when they speak their truths.

The structural disappearance of the stories of the wounds, of the constant presence of danger, of the multiplicity of paper cuts inflicted sufficiently frequently to create painful, enormous holes, serves a larger culture in which such the stories of how these wounds came to be must remain hidden should the rottenness at the core of that larger system be exposed. Just as the juntas of Chile and Argentina disappeared dissenters, tossing their living bodies out of airplanes into the ocean, destroying the records of their torture and death, so have dominant cultures structurally disappeared the truths of trauma. As I write this in early 2024, the stories of how Africans were enslaved and the Indigenous peoples of North America genocidally destroyed by Europeans are being systemically legislated out of textbooks in certain U.S. states because those true stories might make someone uncomfortable or they are defined as being unpatriotic.

This recurrent disappearing act is, I would argue, evidence of the colonization of the trauma narrative from one of ubiquity to one of rarity—and also evidence of attempts to strip any trauma narratives of their associations with social pathologies. For if trauma is rare, unusual, not part of the human norm, then the underlying social rot and corruption creating ubiquitous, normative trauma is never exposed nor challenged, much less spoken of truthfully. If trauma is an individual experience, not the intended effects of a social pathology, then it can be spoken of more easily than if its presence is the evidence that something—many things—are very rotten in the structural and systemic hierarchies of oppression that are the background noise to most of our lives.

TRAUMA IS NOT JUST ONE THING: ANOTHER WAY OF KNOWING IT IS NOT NEW

To decolonize our understanding of trauma and how we engage with healing those who suffer from its presence in their lives and cultures is to overthrow and shift from an individualistic paradigm of trauma as one person's exposure to one, or even many, events that fall within the definitional boundaries of what is considered a real trauma in the worlds of psychiatry and psychology, Criterion A of PTSD. It is to make clear that trauma is not only not new but wired into human responses to the world around us.

Criterion A has itself been a moving target for 4 decades, changing in response to the politics of those claiming its definitional ownership in the American Psychiatric Association and World Health Organization, which publish, respectively, the *DSM* and the *ICD* in their various iterations. That the politicization of these diagnostic documents is rarely questioned, and that they are expected to be bowed to as authoritative, is some of the best evidence of the intellectual colonization of trauma healing by the structural and systemic forms of oppression that constitute the social pathologies of the Europeanized world, aka the Global North.

To name is to hold power over. If I name you deviant or disordered, and myself normal or typical, I create an immediate hierarchy of power with social meanings. Decolonizing the word *trauma* and the constructs that emerge from that word is, in consequence, a potentially powerful, liberatory act. When I do this in my work as a forensic expert, the revolutionary nature of my saying that racial trauma is trauma is reflected in the flurry of activity by which attorneys for the other side frantically attempt to disallow my testimony along those lines—with no success, as it happens. Telling the truth in the most stratified of realms, a justice system that, in the United States, first excluded those who did not own land, then those who were not of European descent, then those born in female bodies; to decolonize the construct of trauma in this setting scares those who were originally admitted to the corridors of power. Those humans who were the deciders of fact—White, male property owners whose property sometimes included the bodies of enslaved Africans—for them, decolonizing power can feel threatening.

To engage in this decolonial activity of naming oppression and colonization as trauma (particularly, for me, in places that have represented those social toxicities) is to validate the lived realities of traumatized people. To tell the truth—that these are traumas—rather than shoving them into the corner of an adjustment disorder, or a personality disorder, or some disorder designated as not trauma, is revolutionary and decolonizing of trauma practice.

As I referred to in passing in a preceding section, in the spring of 2023, I had an exchange with attorneys who claimed that because many of these other forms of trauma have to come into the diagnostic manual via something awkwardly called "other specified trauma and stressor related disorder" and that because microaggression and betrayal trauma are "other specified traumas or stressors" not specifically named in said diagnostic manual, they could not be real trauma. Q.E.D., they wrote, my opinions about these experiences being traumatizing to the people I had evaluated should be excluded, despite my having carefully crafted my testimony so that it would pass through the narrow gate of admissibility known as the Daubert standard for expert testimony.

Because I've worked as a forensic expert in civil rights and discrimination cases, I am keenly aware of the dangers that the narrow gate of Criterion A can create for people, particularly marginalized people, who have been harmed in some way. If a forensic expert cannot say that you have suffered emotionally because you had to sit, silencing yourself, in a workplace where every day aspersions were cast on a central component of your intersectional identities, your sympathetic nervous system (SNS) activating a stress response over and over, while forcing yourself into a frozen dorsal vagal state of numbness in order to maintain appropriate workplace decorum, because hate speech does not meet the definition of Criterion A, how much more critical is it that we decolonize trauma healing to include this person's kinds of painfully traumatic experiences?

Not adjusting, that is, not simply giving in and giving up in the presence of a dangerous social pathology, is not evidence of something wrong with the person. But that is what it means to assign a diagnosis of an adjustment disorder, the one given by the expert on the other side of this case. One is adjusting maladaptively to a nontraumatic stressor. Adjustment disorder, which I once saw as a benign thing, is perhaps one of the most colonizing narratives in the diagnostic manual, implying that a person who is experiencing distress in the face of a psychosocial stressor is disordered, rather than that the psychosocial stressor, the social pathology, being the disorder to which some response is simply human.

Having strong emotional and relational responses to disruptions in one's attachment to other humans is not a flaw in a person's personality, which is the message inherent in the diagnosis of borderline personality disorder, a diagnosis given to a woman who had been profoundly institutionally betrayed for having had the temerity to stand up for the welfare of a vulnerable person in her work setting. A DHCR healer, whether in a directly healing role or, as I have been, in a forensic/teaching role, must ask not "is this a Criterion A event," because that's a question reeking of coloniality. Decolonizing trauma healing with regard to how we identify that which is traumatic to people generates very different questions. Decolonial questions challenge the assumptions of the cultures of oppression, because what kinds of cultures have rules about how to be human, about how to respond to being betrayed, the result of which is to call those expressions of distress a disorder? Calling a person's traumatized inner being disordered is to do further harm to them, to dismiss them, minimize them, other them, cast them out of what is considered human; the diagnosis can itself be a kind of traumatic experience of being psychologically exiled. Decolonizing by expanding our constructs of what constitutes trauma reduces, at the very least, the risk inherent in receiving that kind of invalidating harm at the hands of a professional simply because one has sought surcease for one's pain.

TRAUMA—IT'S NOT ONLY ABOUT FEAR

The ubiquitous model of trauma in the mental health fields is a fear-based one, which makes sense. The assumption that overwhelming fear, horror, or helplessness are causative of the distress referred to in diagnostic manuals is contained in the very criterion for trauma exposure that precedes the remainder of the diagnosis. But is it all about fear? No; it is about, but not solely about, fear of loss of life or physical safety. It is about the activation of fear-based components of human neurobiology, such as the SNS and the HPA axis, which were the systems earliest identified as implicated in trauma response. It is not solely about these systems, as 3 additional decades of increasingly sophisticated neuroimaging have demonstrated, finally putting some biology into the biopsychosocial model of non–fear-evoked traumas.

The fear model is not an entirely inaccurate conceptual framework. It is, rather, an inadequate one. The fear model of trauma ignores the other ways in which our neurobiology can respond as if traumatized and wounded, even in the absence of the kinds of extreme terror, horror, and helplessness that characterize the traumas of the diagnostic manuals. Not all trauma-created distress is due to fear. But the experiences of colonization and oppression, of structural and systemic forms of oppression, engender fear, both immediate and ongoing.

Humans, being primates and mammals, are also wired for attachment (Schore, 2003). In consequence, our species is wired for responding to disruptions in attachment systems as information about danger. These attachment systems and their associated neurobiological manifestations start to work in humans at birth, while our fear systems do not begin to operate independent of those of our caregivers until a human is approximately 6 months old. Thus, the constructs of complex developmental trauma and attachment trauma, which often overlap, start with the preverbal disruptions to attachment before 6 months of age, disruptions that, when persistent, can have devastating consequences for the person who experiences such disruptions. The distress engendered by those disruptions and the person's attempt to manage that distress are still usually misdiagnosed as some form of disordered personality (Ford & Courtois, 2020).

As a consequence of the primacy and immediacy of the attachment and social engagement systems of our neurobiology, any disruptions to connection are themselves forms of trauma for humans and other mammalian species. Fear may not be involved at all (Lahousen et al., 2019). Because of the human attachment system, which allows our species to be born with incompletely developed brains but which requires human infants to depend on older humans much longer than, say, baby horses depend on their dams for other than milk, we are powerfully wired by evolution to sense even the slightest disruptions to attachment, as any parent of a newborn will be glad to tell you with regard to their experiences of leaving their infant's room long enough to take a shower. For a human infant, being attached is being safe; our fear response systems are among those parts of our brain that are not developed yet at birth, but our attachment system is there from our first breath.

Our early primate ancestors relied on trusting first their caregivers and then the other members of their small bands for safety in a world in which humans were still a prey species. If another member of the band was not worthy of trust, humans developed the capacity to quickly detect and be psychically wounded by betrayals of trust (Freyd, 1996). Our attachment systems predispose humans to detect dishonesty and betrayal, disruptions to attachment as the safe place.

Today, when interpersonal betrayals occur at the hands of those on whom we depend, we are neurobiologically equipped with mechanisms that allow us to un-know, forget, or reinterpret as meaningless those betrayals, unless and until we are closer to safe in life or in relationship to the betrayer and can thus know what has been done to us. Dissociation of betrayal in order to maintain attachment occurs not only at the individual level but also in the form of the colonization of our collective consciousness to allow dissociation of the persistence and dominance of social pathologies which are, in effect, betrayals of both our societies and ourselves.

EVIDENCE? OF WHAT? THE OFFICIAL TRAUMA TREATMENT BOX

Colonization Is a Trauma Factory

My proposition is that the project of healing psychic trauma is one that has been colonized intellectually and conceptually in the last century and a half by the same systemic forms of oppression and marginalization that are also the sources of people's pain. Social pathologies are a trauma factory. These social dynamics, which permeate all of the professions, produce trauma through oppression in its many forms, then find ways to marginalize the people who have been harmed, then exclude most of the damage done from formal definitions of trauma.

In our capitalist cultures, one must pay for access to treatments whose intellectual underpinnings are infected with the viruses of social pathologies, including the appropriation of Indigenous and Global South healing methodologies. Poor people get less care than those of means; in the United States, health insurance companies reimburse so poorly for psychotherapy that many therapists refuse to deal with them, which means that people with insurance and not much money have less access. Community mental health organizations might offer one session in a month, if that. The interjection of capitalist values into the way in which trauma healing is done funds the social pathologies of corporations to produce more trauma, and so on and so on, the snake of social pathologies endlessly eating its tail.

The colonization of the field of trauma healing has not only been the case for mental health work imposed on Indigenous people subject to European colonization. The current medicalized constructs defining trauma have led to the creation of a narrow gate for what is considered acceptable care. This gate calls itself an evidence base, with the term *evidence* defined in the most narrow and exclusionary ways as possible and with an emphasis on fear model interventions that lean heavily on the notion that traumatized people must learn to stop avoiding the painful material and be exposed to it in some manner.

This consequently has become a gate through which only a very few methodologies for healing trauma wounds have been able to pass (APA, 2017a). That gate, that narrow place, has become a norm for how the field of trauma psychology speaks of those who suffer from having been exposed to traumatizing circumstances. It has become the tightly woven sieve through which the field defines best practices for responding to those suffering souls. Sitting on the other side of that gate, living in the residue that cannot pass through the sieve, are most traumatized humans and most of the ways in which they heal. A DHCR trauma healer looks to the sides of, beyond, behind the narrow gate, centering the lived experiences of traumatized people. I asked the people who came to me, "What has helped you before I came into your life?" And then my job was to ask myself: how can we build upon that foundation, a process I'll discuss at length throughout this book regarding radical collaboration.

When I wrote *Cultural Competence in Trauma Therapy*, trauma work was also, as a field, still fixated on the notion that human responses to trauma were the kinds of mental health disorders that could be fixed with the right evidence-based, lab-tested treatments, a problematic perspective that I discussed earlier in this chapter. This paradigm, which is somewhat more useful when testing, say, a drug that treats a particular form of cancer, the randomized controlled trial (RCT) model has come to predominate the discourse in the mental health fields about what the "right" things are to do when the trauma-exposed person seeks our help. The paradigm of the RCT is a trap in which the colonized researchers sit.

In this research paradigm, people are carefully screened out of studies if they had any comorbid disorders, that is, other things that humans frequently do to deal with emotional wounding or other ways that the distress of emotional wounding expresses itself outside of the PTSD paradigm. The chosen few would then be randomly assigned to get an intervention, or no intervention, or something that the researchers thought wouldn't have any effect (such as being listened to which, as it turns out, has quite a lot of effects). Leaving aside the people who dropped out of the study, as well as those excluded for lacking purity of distress, some interventions helped some of the people, some of the time, more than the "tincture of time" could (APA, 2017a).

Again, irony because, as some of the founders of the International Society for Traumatic Stress Studies poignantly noted in a panel of past presidents (McFarlane, 2006), the only way that trauma healing was able to come out of the shadows of the mental health world in the 1970s was to be wildly experimental. The baby boomer generation of trauma healers, among whom I was fortunate to take my place, had to take risks with the respectability of our careers, to think outside the frameworks that had dubbed survivors of combat and sexual assault as characterologically weak. We all had to yell loudly in the ears of organized psychiatry to get PTSD into the *DSM-III*. That first generation of trauma workers had to risk being marginalized and subordinated in order to claw their way to quasi-respectability.

We naively believed that if we could just be allowed into the official documents of our fields, then our work would get the recognition it deserved, and traumatized people could get the help we wanted to give them. It was an entirely assimilationist approach, one modeled for us by Freud himself when he sought professional recognition for psychoanalysis from his anti-Semitic Viennese neurology world. Our campaigns to get trauma into the *DSM* fit neatly into the epistemic frameworks held by most of us, the well-colonized and somewhat well-socialized members of the baby boomer generation (well-socialized in that we had gone to medical school or graduate school in psychology or social work), and thus we were trauma healers who believed that if people just knew the truth, it would change the world.

I watched with some dismay as trauma intervention researchers who entered the field through the door of anxiety disorders only after trauma had begun to achieve respectability and grant funding, about 2 decades after the pioneers had created organizations and appeared to win their professional campaigns, proceeded to marginalize the founders and label their ideas "wild and crazy." These practitioners framed their bright shiny new research into what might help traumatized people as though the entire field of psychotherapy process and outcome research, which reaches back a century to the work of Carl Rogers, did not exist and would not apply to what was being done for people self-identifying as trauma survivors. Research on what it was about the relationship between the healer and the sufferer that seemed to make psychotherapy work (Duncan et al., 2010; Norcross & Lambert, 2019; Norcross & Wampold, 2019a) was treated as an annoying intrusion into the study of the trauma interventions, the no-treatment control group of the RCTs. Data about how culture and context and the presence of systemic forms of oppression and social pathologies were even less well regarded.

I can make these statements about what was made official and what was discarded or marginalized and subordinated with some authority and absolute knowledge of how true they are for two reasons. One, I watched the International Society for Traumatic Stress Studies undergo this epistemic and cultural transformation—and I stopped attending its meetings because nothing revolutionary, new, or actually helpful to the people I worked with was happening. I witnessed with some sadness the brilliant, groundbreaking trauma researcher and theorist John Briere's presidential farewell address to the society in the early 2000s. He spoke almost directly to the leader of the faction claiming "It's all about exposure," who was sitting in the front row of the auditorium, and said, with the wisdom of his years working with people who did not fit into Criterion A, in essence, "Great research findings, but what you are proposing doesn't help the people I work with."

I can make these statements also because I was a member of the American Psychological Association's working group to develop guidelines for the treatment of PTSD (American Psychological Association, 2017a). There, for several years, I and two other voices for psychotherapy relationships, along with two other voices for issues of culture and social context, were repeatedly and collectively on the receiving end of the dismissal of three-quarters of a century of research about psychotherapy and almost as much data about culture and context (Brown & Courtois, 2019; Courtois & Brown, 2019). Those of us who were on that group especially because of our expertise about psychotherapy outcome research or cultural and social issues in trauma collectively wrote and submitted to our colleagues carefully researched and referenced pages about these topics, only to have them reduced to a paragraph or two in the final version of the guidelines because these topics were defined by the larger group as tangential to the question of which intervention erased the most PTSD symptoms in RCTs.

The Visible Size of a Wound Is Irrelevant to Whether It Is Hurting

A wound to the soul engendering terrible pain can appear from the outside to be the psychic equivalent of a paper cut or a knuckle skinned while grating a potato. Small, a bit bloody, rarely leaving a visible scar—yet quite painful. The evidence of our body's fragility, those scant drops of blood, are passing reminders of our mortality that can be ignored. The psychic equivalents of these apparently smaller wounds are also dismissed by most of the field of trauma and by the larger culture as well as part of a colonizing narrative that attempts to suppress evidence of the repeated small wounds to bodies and cultures and psyches inherent in colonization.

"Stick and stones may break my bones, but words can never hurt me," goes the old children's chant. Well, no. Not true, not one bit true, simply a colonizer strategy behind which hate speech can hide and be minimized: "Just joking. Can't you take a joke?" Words of hate can cause those psychic paper cuts, and such cuts can open up fragile scar tissue and go to the bone as deeply if they had been made with a carving knife.

I wonder at times whether this particular chant was created by some social pathology or another as a means of indoctrinating children in the English-speaking world, which is full of hateful words and hate speech that "puts people in their place," into ignoring and minimizing the power of hate speech and other forms of verbal abuse to do terrible harm—and teaching those same children to have contempt for those who are harmed by words. These paper cuts are constructed by the colonization of meaning and language as not meeting the arbitrary and continuously changing criteria for what constitutes a real trauma. Those who suffer in the presence of hateful words are mocked by the voices of dominant culture as "snowflakes," "fragile." If one is beaten by one's partner, it's abuse—unless you asked for it, and then it's not abuse, it's some poor henpecked spouse acting as expected. My generation of American baby boomers grew up watching a popular television show which taught that lesson, in which the main character, played by the famous comedian Jackie Gleason, weekly threatened his wife with such phrases as, "One of these days, Alice, pow! right in the kisser," and "Bang! Zoom! To the moon Alice, to the moon!" (Gleason & Satenstein, 1955–1956). My generation was taught to find him funny and to find Alice, the wife, somehow deserving of these continuous threats.

The message about trauma here: if one is verbally battered or denigrated, it's only words to some standing on the sidelines. Or if it's uttered by someone whose official role is comedian, it's only a joke, and those harmed by the words, whether uttered by Gleason in the 1950s or Dave Chapelle today, are exhorted to "get over themselves" or accused of "canceling" someone if they don't want to offer a platform for that particular hate speaker any longer. The colonization of the arts by various forms of social pathologies has been so pervasive as to have been rendered nearly invisible. The celebration of the oppressor in the arts of those oppressors has created a canon that is only now being disrupted by the voices of the colonized, the marginalized, the formerly excluded.

If a Paper Cut Could Metastasize

Imagine not one paper cut but a thousand paper cuts in the same location that are inflicted daily by the toxic conditions of social pathologies present in a person's life as a member of marginalized, subjugated group or six. "Death by a thousand cuts" is a good metaphor for this phenomenon. Where the thousand small cuts of microaggression (Nadal, 2018; D. W. Sue, 2010) or insidious trauma (Root, 1992) are concerned, they add up to the emotional equivalent of the swipe of a sword, ripping through psychic flesh and bones. But because each cut seemed small to the colonized mind of an observer, the dominant culture of the trauma world renders them invisible and excluded from our concerns. Those cut in this manner are, however, being wounded daily, often hourly, and rarely experience a respite that might allow the experience of being closer to safety and healing. They live in some version of what Kaschak (2021) calls "chronic traumatic terror," experienced at varying degrees of intensity. It is as if the small cut metastasizes, invisible until some gaping psychic lesion finally surfaces.

Things Do Not Happen for a Reason

Limiting the officially traumatized to that small subset of people whose lived experience falls within a narrow definitional framework also enables the persistence of an epistemic illusion of colonization, the so-called just world hypothesis (JWH; M. J. Lerner, 1980). The JWH is at the core of the Calvinist Eurocentric theologies and philosophy that infected those who colonized what is now the United States. It is the "everything happens for a reason" rubric, whose subtext is, "Some divine being has ordained this for you, so accept it as your divinely ordained destiny." The JWH is that good things happen to good people, everything that happens makes sense, and life is fair.

The JWH is a belief rendering those who have treated it as fact and as a set of true assumptions about the world particularly vulnerable to the destructive messages of certain social pathologies (Janoff-Bulman, 1992) regarding entitlement, by virtue of one's allegedly superior intersectional identities, to more power, more safety, and more resources than those not possessing the specific intersectional identities. These social pathologies promise a just and safe world to certain groups of people, those not on the margins of a culture, those whose phenotypes and other intersectional identities have been, to date, privileged by the dominant cultural context. The JWH belief system has fueled the uprising of fascism around the globe, both in the past and again today, as working-class, dominant-culture, phenotype-privileged humans, who were promised that their sacrifices on behalf of those in power would protect their phenotype privilege, have raged against the realities showing the falsehood of this belief. Viewed through the lens of DHCR, the rise of global antidemocratic movements is simply the collective, terrified attempts by some people to force the shape of the social world back into the framework that made the world just for them, and only them. Of course, in doing so, other people are made vulnerable, others are harmed. The trauma factory is also fueled by the JWH.

Holding onto the JWH also allows healers, aka professionals, to maintain the illusion that trauma happens to someone else, not ourselves. The JWH has functioned to maintain a fiction that trauma is rare rather than ubiquitous. It has upheld the fantasy that trauma is happening out there somewhere, not, as is actually true, happening to most people some of the time and some people almost from the moment they first draw breath, right in front of each one of us. Decolonizing trauma healing requires those of us doing this work to examine our assumptions about why certain kinds of experiences have been placed within those definitional parameters of real trauma, while others have been excluded even in the presence of reams of documentation about how those excluded phenomena are traumatizing. If at least one-third of all psychotherapists who responded to surveys about this in the middle 1990s are telling the truth, then at least that many healers have been exposed to the traumas that are not really trauma in *DSM* realities.

The Healer's Before-and-After Matters, Too

Questions about the before and the after and the continuous present of trauma are germane and require our careful attention for the DHCR model of healing. We need to begin with ourselves, the healers, so that we begin by disrupting the artificial division of traumatized people into us, the ones who heal others, and them, the suffering people seeking to feel more safety, less pain. What occurred before the official trauma? For the suffering person? For the healer? How did the healer learn to understand, to be in the room with, to engage with the suffering person? How did the suffering person learn to tolerate exposure to another human being in the quest for surcease of pain (Bailey, 2023)? What were their lives, our lives, before, if there was a before, after, if there was an after, and now, in the continuing presence of unsafety?

No one walks into this field without having had a life that guided us here as we became more aware of the presence of oppression and danger in the world and the harm done to others or in which this path was so overdetermined by the trauma residing in our own generational and personal strands of intersectionalities that we could have done no other work. What were the epistemic models that guided the healer's training and their socialization/colonization into their profession? What occurred before for the healer who learned to adapt rather than be responsive, to pursue, as I mistakenly thought possible, competence rather than humility? What happened that we learned to not speak of our own trauma exposures, to be silent, with the exception of a few brave souls (Bryant, 2023; Bryant-Davis, 2005; A. G. Rogers 1995) who have had the temerity to say out loud that they are both healers and wounded.

What came before for the healer—our own intersectional identities, our own participation in dominant cultures as the colonized, the colonizer, or, as is increasingly likely to be the case, some of both, as we have traversed the path to sitting in a room with a person in distress—is as important to the conduct of DHCR practice as are the frameworks that follow in this book, as important as what has happened in the lives of the suffering people seeking our care. We have to engage in a decolonizing of ourselves, evince the willingness to question and at times discard the apparently self-evident truths that colonized our psyches and our training. This is hard, and humbling, and it prepares us to offer DHCR trauma healing.

TRAUMA WATERED DOWN, COMMODIFIED, OR WEAPONIZED BY SOCIAL PATHOLOGIES

This is not to acknowledge that the construct of trauma can, in fact, be overapplied. It would appear that, in the public domain, some people may use the term *trauma* to describe what are, in fact, experiences of no longer being able to assert dominance or privilege over the narratives of human history or over the present-day experiences of other humans' lives. The attempt to take the true stories of slavery (that word itself has apparently been stripped from textbooks in at least one, perhaps two U.S. states at the time of writing this in January 2024) out of public education because knowing that people who looked like oneself (European ancestry) did unspeakable things to people who did not look like them, excused by the lies of phenotype supremacies, will create discomfort which is called "traumatizing" is an excellent example of a misapplication of the construct of trauma.

There is some merit to identifying the pain of loss of privilege as a type of trauma, although some experiences identified as traumatic, such as learning that Europeans enslaved African people in the United States, may be harder to agree to call traumatic through a decolonial lens. Nevertheless, a DHCR healer must squint there and see how the lies of social pathologies harm all. Perhaps here the harm is not in knowing the truth but in learning, later, that truth was willfully withheld from you.

Then there was the so-called false memory movement, built as an act of vengeance against a woman who remembered incest and approached her parents to talk with them about it. The false memory movement said that there had been no incest. It asserted that the accused were the traumatized ones when the adults they had raised told them about what they had never forgotten or recently recalled about how a close family member had incestuously abused them years previously. That was a movement that entirely reversed the narrative of what happened in families where sexual abuse occurred, something that its first target, Jennifer Freyd, a distinguished psychologist and contributor to the feminist and emerging decolonial paradigms of trauma, named "DARVO"—deny, attack, reverse victim and offender.

The psychic wounds of being here in this moment, with privilege appearing to slip away, are for the most part real wounds if one observes the people who are experiencing the loss of the American dream (an illusion) or the American version of the JWH with compassion. The distress being described is not that a child might see a drag queen in public. The issue of subverting socially constructed and mandated gender lines is a metaphor for terror about change.

The trauma and distress, which are very real indeed, are the wounds of those whose understanding of the world has been so profoundly colonized by social pathologies that, for them, up is down. To see up as up would blow their long-standing and deeply rooted view of a just and good world (Rubin & Peplau, 1975) into particles too small to put back together. This is loss of JWH trauma, and it is real, no matter how much it hides beneath what seem to be increasingly dangerous conspiracy theories.

A VIRUS PIERCES THE VEIL OF DENIAL

In the second decade of the 21st century events began to occur with sufficient frequency and transparency that wounds were exposed for long enough that they could not be concealed or at times were no longer allowed to be hidden. These were wounds, such as the extrajudicial murders of George Floyd and Sandra Bland, some of whose origins were millennia or centuries old, generated by convergences of systems of structural oppression, violence, colonization, and disempowerment. Then along came a virus and for a while, every human life was in danger.

An Equal Opportunity Danger at Last

The human population, from the origins of the coronavirus pandemic in late 2019 through the time of my writing this sentence in early 2024, has been in a constant state of danger as it has never been before, given the speed with which people carrying this virus and its mutations can move across the planet, as well as the speed with which the virus itself has mutated and thus evades prior immunities. The supercharged speed of this danger was a creature of our technological age. There were no airplanes during outbreaks of the bubonic plague. There were ships, which could be quarantined in harbors, and while the rats carrying the fleas that are the host for *Yersinia pestis* could ignore the quarantines and slip ashore to infect human hosts, the scale of the danger and death, while enormous in the context of that time in history, was not what we have experienced with COVID-19. Populations moved slowly about the planet then. *Yersinia pestis*, a bacterium that did not need to mutate in response to antibiotics, did not change shape. Humans also moved relatively slowly in 1918 and 1919 when the flu pandemic appeared, although that pandemic was potentiated by the movement of populations in the aftermath of the First World War.

The more quickly and easily human hosts for new diseases can move about the planet, and the more quickly and easily the source of the disease can shape-shift, the more dangerous those diseases are to us. We are thus in a continuous state of risk about which most of us try to be in denial, which is probably why now, in the early months of 2024, people I know who practice denial to one degree or another keep coming down with a COVID infection.

Thus, 4 years into the emergence of this equal opportunity risk many humans continue to experience reminders that the life they knew before 2020 shows no signs of returning. Those who are staring unflinchingly at the biological realities in which we now live are grieving for that life and wounded by its loss. Other people, however, are proceeding precisely as they would have before the pandemic, infecting themselves and others once again, because of being informed by social pathologies and colonial mindsets that create false feelings of invulnerability in those whose intersectionalities are primarily dominant. The day I edited this paragraph for the fifth time, in December 2022, a friend and colleague shared the story of her disrupted holiday plans: one part of her family has steadfastly refused vaccinations and was collectively exposed by another family member who walked in the door to cheerfully announce that he was positive for the virus. All were people who I know, from her telling over the years, are afflicted with the social pathology of White supremacy that lies to them that their skin color makes them immune. All, for the holiday season of 2022, were ill, including one very sick young child who has fortunately since recovered.

These dangerous ideologies of invincibility, applied to a speck of protein that does not care about a person's position in the social order, have led to similar approaches to other kinds of risks, both physical and psychic. These social pathologies promote a narrative that, if there had been any danger, it is all gone now—which, in turn, brought the rates of illness and death up again in the early winter of 2022 and each winter since. The official COVID-19 emergency has been declared over by governments, which means mostly that statistics about case counts and deaths are no longer being accurately collected and reported. The parallels between how the larger culture deals with the virus—denial, minimization, killing the messenger (death threats against public health officials have so far not been acted on, but they are persistent tropes promulgated by purveyors of social pathologies)—and how it addresses psychic trauma are striking.

Trauma is like this virus. It is ubiquitous and, unlike this particular speck of protein, always has been. It has always been an equal opportunity phenomenon, affecting all of us some of the time and some of us all of the time whether that truth was convenient to the social order or not. The human nervous system is, as the science of trauma is discovering more all the time, designed to assist us in responding to the possibility of a trauma and in coping with its aftereffects so that we may continue to perform activities necessary to sustain life, even when those coping mechanisms come at a considerable price. We are hardwired for responding to trauma and seem to be living more consciously immersed in it than ever—while, at the same time, social forces push for a new dissociation of its ubiquity and a repathologizing of our very human nervous system responses. The colonizing of the trauma story to "rare, not here, not us" lives in those dissociative forces of colonized realities.

My colleague Ellyn Kaschak (2021), who has thought in great depth about these matters, has recently coined the term *chronic,* or *contemporary terror disorder,* to describe the persistence and ubiquity of trauma. She wrote:

> Yet the terror does not abate or even lessen. It instead takes up an underground residence in our very psyches and in our bodies as well. We are more nervous, irritable, and perhaps angry and aggressive. Some of us look for someone else to blame and hatred rears its ugly head. We begin to go outside of our homes less, only when necessary. Some of us emerge only with guns in hand. We begin to fear each other, and the social fabric begins to tear apart. There are as many iterations of buried terror as there are of the overt variety.
>
> The terror does not become "post." It instead becomes perpetual as it hides from our own consciousness, as we try to carry on in the new normal. The various threats to our very beings come together to unite as a threat to our very existence, all of us. A threat many of us are perpetuating unconsciously by choosing sides, designating enemies, fighting over every issue from vaccinations to masks to voting to shooting others in "self-defense." Not discussing, but shouting, attacking, and demonizing those with whom we disagree, or whom we have chosen to represent our own personal terrorists. (Kaschak, 2021, paras. 7–8)

IT AIN'T OVER UNTIL IT'S OVER—AND IS IT EVER OVER?

I first heard the notion that it was kind of quaint and privileged to think of PTSD as "post" and a "disorder" at an international trauma conference held in Amsterdam in the early 1990s, in conversation with an Argentine psychiatrist. We started out talking about being Jews, the "six degrees of mitochondrial DNA separation" conversation that Jews whose families came from Europe frequently have when our phenotypes wave to one another.

His family had fled Germany as refugees to Argentina just before the Nazis shut the gates out of Germany forever. Like many Jews, we engaged in a spirited discussion of how the thorough assimilation of German (and Dutch and some French) Jews before the Nazis came to power made the trauma of what came next seem much worse, given how those Jews had seen themselves as German or Dutch or French first and Jewish only because their grandparents were. This is a lot like the Jews of the United States, I might add, until the past few years—assimilated, Americans who happened to celebrate Passover instead of Easter.

Then he said something to the effect of how we Jews didn't get to have posttraumatic anything because it was all still going on. This was before a terror group acting on behalf of Iran blew up the Jewish center in Buenos Aires, sending large numbers of the Jews of Argentina fleeing elsewhere, second- and third-generation refugees. And, he said, no one in Argentina—

which had at that point just finished up a dirty war of the generals that had led to the extrajudicial murders of so many people, the theft of so many children and their placement into the homes of military loyalists, the slow return from prison camps of the tortured—no one was post anything either. It wasn't over. That was the early 1990s. It's apparently still not over in Argentina, where DNA is now allowing stolen children to be found by their grandparents and the bones of their parents to be identified in the unmarked mass graves.

It's also, to reprise my reference to Kaschak's brilliant essay, written in December 2021, not post anything anywhere. Trauma and terror, the actions and actors of social pathologies, are endemic. It is consequently disingenuous to refer to a kind of distress as posttraumatic, because that is, in some ways, evidence of the colonization of thinking about trauma as something bad that happens to an individual and then is over.

My preferred terminology is thus *trauma exposure*, indicating the many layers of trauma and absence of safety that occur in people's lives, because the conundrum of creating something resembling safety when there may be none is one of the great challenges confronting every trauma healer who is awake to the realities of our social environment (Brand et al., 2022). I think I can safely say ("safely," a joke because one must have a sense of humor when facing horror) that the challenged people likely include anyone picking up this book with its title. The distress starts to happen before we are born, continues during the trauma, and after its immediate acute phase, if there is one, or continuously as the social pathology marches, jackbooted, onward.

3 DECOLONIZING TRAUMA HEALING

SOME COMMENTS ABOUT TERMINOLOGY

I have already discussed using the term *social pathologies* to refer to systemic and structural forms of oppression that are endemic sources of traumatization. As another decolonizing strategy, I would like to challenge the duality of the roles of the trauma healer and the official suffering trauma-affected person. A path toward that not quite nonduality will be, going forward, to use the terms *trauma healing* and *trauma healers*, not treatments or psychotherapists, unless I am referring to past practices or usual versus decolonial methodologies, and *suffering person* or *trauma-exposed person*, not client or patient.

Why? What's in a name? Isn't this simply splitting hairs? I think not, because language is powerful: the subtexts of words—the ascriptions that have been draped on them as they have come into use—matter, and all of these words convey the colonizing messages of "normal," "pathological," of the healer as not trauma-sufferer, the sufferer as not self-healer. As we name a thing, so we understand it. Psychotherapy, as practiced since Freud presented psychoanalysis to the Western world, has been colonized and

https://doi.org/10.1037/0000421-004
Decolonizing Trauma Healing: Toward a Humble, Culturally Responsive Practice,
by L. S. Brown

corrupted from its inception by the pressures both external and internal that anti-Semitism placed on its mostly Jewish founders. Freud and his students, a group in which Jews were overrepresented in relationship to their numbers in the pre-Nazi European population, were actively persecuted during the course of their lives. The term *psychotherapy* brings with it the ghosts of the traumas that shaped its creators, and so I choose to abandon that word.

There is also the problem of how the work of healing wounded souls and spirits has become a colonial walled garden owned by professions. The less I pay homage to the construct of psychotherapy as the sole source of healing from wounds to souls, spirits, and communities, the more I can weave some truths about psychotherapy's roots and history into a decolonial trauma healing framework, as well as develop the more expansive vision that is decolonial, humble, culturally responsive (DHCR) practice. Understanding what is deeply wrong with the edifice of psychotherapy, with the notions of mental health and behavioral health, the rejection of practices that are indigenous beyond the narrowest construct of that term, as well as the medicalization of work with traumatized people, all of these aspects of coloniality in trauma healing seem central and deeply germane to generating a humble approach to standing in the presence of trauma.

I am also going to use these different words because the decolonial truth is that humans have been assisting other humans with healing from trauma for millennia. We did so before there was a thing called psychotherapy that separated this healing work into that done with minds from that done with bodies, as if the two were unrelated one to the other, the Cartesian fallacy that misdirected the thinking of the Christian European colonizer cultures.

This other trauma healing work did not disappear when psychiatry and then clinical psychology, clinical social work, counseling, and hypnotherapy each came along in turn to claim the right to be soul healers, erecting barriers to entry to healing practice as their sphere of influence metastasized. Parallel, sometimes underground, sometimes illegalized practices of various trauma healing arts persisted, never legitimized although often appropriated when stumbled upon by members of Christian Eurocentric cultures.

Healers of wounded souls and communities have continued to go about their work alongside those who thought that there was only one path, that of the helping professions. These healers didn't get insurance reimbursements. The *curanderas*, the wonder-working rabbis, the meditation teachers, and those who passed on traditions of sacred plant medicines simply did their jobs, and perhaps did more for suffering people than many of the legitimated, professionalized, and therefore colonized, modalities. These folks, operating in a parallel universe that has looked benignly and with some humor at the efforts of healers such as myself to jump through the hoops of the dominant culture that signify legitimacy, while hiding from us for fear of being exposed to ridicule or punishment, have offered healing in ways that have nothing to do with psychotherapy as it's usually conceptualized. They are the healers to whom the first writings on decolonizing trauma work frequently refer; medicine people, elders, *curanderas*, vodun and Santeria healers, 12-step sponsors (Comas-Díaz & Jacobsen, 2024).

Traveling into that parallel world, as I have been doing with increasing frequency after having attained my legitimacy credential, has brought into very sharp focus the problem of how psychotherapy as a discipline lacks humility with regard to the appropriated healing methods for which psychotherapists have been taking credit and charging money for the last century. Not a small amount of what Western and Eurocentric folks refer to as evidence-based treatments for the suffering that arises from exposures to trauma are in fact appropriations of healing methodologies that some colonized Indigenous culture of the Western Hemisphere or the Global South, or of some group of marginalized and subordinated people, have been doing with and for one another without needing the permission or the imprimatur of a Western organization.

In this way trauma healing's coloniality and need for decolonization is a bit like the whole process of assisting babies into the world. Until Western medicine, which was almost entirely populated by people who were genetically and physically incapable of giving birth (natal men), decided to appropriate and medicalize childbirth in the Global North toward the end of the 19th century, women birthed with the help and accompaniment of other women—midwives, family members, friends, usually those who had given birth themselves. Some women and infants died, as some do now in the hands of Western medicine, because pregnancy and childbirth are full of dangers. Some mothers or babies died for a new reason, because the men who had appropriated the job of delivering an infant didn't wash their hands between births and passed infections along from one birthing woman to another. Some women and infants still do die during the birthing process, no matter how medicalized it has become, with Black, Indigenous, and people of color (BIPOC) women and their infants dying at higher rates than all others because of the concatenation of failures of care offered to them from the moment of conception to the post-partum period. Even BIPOC women who have access to wealth and high-quality care, for example, the tennis giant Serena Williams, have the kinds of worse quality care during the labor and delivery process that many of their BIPOC sisters experience.

Not until the women's health movement of the late 20th century was this appropriation of catching babies by the medical establishment challenged. Some of the power to run the process of having a baby was taken back by birthing women themselves who wished not to be rendered unconscious while their infant was pushed outside the womb and who wanted to be perceived as the agents of this experience, not its passive recipients (Boston Women's Health Book Collective, 2011). Those catching the babies have become increasingly among those born with the ability to give birth themselves, midwives once again taking their place alongside obstetricians, the ranks of obstetricians changing from mostly those who could never give birth to those who could, and often had.

No one would say that childbirth or the process of reproduction is decolonized—in fact, attempts by governments to recolonize the womb and tear away bodily autonomy from birthing women, as well as nonbinary and trans people with wombs, are expanding exponentially in the year after the 2022 *Dobbs* decision nullified those rights in the United States. The enslavement of the womb has been creeping in for several decades via the policing of indications of substances in the blood of those giving birth so as to allow states to preemptively steal infants at birth in the name of child protection. Patriarchy fights back hard against any attempts to cede power to those who carry a pregnancy. Even the words *legitimate* and *bastard* refer to whether a child is officially claimed or possessed by a man, patriarchy baked into the notion of whether a child is legitimate rather than an illegal immigrant into the species.

But the process by which childbirth was professionalized in the Eurocentric world since the middle of the 19th century, beginning with the expulsion of midwives from the births of the ruling classes and rolling out into the birthing rooms of all women, a process that has put birthing women into more danger under the false promise of the mantra that a doctor is safer than a midwife, and then the ways in which that professionalism was challenged, which in turn brought more agency and empowerment to some birthing women and, for some, opened the door to a vision of childbirth as an active collaboration between the birthing mother and those assisting the process, serves as an example of how trauma healing might also be decolonized, deprofessionalized, the suffering people empowered to be the agents of their change and healing rather than the recipients of the rules and norms of those accompanying them. It also is a cautionary tale of how social pathologies attempt to sabotage such efforts to decolonize and return control to those most affected, whether it is giving birth or experiencing and healing from trauma exposure.

As noted earlier, I'm using the descriptive terms *suffering, trauma-exposed people*, and *people in distress*, so as to indicate that here is a human having particular experiences rather than a class of distanced or pathologized others. Healers and suffering people: this describes how a person is being in relationship to the other, sometimes the same person, sometimes not.

Trauma healers sometimes have specialized training in addressing the suffering that trauma brings. Sometimes they do not. Some trauma healers simply know how to be healing in the presence of a suffering wounded soul or on behalf of a suffering wounded community. Just because some of us who have the honor to sit with suffering people have had some specialized training or received a certificate attesting to same doesn't allow us, if we wish to be decolonial, to distance ourselves from the suffering people who honor us with their stories and their pain by labeling them as other than what they are—humans in pain, or humans causing pain, or some combination of both.

Nor should our training give us special status in relationship to those people. We are honored by their willingness to let us witness their pain, not by the certificates we have accrued. So there shall be no diagnosis language in this volume except where I use it as an example or to deconstruct and critique it. *Suffering, wounded people, traumatized people, people with distress, people whose behaviors cause distress, suffering communities,* all of these are terms I will use here.

A decolonial epistemic framework requires us to rethink the exclusion of the myriad experiences that may be labeled "not really trauma but sure feels like one" discussed in the previous chapters and to inquire into how that exclusion might have assisted in the propping up and normalization of toxic cultural dynamics, of the social pathologies promising a just world to the chosen few and otherwise doing harm to most people's abilities to feel safe enough in the world. To quote Brand et al. (2022), "for individuals who may have never known safety, the idea of getting safe can feel entirely unconceivable, and 'getting safer' like a trick, and/or feel impossible" (p. xiv), a problem that we'll discuss at much greater length later in this book, since getting to something resembling safety is, I contend, the core of trauma healing.

Decolonizing trauma healing requires a critical examination of the epistemologies that we who practice this work have held to be true. Decolonizing is a heretical and radical exploration and deconstruction of what we as professions of trauma healers have been willing to know. Adopting a DHCR standpoint invites a deep and honest interrogation of what we and the field of trauma healing have quite literally dissociated, of what we have collectively unknown and disowned. Decolonizing asks us instead to open our hearts and minds and healing paradigms, allowing the broadest possible lens for knowing fully what trauma can be and what it does in the bodies, minds, spirits, and communities of humans.

Decolonizing the Us and Them of Trauma Healing

Something else that I failed to say strongly enough the last time I wrote on this topic, but which I had the opportunity to say when I gave my presidential address for the American Psychological Association (APA)'s Division of Trauma Psychology in 2010 and which I now say every time I teach about trauma to any group of people, is that most trauma healers are also humans who have experienced trauma as decolonially described. Nothing about DHCR practice is about us—the healers—and them—the traumatized people. This is about a humble, culturally responsive collaboration between two people. One person in that particular relationship is offering what they hope to be healing, based on their emerging understanding of the other person in the room. That person is without the illusion that they are not also healing themselves in the process of their work.

That last point is considered to be almost anathema by those practicing trauma therapy as usual, referred to as role reversal or poor boundaries. DHCR practice insists that healing is bidirectional, even though it is rarely equally weighted; the DHCR practitioner does not first do their own work and then plunge into being a healer. The DHCR paradigm knows that healers are always being healed by our work, always being trauma-exposed by our work and by our worlds, and bringing all of that back into the healing process, being vulnerable with ourselves rather than armored in faux competence.

This paradigm of reciprocity in healing, first written of by Saks Berman (1985), Surrey, and other feminist therapy theorists in the last century, is a profoundly decolonial perspective. In this healing modality there are no experts and seekers, no neutral, abstaining, invisible doctors and exposed, interpreted patients. There are humans in collaboration with one another with the stated goal of the healing of one, and the possible additional healing of the healer, and with the decolonial goal of healing the communities of both through this practice. Because each person in a community traumatized by colonization who heals from the wounds to themselves, their ancestors, and their world is a part of that community itself more healed, what Comas-Díaz and Jacobsen (2024) describes as the *ancestrality* and *vincularidad* points of her decolonial psychotherapy medicine wheel.

The wounded healer, who over time is every one of us, does not pretend to have a fixed set of official things that we know will work to unbreak the brokenness of the other person's inner and interpersonal worlds. We instead offer whatever wisdom we have available, which includes knowing how colonized all of us have been, and some ideas about how to address the experiences of being traumatized, how to hold a space in which another traumatized person can be seen and heard and known, which is the first step in the healing process.

This contrast between the official stories propped up by social pathologies, lately with increasing vigor in some parts of the world, and the story that is the truth as told from the 30,000-foot perspective where the colonizing reality is no longer defining the terms of the narrative, is an analogy to how experiences are defined or excluded from being brought under the mantle of trauma. There is a parallel here for how approaches to healing trauma's psychic wounds are legitimated by the narrative of evidence-based interventions while relational, somatic, and Indigenous modalities that are unlikely to be the subject of the randomized controlled clinical trials are subjected to various delegitimizing narratives. Trauma healers at work when Francine Shapiro first offered eye movement desensitization reprocessing (EMDR) to our field may recall that an entire website was built devoted not to intellectually critiquing that healing modality but to actively and, in this author's opinion, viciously mocking it and mocking Shapiro. Never mind that EMDR now, 40 years on, has the evidence base; in the minds of many, it is still remembered as the subject of ridicule and scorn.

The world of clinical trials is a study in the colonial walled garden of knowledge at work. To conduct such a research trial, one must be in an institution that supports doing this kind of expensive research, which means a research university or other large institution with a grants office, rarely a small liberal arts college, and certainly not the office of an independent scholar with no institution at all. One must have grant funding, and quite a lot of it, in the tens and hundreds of thousands of dollars. One must exclude from the participant group everyone with comorbid conditions, in other words, all of the traumatized people who are trying to regulate their neurobiology in ways that get diagnosed as something other than posttraumatic stress disorder (PTSD). One must thus be so deep in the colonized world of academia, institutions, and official science that a more difficult-to-study group of people, those who are trauma-exposed and respond in infinite factorial combinations of manners to that exposure, nor a less tightly defined and easily studied intervention cannot even be imagined as a possible focus of curiosity and inquiry.

WHAT OCCURS BEFORE

Something I wrote at the beginning of *Cultural Competence in Trauma Therapy* (Brown, 2008) remains true to me:

> Even such an apparently neutral trauma as a natural disaster or a car accident can have this sort of complex and multidetermined meaning structure because the emotional impact of trauma is not merely about what happened in the moment, but also reflects what occurred before and what transpires next (p. 3).

From a decolonial framework, "what occurred before and what transpires next" are the lineaments of the big picture of what trauma healing has to include in order to be effective in reducing human distress. As I have touched on earlier in this book, the before and after are salient to decolonizing trauma healing because they offer that 30,000-foot view that a DHCR trauma healer needs.

One of the mystery novelist Elizabeth George's most poignant and painful books is titled *What Came Before He Shot Her* (2006). The denouement in the novel is the murder of Helen, the beloved pregnant wife of the wealthy aristocratic protagonist of the series, Thomas Lynley. But the book is almost entirely about the complex childhood trauma experiences of the child who shoots her. Her death, although a tragedy that is central to the narrative of Lynley's story for volumes of this series both before and after this particular book, is an inflection point in the lives of two characters. Fiction not so far from truth.

One of these characters is an aristocratic, privileged, White English woman, married to a powerful member of the law enforcement world who is himself a British lord with ancestral lands and title. She thus believes in her safety at the door of her home in an expensive London neighborhood, her detective chief inspector husband's longtime residence, the location at which she is shot and rendered brain-dead. The other person is an adolescent, a young man of color, depicted as growing up in not only financial but also emotional poverty, abused and neglected, allowed to vanish from the view of those who should have ensured his care, and consequently never having known that anything resembling safety was possible.

He is also incapable of appreciating his power to end a life because his sense of his own powerlessness is so profound and pervasive that he is utterly surprised by having committed this act. The trauma of Helen's death, and the death as well of her unborn child, are inextricably woven into the trauma of the child who commits the act ending those lives, as well as the utter loss of the just world hypothesis (JWH) for Thomas Lynley. The child who killed likely would not have been vulnerable to killing another human being had he not been abused and neglected, dehumanized and cast off his entire life. Helen would not have felt safe enough to be heedless of her surroundings if she had not come from centuries of privilege. Lynley would have faced terrible grief, but not the trauma of utter loss of existential meaning, were he not an English lord. What came before matters for how trauma occurs, for how trauma is experienced, both in fiction and in real life. There is a trauma-to-prison pipeline; while only a small percentage of people exposed to trauma end up incarcerated, most of those who are incarcerated have extensive histories of trauma exposure.

WHAT COMES AFTER ALSO MATTERS

When we encounter a person who has been exposed to trauma of any form, whether a person entering a therapist's office, an incarcerated person sent into prison because of crimes of violence or crimes of coping, a person seeking asylum, or someone who is "merely" the receptionist at our dentist's office whose path we cross without thinking much about that person's life and story, what we as healers do next, and how we do it, matters. What we do as citizens matters every bit as much. When we vote for laws about gun ownership, bodily autonomy, or how law enforcement is or is not held responsible, or when we, without pausing to think about it, support a system in which traumatized military members are punished with dishonorable discharges for manifesting the effects of their trauma exposure, or when we passively participate in a carceral system that is about retribution and incarceration rather than about restoration, repair, and consequences that might heal, we are in the *after* of the larger society in a way that matters, an after of coloniality.

CHANGING THE COLONIAL NARRATIVE IS DISRUPTIVE TO THE STATUS QUO ANTE

Status quo ante: the way things were before. Nostalgia trauma. Recall the two stories about Columbus and 1492 discussed at the beginning of Chapter 1. If we observe what, in the factual story, is experienced as wounding by some members of the cultural dominant through our own compassionate decolonial and liberatory lens, we can see that often the manifest content of things reported to be traumatic in those facts are distractions from the trauma of loss of a JWH. These distractions (e.g., a certain governor's infamous "war on work") spring from various social pathologies that, while claiming certain people as their beneficiaries, assert that those people are harmed by decolonial narrative and facts. These slogans are distractions from an emotional reality for colonizers.

Psychic wounds lie beneath the thin veneer of privilege, wounds that were soothed by how things were in some before time that never really existed. Jones (2023), a scholar of the White evangelical movement, which is woven almost inextricably into the Christian Eurocentric colonizer narrative, has found that this intersectional identity includes a belief that the United States was to be a divine gift to White Christians, a belief that persists into the present time. How terribly traumatic it must feel to someone who holds such a belief to see the United States becoming less White and less Christian, decade by decade. The just world of this intersectional identity is being exploded by demographic and social realities. This is trauma, not fragility.

A DHCR healer needs to not be distracted by the manifest content emitted by this kind of trauma for people with this and related intersectional identities, even though what is being said may be something that the healer finds offensive, easy to dismiss, or difficult to comprehend. We do not, after all, want decolonial work to become the new epistemic hegemony, or we shall have failed at our ultimate goals of liberation. DHCR trauma work is culturally responsive to both the colonized and the colonizer.

There is trauma living between the lines of the slogans. It is trauma that is denied and obscured by the recruitment of vulnerable people, clinging to the fringes of a dominant identity, into the colonizing narratives of certain forms of systemic oppression and social pathology in which these folks are the real victims, victimized by wokeness (developing a raised consciousness of injustice) and the theft of what they perceive to be their divinely given sovereignty. These are the believers in the first version, the mytho-history version, of the Columbus story, and they insist that it is true, because if it is not, well then, who are they? People who think of themselves as moral, yet who have benefited, albeit usually indirectly, from harm done to others. They are angry that a day once named for a colonizer and enslaver has, in some places, been renamed as Indigenous Peoples' Day. Their nostalgia hurts them. The fantasy of what was, and thus what was lost or stolen, becomes an experience of trauma, even when the details on which this experience is based are confabulated, to one degree or another.

The second story about what Columbus and his ilk did, which is the factual story, feels terribly dangerous to these folks—thus the laws against speaking of slavery or the genocide of Indigenous people in any textbook described earlier, which outlaw any publicly funded organization in the state of Florida from teaching, at any educational level, about inclusion, equity, or, even worse, diversity.

If the truth is dangerous, it can, when inescapable, be traumatic to confront, not because exposure to truth intends harm but because truth exposes being lied to, institutional betrayal at a massive, societal level, committed by those most powerful in the hierarchy of oppression. Truth exposes complicity, witting or not, which can create moral injury, but it also reveals our collective credulity. There should be no shame in either, as people are recruited into both complicity and credulity before there were words or the capacity for critical thought. Nor should there be guilt for the sins of those who came before us. However, we cannot heal wounds of social pathologies that are hidden and covered up; betrayal blindness always precedes the pain of knowing betrayal trauma.

When I put on the hat of a DHCR trauma healer, I know that what these folks are saying, if one skips past the distracting content about wokeness and drag queen story hours. They are in fact being terribly wounded and frightened. They are terrified by manifestations of some changes to dominant forms of systemic and structural forms of oppression by the social norms and institutions that harmed others but made their worlds seem safe and just for them, at least for a moment. These structural forms of violence and disempowerment for others, couched in the terms of a divine gift, offered the comforting lies told to these people and their forebears that upholding those forms of structural oppression would keep them and those resembling them safe from the usual vicissitudes of life (Hannah-Jones, 2021), blessed by the divine (Jones, 2023).

DHCR Disrupts False Binaries

Just as DHCR practice challenges the duality of the positions of healer and sufferer, so the decolonial project also disrupts the false binaries of Eurocentric coloniality. A good example is that of people whose gender orientation and sexual phenotype are out of synch: trans, nonbinary, gender-nonconforming people. Eurocentric culture is quite insistent on the gender binary, often embedded in highly gendered languages, such as French, in which every object is assigned a gender.

To cease to be distracted by the attempts made by people whose gender orientation is not that of the bodies into which they were born to live lives of congruence, however they might accomplish that, means examining the price, and losses, of the imposition of a gender binary, an offspring of toxic masculinity and systemic misogyny, arising from the colonizing European cultures. Many of the Indigenous people of the Western Hemisphere did not have a gender binary. The Talmud, the first great interpretation of Hebrew scripture, described at least six genders, some of which we would recognize today as nonbinary and trans, despite the fact that in Hebrew it is impossible to say the words *you* or *them* without gendering these pronouns.

Unlike past iterations exploring marginalization and trauma, DHCR epistemics necessitate examining the price carried and paid by people who uphold structural forms of oppression, of which that binary is one example, in order to avoid the pain and grief, and even trauma, of knowing truth. This is truth about how patriarchal body phenotype systems of oppression have hurt those who conform to them as much, if not more, than those who do not or cannot twist themselves into a binary pretzel. There are real differences among human bodies, although many of them do not occur in a binary fashion. DHCR trauma healing work interrogates not only this but all imposed categories arising from Christian Eurocentric colonizer epistemics.

Not everyone is ready to leave behind their protective mythologies, those that shield them from knowing how they and their ancestors have been wounded by wounding others. Another manifestation of DHCR trauma healing practice is deepening compassion for those hiding their pain under the thin veneer of White skin privilege, particularly when, as we shall discuss later in this book, they have other intersectional identities making that veneer frail, only microns deep around their other marginalized and traumatized strands.

In all of the above I am simply asserting that DHCR trauma healers—who as a group have rightly privileged the voices of those who are marginalized, subordinated, and targeted in today's world, a preferential option for the pain of the marginalized, subordinated, and oppressed because those voices have been so excluded until recent years—need to not be too distracted by the manner in which members of dominant groups who live with some forms of structural privilege express their experiences of trauma. There is no binary of traumatized and not-traumatized people. There is a continuum of knowing how badly one hurts and a continuum of awareness that the roots of that pain grow in the soil of social pathologies for colonized and colonizer alike.

Somatic Does Not Equal DHCR

There are also generational trends in the field of healing work. In the past few decades the body as a location of trauma has been discovered much in the way Columbus allegedly discovered the Western Hemisphere, and a plethora of somatic healing approaches have come into fashion. A colleague who recently completed training in one of those approaches told me of her frustration about how the topics of culture, context, and oppression were never once mentioned by those teaching the course and how attempts made by her and one other politically aware student, both of them experienced trauma healers, were politely sidelined (A.K., personal communication, June 2022).

This is all to say that it matters not which intervention you're employing if it's offered without an awareness of the social pathologies that are the root causes of the pain that people bring to your work as a trauma healer, and if it cannot meet the criteria for DHCR trauma healing work described later in this book. Somatic work is great; trauma is a biopsychosocial/existential-spiritual thing, and the place where we enter the healing process is less important, in my opinion, than is the epistemic framework through which we enter. Branding how healers work with the body, requiring a person to get the official credential, and touting one methodology as superior to others are all manifestations of the intrusion of rogue capitalism into the trauma healing space and are distractions from the question of how such training operates to uphold or overthrow colonial epistemics in healing trauma. A decolonial, decolonizing, humble, culturally responsive framework can go through any of these doors, and all of them.

Not the Trouble With Trauma, but the Trouble With Diagnosis

In a DHCR healing paradigm, psychopathology texts and diagnostic manuals might be considered the holy scriptures of how to colonize the minds of both suffering people and their healers and show people how to pass for normal. Let's take a look at that before we circle back to the question of how marginalized and subordinated humans attempt to stay invisible to the all-seeing and all-knowing eyes of hierarchies of structural oppression.

When J. R. R. Tolkien created the metaphor of the Eye of Sauron as stand-in for the apparent inescapability of evil and the colonization of the hearts and minds of the good and the innocent no matter how much they resisted the pull of the Eye, he could not know how pertinent that metaphor would remain decades onward. He served in the trenches of Belgium and France in the First World War. He knew the trauma-affected veterans of this war.: he was one of those men. Bilbo and Frodo Baggins, his hobbit protagonists, exemplify all of what I will be discussing in this book: the effects of betrayal, of lost relationships, of extreme danger of death, and of the costs of attempting to pass for normal when one has returned from the war. They were brave. They were wounded terribly in spirit. And so, after returning home, marked by what had happened to them and by their own struggles with moral injury, they faded, quite literally.

Most fans of *The Lord of the Rings* trilogy do not think of these books as studies in the effects of trauma. If it's been a while (or never) since you read them, I invite you do to so with the eyes of a DHCR trauma healer. Or not. There are many other stories, written by traumatized people from many standpoints, with many different intersectional identities and experiences of colonization. Find the story that speaks to you, because it will assist you in decolonizing yourself of the notion that trauma belongs in the realm of the psychopathology texts.

Social Pathologies

Putting disorderedness where it belongs and ascribing it to social pathologies, to cultural phenomena meant to oppress and colonize, rather than to locate it in humans as is currently the norm, is an essential step in doing DHCR, and thus liberatory, trauma healing work. Why? Because, for starters, the neurobiology of trauma and attachment, of fear and connection, lead people to have the precise responses and forms of distress that are generally the ones that have been labeled as disordered. But what if these are the responses for which our nervous systems are naturally wired, no matter how our lived experiences and intersectional identities shape the expressions of our bodies? What if these responses are simply how human bodies are supposed to respond to danger, to disconnection, to loss, to betrayal, except as our bodies naturally will do? What is disordered about that?

An analogy can be made to the human gastrointestinal (GI) system, a complex, multiorgan system that does an excellent job of pulling nutrients out of food, processing them as needed, and allowing that which is waste to be regularly ejected. It is the home to our commensal, the gut biome, a sophisticated collection of bacteria that work in tandem with the organs of the GI system and the enzymes and hormones that it produces to allow the process of digestion to proceed apace.

What happens when a toxin is ingested or a dangerous bacterium enters the gut, *E. coli* hitching a ride on a piece of lettuce perhaps? The GI system signals that something is wrong—I will spare you all the gory details, you know them yourself. The point here is that by being in palpable, odoriferous, visible distress, the gut is signaling the presence of a toxin. The gut is not disordered at all, although it and its human are suffering. The gut is poisoned. Healing the gut requires vanquishing the toxin and also respecting that it did the human in question the favor of signaling, in an inescapable manner, that the toxin or dangerous bacterium was there. Because many of the ways in which modern medicine vanquishes the toxin wreak havoc on our commensal gut biome, healing the gut does not stop with doing away with the intruder, which is the point at which symptoms, that is, the gut saying something is wrong in here, show up. Healing the gut also includes steps toward the restoration of the commensal gut biome.

So too with exposure to trauma, to the toxicity of social pathologies, to disruption to senses of safety, predictability, and connection, all of which lead our neurobiological systems to send out information that trauma is near or still here. Neither these natural responses of human bodies to trauma nor the metadistress evoked by such natural responses, which is about trying to manage these neurological cries for help that are as difficult for humans to coexist with as is a gut visited by *E. coli,* are disordered. They are simply a human body responding to danger or threat to attachment or some combination of both, acutely or chronically. As is breathing, as is the beating of the heart, these neurobiological responses are natural. A DHCR healing practice says there is nothing pathological in the expressions of distress. Pathology is in what is causing the distress.

So What Is Trauma Doing in Psychopathology Texts? Still?

At the risk of being repetitive, it's there because the social pathologies have colonized our conceptual and epistemic frameworks. I'm going repeat this line in one form or another throughout this book because the pull to name psychic pain a disorder is a powerful one, the professional Eye of Sauron. Every time one of us who works as a healer in the United States has to fill out the bill to the insurance company on which we are required to state that it's a disorder that we're treating and that in consequence this treatment we're billing for is medically necessary, there's that eye. This is a form of hypnotic induction by superbill, the Eye of Sauron of an insurance company, an act of betraying our own values whose cumulative effects on even trauma healers with the best intentions cannot be underestimated.

The mental health professions, to whom the healing of traumatized people has been consigned in the modern world, are deeply steeped in the narratives of normal and abnormal, natural and unnatural. The general message is that if your soul and psyche ache in some way from having encountered the reality of death, the fragility of life, the disruptions to safety and connection that are part of trauma exposure, then you fit into the abnormal psychology textbook or the latest version of the *Diagnostic and Statistical Manual of Mental Disorders (DSM)*. Because, as some of my colleagues have been only too eager to point out, only about 20% of people who are exposed to a Criterion A trauma develop PTSD (Briere & Scott, 2014), so, their logic goes, to have this distress in this form is abnormal. Q.E.D.

Two problems can be found in this seductive illogic. First, as we shall explore in depth in this volume, the harm done by trauma does not stop at the boundaries of the *DSM* definition of PTSD. Second, as John Briere (Briere & Scott, 2014) has so inconveniently pointed out with his in-depth research on trauma-exposed people, the other 80% aren't fine. They are in distress. Their distress simply doesn't fit neatly into the confines of PTSD, which is the official disorder for how one should look if affected by exposure to trauma.

When we apply a DHCR model to understanding both what trauma is and also how it does harm and is a source of pain, Briere's data and analysis are foundational to my undisordering project for the distress of the trauma-exposed. Trauma is not Criterion A. Criterion A describes a small subset of the experiences that humans feel as traumatizing. Trauma's effects, as well as the ways in which humans struggle not to know how we are affected, are simply the human condition, I say again and will repeat in the remainder of this book. This pain and the attempts to escape it, to numb it, to not know about it, are not symptoms of disorder. They are distress signals sent up by human neurobiology about something dangerously wrong in the world.

BEFORE PSYCHOTHERAPY

People healed from the suffering created by trauma exposure long before there was something called psychotherapy. They have continued to heal without it since Freud discovered the thing that many people, most of them assigned to a lower social status, had learned millennia before him. This discovery of Freud's, which he borrowed without much attribution from Pierre

Janet and Jean-Martin Charcot, that listening to a person helped them, was revolutionary in that in essence it told the professional, in this case a physician, to sit down and close their mouth (for a little while, at least). As Europeans did not discover the Western Hemisphere but rather only colonized and laid waste to it, so psychoanalysis and its successor psychotherapies did not discover that listening to suffering people could be of help. It was simply colonized and turned into something that one could only do after many years of specialized and supervised training.

It was radical at the time for Freud and his followers to actually pay attention to what suffering people—in particular, suffering women—were saying, given how uncommon that whole listening thing seemed to be among the medical professionals of the Western world. This failure to listen carefully was quite culture-bound and flavored with misogyny in the Western world. In Asia, practitioners had been listening to the bodies of suffering people through their pulses and tongues for millennia. Among Indigenous peoples in the territories colonized by Europeans, healers listened to, sweated with, and walked though visions alongside suffering members of their communities. Healers knew which plants were the medicines that would allow suffering people to go to the bottom of the wells of their grief and pain and emerge more healed: psychopharmacology without Big Pharma.

But in Freud's cultural and social milieu of fin de siècle upper-class Vienna, it was revolutionary to listen to people, particularly those natal woman who constituted the bulk of those who first sought his help. That is, sadly, until listening stopped being what psychoanalysis was centrally marked by, listening occurring only to impose interpretation, a loss and transformation that I will discuss at length in a number of places later in this book. The notion that a healer of souls should listen to suffering people was shoved to the side, to be rediscovered by Carl Rogers, who came very close to proposing how to decolonize the healing of souls at the end of his career (C. Rogers & Stevens, 1971).

Freud lost the revolutionary thread of simply listening when he put into the mix the unnecessary overlay of requiring an expert interpretation, made by the expert professional, of what the suffering person said. One cannot blame him for being assimilated into the culture of expertise as he attempted, with varying degrees of success, to distract people from the inconvenient fact of his own membership in an oppressed group. The interpretation, rather than what the suffering person said, then became the truth of what was happening: "You are having this dream, and it means this thing, and thus you are this other thing."

In this way Freud and his followers, and all psychotherapists since then, could have the illusion that we were doing something other than having a relationship with a suffering human being and that our expertise, whether it was how we interpreted or the intervention we used, was what mattered. This is trauma therapy as usual. It could be interpretation of free association. It could be challenging an irrational belief in cognitive behavior therapy. It didn't matter. Therapy became a means of colonization of the suffering person with a particular epistemology of their suffering. These ways of knowing have had the effect of upholding social pathologies by making the suffering person's suffering into a problem. It has also defined people in emotional pain as those who could not accurately know themselves without the expertise of a professional. This is the opposite of the DHCR epistemic of analyzing power, utilizing the healing process as a liberatory one in which connections between distress and oppression are made explicit.

Ironically, the DHCR standpoint reflects long-standing findings about psychotherapy outcomes. The closer to a DHCR approach a healer can get, the more likely they are to be following, knowingly or not, the findings of that body of knowledge. As Norcross and Wampold (2019b) lamented in their thoughtful and piercing critique of the APA's *Clinical Practice Guideline for the Treatment of Posttraumatic Stress Disorder (PTSD) in Adults* (APA, 2017a), all of the evidence-based interventions that the guidelines were recommending be applied to humans suffering after trauma exposure only accounted for a minuscule sliver of what might be reducing that suffering. The enormous portion of that which was healing for the suffering person, everything about the relationship of humans sitting together in a room with the goal of reducing suffering, was ignored entirely. Thus those guidelines represented, as they said, a tragic lost opportunity to tell the truth that it's the humans in the room and their relationships, not the expertise, interventions, or interpretations (p. 1).

Some of the suffering humans who have healed their trauma-created suffering have done so through deep engagements with nature or with other nonhuman living beings or in relationships with a divine being whose presence they perceive to accompany them. Some do it on the mats of martial arts or yoga, healing systems which come to us from several different Asian and South Asian cultures. Some have done so by writing stories and poetry. The late great poet Mary Oliver, whose words, "Doesn't everything die at last, and too soon? / Tell me, what is it you plan to do / with your one wild and precious life?" (2005, p. 94) and whose poems have been read in many a trauma healer's office and many a suffering person's healing spaces, was herself a person who suffered through a childhood in hell. Her healing was in her writing, not in the office of any psychotherapist.

The effects of exposure to trauma hurt like hell. They can be debilitating, exhausting, confusing, overwhelming, consuming everything in and around a trauma-exposed person. If not healed, they pass on their effects for generations (Danieli, 1998), and sometimes they are passed on by creating experiences of trauma for others. This pain is not the disorder; it is the body telling us about something disordered in the world around that body, or around the bodies of their ancestors, or in their cultures, and about the ways in which social pathologies have guided those expressions of pain, given them meaning, assigned them a rank in the social hierarchies of a particular culture.

Activation of the trauma and/or attachment systems, of the unknowing/dissociative and coping systems in the dorsal branch of the vagus nerve, that occur in response to a disruption in the force of connection or safety are responses that are all naturally part of human neurobiology and do not deserve to be referred to as illnesses if we apply a decolonial model to our work. We cannot be biologically reductionistic; DHCR work is not simply intervening with these bodily systems while ignoring the structural and systemic social realities that are activating the body.

While all of these phenomena are the sources of great emotional pain and confusion, expressed variously as dissociative experiences, nightmares, or flashbacks and the desire to numb with substances, food, or overwork, expressed as agitation, impatience, or lashing out in violence against the self and others, all of this is distress occurring naturally in our nervous systems in the manner in which our nervous systems were designed to respond to certain kinds of experiences. A DHCR epistemic takes this information and places it into the contexts of colonization—current, past, large, and difficult to detect.

ISN'T THIS ALL JUST POLITICAL? YES, AND RIGHTLY SO

Yes, as Judith Herman (1992) said: Trauma is political, and knows no parties, only abuses of power, experiences of powerlessness, disruptions in existential systems. But why then does it follow that social pathologies should be considered forms of illness rather than simply political matters? That's an interesting and worthwhile question that deserves my thoughtful response. The personal is political, in that it always has meaning within the larger politics of structural forms of oppression. When it's possible to make public health measures in response to the COVID-19 pandemic political or, looking back in time, weave outbreaks of the plague into already extant anti-Semitism, it's not hard to notice that social pathologies do a good job of turning biological facts into the mythological truths of oppression.

The social pathology of patriarchy, built on the scaffolding of those biological realities, has no reason for continuing to exist, yet it continues to shout from the mists of prehistory that natal men and current social constructs of masculinity are supreme and ever and always have been. This is an example of a politicized explanatory fiction that refers back to biology to excuse its depredations. Patriarchy, like a virus, has no value. It infects minds as viruses do cells, simply to perpetuate itself and give more power into the hands of testosterone-affected bodies, and to treat those who are not testosterone-affected—or even if so biologically organized, do not meet a current cultural context's criteria for how such a body should dress and look—as targets, as lesser than, as acceptable recipients of severe of punishments. These penalties have been leveled, officially or not, against those who violate patriarchy's rules—dressing in the clothing of the wrong sex, being gender-nonconforming, or being a woman who won't smile or who talks back.

Similarly, there is no good reason for White supremacy or any other kind of phenotype supremacy to exist except to perpetuate itself. The excuse for lynchings, beatings, pogroms, genocide, and the smaller punishments of varieties of social exclusion is that someone has violated the rules of this social pathology.

There are no good reasons for systemic misogyny or toxic masculinity, the evil twins of patriarchy, to exist except, like a virus reproducing in a cell, to make more copies of themselves. There is no good reason for xenophobia (although I suppose that some evolutionary psychologists would argue that fear of the other is as wired into us as is the need to attach, an argument that I reject as having outlived its utility, if it ever had any—and we can't go back in time to ask early *Homo sapiens* if this was in fact true for them).

There is no good reason for sexualizing children and sexually violating them, for sexual assaults against people of all genders, those with vulvas and those without. There is no good reason for colonization other than the desire to own what is not one's own and grab it without compensation. There is no good reason for forced conversion to a particular religion or killing people who aren't a particular religion or phenotype or who hold a particular political viewpoint, simply because they are that thing. There is no good reason for not wanting some limits on the availability of assault weapons (in fact, the absence of bans runs counter to the survival of the species), no good reason to ban children from access to certain ideas, such as the fact that some of the European colonizers of this continent enslaved African people and that a war was fought to protect the ability to do so—other than to uphold some form of social pathology that gives power to those promoting that pathology. Social pathologies are viruses that replicate in order to keep on replicating.

No good reason at all for any of this, other than to allow power to continue to accrue to those who create and uphold the ideologies of these social pathologies. Social pathologies could thus be seen as making some mind viruses seem benign or even rewarding for some people some of the time—until the virus turns on them (e.g., the French Revolution of 1789, or the Russian revolution, or the victory of the Indigenous people at Little Big Horn). For some people structural power in a society flows from their promotion of social pathologies as truth and as protection for some groups of people from losing their privileges in a particular culture. The strong man leaders of fascist nations draw upon their fluency in a social pathology to attempt to create unlimited personal power for themselves—until they lose their grip and, like Benito Mussolini, end up hanging from a lamppost or, like Nicolae Ceauşescu, lined up against a wall and shot.

The only thing that I think these social pathologies accomplish is, like an uncontrolled pathogen, doing some form of harm to almost all human beings, including to most of those who think that they benefit from promulgating and upholding these ideologies. Only a very few humans benefit, and even those, I would argue, do so at great cost and usually temporarily, excepting the sociopaths in our midst whose social power derives from their exploitation of the themes of the social pathology. DHCR trauma healing acknowledges how vulnerable humans are to the grip of social pathologies when we are not their targets or even, in the form of internalized oppression, when we are.

Systemic forms of oppression are thus, to me, obvious candidates for being labeled pathological. Like a virus, they sicken minds and cause harm, even death, to people. Such harm to people is long-lasting and difficult to repair. The harm done can be transmitted from generation to generation through modifications of gene expression, the epigenetics of trauma. Social pathologies destroy cultures and languages that were of value to those who were members of those cultures and spoke those languages.

Social pathologies kill when they put the financial well-being of the very few over the survival of the planet; the social pathology of rogue capitalism, which places the making of money for the few as the highest good, stands behind the resistance to all attempts to stop pollution that is inexorably changing the planet's climate. Social pathologies do zero net good for humans as a species. The history of humanity is replete with the stories of how some version or another of a social pathology has caused tremendous harm, has damaged the body of the human species, left us and our planet collectively wounded and in distress. How is that not an operational definition of a pathology? Like a virus, only not merely a speck of protein but rather a hierarchy of value, an ideology, an infection of epistemologies, of self-concepts, of ideologies.

Trans Hatred: An Example of How Natural Disaster and Social Pathology Overlap

Social pathologies also make purely natural disasters much worse for the humans living through them. Take the example of trans people, whose lived experience of their gender orientation does not fit into the box created by Eurocentric rules for a person of their sex phenotype. If a trans person living life fully in their gender orientation is using hormones and presents in their congruent gender but has not had surgery to modify the genital expression of their sex phenotype, either by choice or due to lack of financial means, they may not be able, during a tornado, to get a safe bed in the section of an emergency shelter for people of their gender orientation.

This would be because a government has passed a law requiring them to bed down among people who share a genital sex phenotype with them. These rules are manifestations of the social pathology of the idea of an invariant gender binary of Western cultures. This social pathology, with rules that place genital expression of sex phenotype over lived experience of gender orientation, make the tornado worse for that trans person. The social pathology of trans hatred has placed them in the path of interpersonal danger on the spurious grounds that a trans woman might be entering natal women's space in the shelter in order to commit rape, an urban legend for which there are no supporting data.

Until the emergency shelters, public restrooms, and locker rooms of the world have single-person options available, the gender binary—an expression of Eurocentric flavored patriarchy's rules about sex phenotype—puts people at risk of sexual assault, and this includes risk to masculine of center natal women who are socially constructed by others, due to how they present in the world, as being natal male, despite a female gender orientation and genital sex phenotype. I've witnessed some of these women being screamed at and having security called on them in public restrooms; I was married to one and was her restroom bodyguard, vouching for her genital sex phenotype.

This is not a hypothetical tale of possible harm but rather the recounting of real dangers laid on top of the losses of a natural disaster. The most recent U.S. Department of Justice statistics suggest that around 60% of trans women are raped in their lifetimes; this contrasts with the feminist Rape, Abuse and Incest National Network's numbers estimating that around 16% of women are sexually assaulted in their lifetime or higher numbers, around 25%, from the National Sexual Violence Resource Center (Truman & Morgan, 2022).

No one should be sexually assaulted. Sexual assault is a weapon of patriarchy which is apparently used more frequently to punish gender nonconformity in people who were born with a penis than in natal women, perhaps because the violation of patriarchy's rules committed by a trans woman in her rejection of the notion that her genital sex phenotype defines her is coded as unforgivable. In the enormous form of structural oppression that is patriarchy, a penis is overvalued, and the notion that a person born with one finds it discordant with their lived knowledge of who they are is, in the Eurocentric gender binary, treated as dangerous. Thus the gender binary can turn a natural disaster into one fueled by toxic social pathologies.

Trans people in the United States and elsewhere in the world live in many jurisdictions whose laws require that their gender orientation must be ignored in favor of their natal sex (many trans people refer to as "sex assigned at birth," but I prefer "natal sex" or "genital sex phenotype") and are placed, by those laws, in situations of increased danger every single day by such laws. If the social pathologies of gender binaries and trans hatred were not in play, the trans person could safely go to a bed in the section of the emergency shelter for people of their gender expression, with their genitals covered by clothing just as those all around them, or there might be safe enough places for people not in the gender binary, such as my former spouse, to take refuge. Simply building the physical structures in which people seek refuge in times of disaster could make having lost their home and possessions and medications in the tornado or the flood just a tiny bit less worse for these extremely marginalized and subordinated people.

More recently, legislative bodies have committed mass trauma on young trans people and their family members by outlawing any form of care that would assist these young people in affirming their gender orientation. This means emotional care as well; while the new focuses on how these laws forbid the use of hormones or surgical procedures in the care of such young humans, "gender-affirming care" is a phrase that includes the resistance of a healer to participation in some new, twisted version of the so-called conversion therapies that were thrust on lesbians and gay men, which did harm and were themselves traumagenic. The steady drumbeat, led by self-serving politicians, of antitrans hate speech masquerading as lawmaking, has been enlarging the social pathology of trans hatred such that its pervasive traumagenic effects harm not only the people living in the jurisdictions that have outlawed their care but, via the process of insidious traumatization, are wounding the souls of any young trans person and those who love them no matter where they reside. It is sending these trans youths and their families into exile, another trauma layered on top of the rest.

What I think is true is that by rejecting genital sex phenotype as a lifelong, utterly defining characteristic of self, trans people are exploding the very basis of patriarchy. If we admit that the presence of a penis means nothing other than that a developing fetus was affected by in utero testosterone, so that the previously undifferentiated genital bud tissue grew large, then the entire edifice of patriarchy collapses. A penis is a large clitoris: same tissues, same structures, just an average difference in size.

CONSIDERATIONS FOR TRAUMA HEALING

For a DHCR trauma healer, bringing this perspective to their work with a person punished and traumatized for being trans may be essential to the healing process. As we'll discuss at many places woven into the discussions found later in this volume, critical consciousness, the awareness that one is not the problem, is core to DHCR trauma healing. DHCR trauma healing work does not exist in the absence of the idea that the personal is political, of bringing attention to the sources of trauma in colonization and subjugation at some point in the healing process. Considering that one's existence is the greatest threat ever to Christian Eurocentric patriarchy, which is wedded to a gender binary based on genital sex phenotype, is potentially liberatory, empowering, and fertile ground upon which critical consciousness might grow. Seeing that one is so enormously powerful that the attacks on one's personhood are coded messages about one's power is a very different way of helping a traumatized trans, non-binary, or gender-nonconforming person take power back from pain.

The same way of thinking holds true for neurodiverse people, such as those on the autism spectrum, who are often very affected by social or sensory over-load and stigmatized for being so. An autistic natal woman who has lived by herself, happily doing a well-paid, online job and being able to control social and sensory input, who finds herself after a natural disaster in a shelter, with-out her noise-canceling headphones, neurologically overwhelmed because the neuro majority does not create safe spaces during natural disasters for people who are harmed by the shelter environment itself, is a different example of how social pathologies—in this case, ableism—turn a natural disaster into a more enduring source of harm. When such an autistic person has a meltdown, yells and throws things, they risk being ejected from the shelter or even incar-cerated by law enforcement personnel, who are among the biggest risks to the lives of autistic people even in the absence of a disaster. Social pathology turns a natural disaster into the risk of oppression and increased trauma. The absence of these social pathologies, the presence of spaces that would make humans like them safe enough during times of terrible loss, could mitigate the suffering rather than amplify it in a context where the specific source of the suffering was meteorological or geological.

So now what do we do? In the following chapters we'll continue our discus-sion of what constitutes the evidence of the epistemic colonization of trauma healing in the Global North, contrasting it with a DHCR approach as we go.

4

WHERE WE'VE COME FROM

The Heritage of Decolonial Healing

Despite the colonizing influences that have plagued most of the field of psychotherapy, a look at the past allows glimpses of earlier moves toward integrating an awareness of systemic oppression into the psychotherapeutic process (Brown, 2017; Comas-Díaz, 2012), as well as efforts to center the humanity, not the pathology, of the suffering person. Some of these attempts have persisted, although in a form where their social justice orientation is much less visible. Others are historical curiosities, known to few. Still others constitute the attempts at decolonial practice developed in the past 5 decades by feminists, womanists, and mujeristas, multiculturalists, queer theorists, and critical psychologists. To understand decolonial psychotherapy it behooves us to know on whose shoulders we stand. The thinkers I refer to here have influenced my own work; there are likely many earlier liberatory and critical theorists whose work has affected psychotherapy practice of whom I am unaware, and this is consequently not an exhaustive review. It is a plunge into my own library.

First, though, we must begin with Sigmund Freud, the colonized man who created a healing modality that came very close to the edge of being truly revolutionary—and who then had to pull back because of who he was. What

https://doi.org/10.1037/0000421-005
Decolonizing Trauma Healing: Toward a Humble, Culturally Responsive Practice,
by L. S. Brown

follows are my thoughts on this matter, not truths, simply an attempt to make sense through my own lens of what led the field of healing wounded souls and psyches so far astray.

WE BEGAN COLONIZED: HOW SHLOMO BECAME SIGMUND

This corruption caused by colonization at the heart of the arts of healing wounded souls and psyches has its seeds in the life and struggles of Sigmund Freud, Hebrew name Schlomo ben Yakov. He was a man who attempted to make himself more respectable and accepted than who he was—a Jew whose parents came from Galicia in Ukraine, whose grandparents were Hassidim and thus at the margins even of Jewish society. He married a woman who was the granddaughter of the chief rabbi of Hamburg, then forbade her to light Shabbat candles in their home. He attempted to avoid having a Jewish wedding. It appears that he did his best to make the fact of his being a Jew recede as far as possible into the background of his own consciousness because to allow himself to know just how much of a Jew he was would have been an intolerable intrusion of the "you are not safe" story.

Freud was born in Moravia, in what is now the Czech Republic, while it was occupied by the Austrian Empire. Thus Freud was a triple, perhaps quadruple alien and outcast in Vienna, the capital city of that empire, the place where he built his life and his theory. He worked mightily to craft a narrative about the nature of suffering and its amelioration that would be accepted by the powers that be in his world.

He fawned and assimilated and took back some of what was most revolutionary in his earliest work, truths about how repeated violations in childhood were at the root of a great deal of pain for the people who sought his help (Masson, 1984), because at the hidden core of his intersectional identities was Jewishness. With that came intergenerational trauma and its epigenetic expressions in neurobiology, trauma that likely went back at least a millennium, and perhaps longer. His development of the construct of repression, which is a way of unknowing, speaks volumes to me about his life of being never safe enough, of himself having to unknow—repress—the reality that his colleagues disdained him and that his life was at risk from the many virulent anti-Semitic movements that were part of Viennese politics while he lived there, well before the Nazis marched in.

Freud has not been a sympathetic figure to most modern decolonial thinkers in psychology until the work of Daniel Gaztambide (2019, 2020). Gaztambide's trenchant analysis opened new doors for people who had not read Fanon

(1967), one of the earliest decolonial thinkers and himself a psychoanalyst, to understand Freud not as a White man but as a Jew in danger who had radical ideas and then needed to bury them deeply so as to make himself less of a target. And what creative thinker, which Freud was, does not want their creation to be applauded? He believed, perhaps accurately, that in order to make ability to see and hear what others around him did not, to detect the whisperings of what lay beneath the surface of the mind, to discern the patterns he was able to draw in the words and actions of people around him, that he had to make his vision palatable to the powerful. He was probably correct in this belief, given the responses to the initial publication of his findings about sexually abused women.

To understand Freud's path toward the betrayal of suffering people we must apply the tools of liberatory analysis to the suffering person he was. Decolonizing psychoanalytic and psychodynamic practices so that they can meet the criteria for decolonial, humble, culturally responsive (DHCR) work, an example of which can be seen in the writings of Gaztambide (2019, 2020) and Tummala-Narra (2016), who has written extensively about being a Black, Indigenous, people of color (BIPOC) psychoanalyst working with other phenotypically marginalized people, asks psychoanalysts to see Freud through his intersectional identities, through his own experiences of oppression and danger, his own suffering.

Interrogating Freud's intersectionalities in this way, a first DHCR step means asking, How is any precept of psychoanalytic theory and practice that I was taught to be necessary and sacrosanct most likely simply an artifact of the founder's disowned lifetime of terror, his repression of the knowledge that killers quite literally lay in wait beyond every door through which he stepped onto the streets of Vienna? If this methodology, with its focus on the unconscious, was a means for him and the many Jews among his students and analysands to unknow the dangers amid which they lived, a safe detour away from the dangers of their social realities, or a way to interpret fears from realities into symbolic products of the unconscious mind that could know and not know at the same time, then what of the classical psychoanalytic frame, particularly that of so-called neutrality, remains necessary or healing? If self-disclosing opened the door to danger, that is, to being known to be a Jew, then why not put it off limits?

Understanding how people unknow, repress, or dissociate, or how they represent the unknowable dangers of their worlds in unconscious symbolism, in dreams and free associations, can be of tremendous value to traumatized people. But the interpreter, the arbiter of meaning, cannot be the healer, as is invariably true for psychoanalytic paradigms. DHCR trauma healing simply cannot begin and end with the unconscious mind.

It's not hard to decolonize psychoanalytic and psychodynamic epistemics when we return to their roots, which are about regaining access to that which has been repressed. Assumptions about power dynamics and the role of the healer can be rolled back past the layers of colonization that grew on top of the original power of being heard and being known.

DHCR trauma healing is about knowing, but, in contrast, not only the kind of knowing that is a stated goal of psychoanalysis, where the process intends to uncover unconscious motives and defenses—in other words, some of the ways in which people do not know. A DHCR healer simply cannot make the unconscious more important than also knowing the truth of social patholo-gies that are the sources of distress, of knowing where safer might be. Trans-ference and countertransference must be reimagined through the lens of intersectionalities, the ways in which healer and sufferer represent things to one another in the context of real social and political worlds. Distress is no longer a neurosis but rather, as discussed at length in this book, seen as a reasonable response to the feelings evoked by exposure to social pathologies. Psychoanalytic methodologies applied to unknowing of dan-ger and distress can, when utilized with the kind of critical consciousness demonstrated by Gaztambide (2019, 2020) and Tummala-Narra (2016) or the relational focus of modern analytic thinkers like McWilliams (2004) or Stark (1999), can absolutely meet the criteria for a DHCR healing methodology.

DHCR trauma healing can, by decolonizing the origins of our field, con-sider psychodynamic practices as forms of trauma healing. Listening carefully to what is said and not yet said and attending to the relationship between healer and sufferer are practices that can be core to integrating almost any other healing modality into DHCR work. But the notions of neutrality, the illusion that the intersectional identities and social positions of the healer are invisible to the distressed person, and the concept that the healer should abstain from offering overt expressions of care and concern are all compo-nents of what psychoanalysis developed into that reflect Christian Eurocentric colonial epistemics and thus do not support a DHCR paradigm.

Remembering Freud the Colonized Man

Critical and decolonial thinkers who have not read Fanon (1967; and I am surprised by how few of my colleagues in this wing of the field have read him) and only think of Freud as the betrayer of sexually abused women often forget that Freud was a Jew who spent his dying days in exile in England, having had to flee from the Nazis at the end of his life. Most refugees, from anywhere in the world, at any time, don't get to bring their furniture and rugs, as he did. Freud had some phenotype privilege as a natal man and social privilege as a highly educated and socially well-connected person, like various other analysts, artists, and intellectuals among European Jews who were rescued and slid past quotas to something closer to safe in Great Britain, the United States, Argentina, Cuba, Canada, and Shanghai. The fear of being persecuted as a Jew, from which he had spent a lifetime distancing himself, followed him into exile and death every bit as much as that persecution followed his compatriots who made it out alive with only the clothing they wore.

The Power of the Political Context and the Fragility of a Bestowed Privilege

Freud's experiences in the years leading up to his death are a master class in understanding how context changes everything about the meaning of a person's intersectional identities. Before the rise of Nazism, he was the respected rebbe (teacher, in Yiddish) of psychotherapy. There he was, the rav, as he would have been called in a Jewish learning setting, with his favored students, with an insistence on loyalty to his teachings and expulsion of those who offered different interpretations, just as happened in the Hassidic courts of Eastern Europe. (Among the Hassidim of today, one group won't recognize the kosher seal of the others, if that gives you any flavor of what I mean here; with psychoanalysis, it's whether you got your training from the orthodox or a renegade institute. Hassidic or psychoanalytic, it's about your lineage.)

After the Nazis absorbed Austria into the Greater Germanic Reich in March 1938, Freud was, in his own city, only a Jew once again. He was a man with a target on his back, a man whose books were burned by the government and whose daughter Anna was arrested and kept overnight by the Gestapo, an event that seemed to finally break through his unknowing of his own danger and allowed him to give in to the attempts of some of his non-Jewish followers to get him out of the Reich alive.

The neurobiology of the many layers of his trauma from before the time that he lost his illusions of safety waves to us from the background of his life story like bright flags. Freud soothed himself with cocaine. Think about what it means that a person soothes their distress with a powerful substance when that person's intersectional identities are complicated: a man who valued women yet enshrined some aspects of misogyny, never subjecting them to the kinds of interrogation that he applied to so many other dynamics of life; a man with White skin, not considered White by those around him because he was a Jew, who made devil's bargains with oppressors, with anti-Semites, with the medical powers that be of Vienna, one of the most anti-Semitic cities of old Europe, in support of the social pathology of misogyny and toxic masculinity.

DHCR trauma healers need to study what it was about Freud's inter-sectional identities that laid the foundations for all of the complicated and confusing origins of the fields of healing souls and psyches, whether or not the focus is on the healing of trauma. Freud made compromises in the attempt to save himself and his discoveries from being cast aside. He assimilated and fawned. Freud's refusal to acknowledge that he had any identities replete with trauma planted colonization and a form of corruption in the roots of the tree from which psychotherapy then grew.

In so doing, he modeled for the rest of us who write about and practice the healing of suffering souls that such compromises might be necessary in order to achieve professional survival, much less success. His was a narra-tive of dealing with oppression by surviving as best one can because there is no hope of liberation. That narrative, the trance of despair in the face of colonization, corrupted psychotherapy, focused it on adjustment rather than liberation, a dilemma we are attempting to resolve within the DHCR trauma healing model.

Freud was very uncomfortable about being a Jew. To embrace his Jew-ishness more fully and joyously would have been dangerous for him, and he both knew and unknew it continuously during his lifetime, documented in his correspondence and journals. To live too directly with conscious knowledge of his risks would have impeded his desires for professional recognition. So he knew and unknew when his professional position might be threatened.

It took having the Gestapo arrest his beloved daughter Anna to break through his trance of unknowing long enough to cooperate with those who helped him leave Vienna. The parallel to the coming-to-know experiences of some incest survivors who unknow their abuse until their children are born (ironically, this describes the group of women who were among his first analysands, whom he betrayed in order to make his new theory more respectable and protect himself professionally) is striking.

The irony of this parallel—finally knowing one's own danger to protect a beloved child—should escape no one. It should create compassion within DHCR healers for Freud as a suffering, trauma-exposed person facing the same kinds of dilemmas and impossible choices as the living suffering people with whom DHCR healers work. Sadly, because he created modern psychotherapy, Freud's unknowing strategies of conformity, status seeking, and denying one's own marginalized and subordinated intersectional social positionalities were baked into the thing he created.

There are similar tales likely to be discerned in the founding stories of nearly every model of psychotherapy, stories of unknowing, of having parts of intersectional identities needing to go underground. Unlike Ignacio Martín-Baró (to be met later in this chapter), there aren't very many progenitors of theories of psychotherapy who could both know and dissociate themselves from extreme danger. Most founders of schools of psychotherapy aren't as much at risk of dying for their beliefs or for some aspect of their intersectionalities as was Martín-Baró. I certainly could not have demonstrated whatever it was that he had—courage, foolhardiness, unknowing danger to speak truth. I haven't been bold enough to write this book until I entered my eighth decade of life and knew that I had nothing to lose by writing what seems true to me, after nurturing less radical versions of these ideas for my entire professional life. So now let's meet some other protodecolonialists.

ADLER AND THE SOCIAL CONSCIOUSNESS

Alfred Adler, a student of Freud's who began as an orthodox analyst, was the first modern-era psychiatrist to focus on issues of personal power and social realities. In my doctoral program, he merited less than a day's worth of attention. Despite this, I can recall how, as a budding feminist therapy theorist, I was struck by his attention to constructs that were becoming central in nascent feminist therapy—issues of power, powerlessness, and social inequality as sources of psychological distress.

Adler is best known to the casual student of psychology and psychotherapy as the originator of the construct of the inferiority complex. A present-day analysis of this paradigm suggests that what Adler was describing were the effects of internalized oppression and systemic exclusion, represented intrapsychically. His own struggles with anti-Semitism appear to have functioned to heighten his awareness of the ways in which power and powerlessness could be the etiologies of well- and ill-being, this despite his having responded to his own internalized oppression by converting to Protestantism.

Adler was also the first modern psychotherapist to point to social inequality as a source of emotional suffering and to have argued that in order to treat people's psychic pain a psychotherapist also needed to engage with the inequities in their social environment. His work identified social justice as a necessary component of the healing environment and a goal of the practitioner. He worked to provide emotional health care in communities of blue-collar workers by establishing mental health clinics in workers' communities in Austria at a time when psychoanalysis, then the only psychotherapy, was primarily serving the economically privileged. He thus demonstrated an awareness of the importance of including the perspectives of people across the social class spectrum in the development of psychotherapy theory and practice.

Foreshadowing the work of Rogers, and consistent with the DHCR model, Adler emphasized the communitarian and interpersonal nature of healing and rejected the patient-on-the-couch model, insisting that psychiatrist and patient face one another, seated, as equals. Unlike Freud and his loyal followers, especially the latter, who erected increasingly stringent barriers over time to participation in the work of healing by anyone other than physicians, Adler believed and taught that lay people, teachers, and community organizers, among others, were important actors in the process of recovering from psychological pain. This is proto-DHCR thinking.

Unfortunately, Adler's work became marginalized and subordinated within the mainstream of psychotherapy education over the years after his death in 1937 to the point where he is routinely misrepresented simply as a rebel student of Freud, relegated to a minor mention of the inferiority complex, rather than as a peer to Freud who sampled psychoanalytic thought and found it wanting, then took the best he could from it, added the social justice orientation, and created something different.

Today Adler is also identified as a founding thinker of the community psychology movement, which focuses on healing communities and the prevention of distress rather than treatment of individuals, because of his work's emphasis on the relationship between the well-being of the individual and that of the community and on the prevention of psychological problems through early interventions in the parent–child relationship and on the social environment. Community psychology has itself been an attempt to deindividualize and render communitarian the work of healing; like Adlerian psychology in the form envisioned by its founder, it has fallen to the sidelines of the field over time, reflecting the colonizing power of individualism and the notion of the pathology of the person.

Why, one wonders, did Adler's decolonial insights become sidelined after his death? I would like to suggest that his invisibility in the psychotherapeutic mainstream, in contrast to the dominance of psychoanalysis through the middle of the 20th century, and then the new dominance of cognitive behavioral paradigms, was precisely due to the decolonial focus of his work and his emphasis on social justice and gender equality. Because Adler's work had such a strong social justice orientation and paid so much attention to the harmful effects of inequity, it could not be co-opted by institutions of the dominant culture in the manner in which mainstream psychoanalytic thought has been; it could not participate in oppression of marginalized and subordinated persons.

Additionally, because Adler and his students, such as Rudolf Dreikurs, welcomed persons holding no advanced degrees into their fold for training, acknowledging that the capacity to heal was not linked to the possession of additional letters after one's name, the hierarchical and exclusionary structures that came to pervade psychoanalytic and eventually most psychotherapy training in the United States were absent from the Adlerian world. It is distinctly possible that Adler's radical egalitarianism has played a part in his becoming nearly invisible to most psychotherapists today.

Consider that even cognitive behavioral psychologists have a familiarity with psychoanalytic constructs such as transference and countertransference, even if only to disavow their presence in cognitive behavior therapy (CBT), yet rarely note that Adler's work had a profound influence on early cognitive behavioral practitioners such as Albert Ellis, whose rational emotive therapy was an early iteration of what became CBT. Much of Adler's work and ideas have been integrated and subsumed into near-decolonial approaches (e.g., existential and humanistic psychologies), and in that integration his decolonial and social justice emphasis has been watered down or made less important. Yet DHCR practice stands on his shoulders.

THE WRETCHED OF THE EARTH—FRANTZ FANON AND THE PATHOLOGY OF RACISM

In January 1972, prior to identifying myself with feminist ideologies but in the midst of my engagement with social justice movements to end America's war in Vietnam and to give economic justice to farmworkers, I enrolled in a course called Radical Psychology. That course introduced me to Frantz Fanon's work; the now yellowed paperback on which I scribbled notes from our lectures, his foundational book *Black Skin, White Masks* (1967), has been in my library for 52 years now.

Earlier I had been exposed to the radical idea that psychotherapy needed to give way to prevention in coursework with George Albee, who taught the undergraduate abnormal psychology class that I took in 1970. He used that course, and the power of his role as chair of the department and president of the APA, as a means of subverting everything the class title stood for. Albee, who became a mentor and then a friend, firmly located the problem of human distress in social disorders. He taught that discrimination might have mental health consequences and that sometimes people were given diagnoses when they were simply behaving in ways not approved of by dominant society or might have no problems at all were their social causes prevented or eradicated. To use a phrase from that time, it was mind-blowing. But it took Fanon's incisive and penetrating political analysis to make the relationship between racism and psychological suffering strikingly clear, a truth from which I could never after turn my head.

Fanon, a Franco-African psychiatrist born and raised in what was then the French colony of Martinique, pioneered the psychological understanding of racism as a form of pathology. The epigraph in *Black Skin, White Masks*, a quote from author, socialist activist, and politician Aimé Césaire, one of Fanon's intellectual and political mentors, pithily summarizes his message: "I am talking of millions of men who have been skillfully injected with fear, inferiority complexes, trepidation, servility, despair, abasement." Césaire, writing about the effects of colonialism as a political scientist, is cited by Fanon as the latter explored in depth the ways in which this form of systemic and structural oppression and inequality functioned intrapsychically to damage those who are colonized. Note that this quote refers to Adlerian constructs such as the inferiority complex and describes how, in order to survive in a colonized world, the colonized human assimilates what is seen in the mirror of colonization.

In a decolonial psychotherapy we can extrapolate the construct of actual colonization and its various manifestations in the French colonies of the Caribbean and colonization's ill effects as described by Fanon to all marginalized, subjugated, and subordinated persons who have internalized degrading and dismissive constructs about their group as a means of surviving the colonizing, traumatizing world in which they must function somehow. We can also use the term *colonization* to refer to ways in which people who are technically not marginalized and subordinated but nonetheless denied access to the entirety of their phenotype privilege due to, for example, poverty or educational or occupational disenfranchisement have been socialized to fear social equality and consequently to require the subjugation and disenfranchisement of the other in order to maintain a brittle sense of worth.

Fanon noted the myriad of ways in which racism and the colonizing of the homelands of Indigenous people of color by Europeans had the net effect of infecting many people living under a colonial yoke with forms of self-hatred and powerlessness. Importantly for the DHCR construct, Fanon observed that this internalization of oppression was not unique to colonized people of African descent. Rather, he also noted its presence in members of socially constructed marginalized and subordinated stigmatized and despised groups no matter what their phenotype. He also spoke of the colonization of the colonizers, the colonization of the mentalities of putative members of the dominant who are in some manner defined as outside the pale.

While Fanon's awareness of the dynamics of gender was poorly developed and, sadly, replete with misogyny, his insights about the idealization of the colonizer/oppressor by the colonized/oppressed seem to apply clearly to the ways in which many natal women have deidentified with their gender and practiced assimilation to the degree allowed in patriarchy, attempting to avoid being seen as fitting anywhere within stereotypes of femininity and adopting masculine-identified behaviors when attempting to succeed in patriarchal societies, including expressions of contempt for and competitiveness with other natal women.

Fanon was able to see that for heterosexual women of color, colorism (a subtype of racism, an internalization of the colonizer in which phenotype supremacy is practiced within the colonized darker-skinned group, and lighter skin is socially constructed as evidence of more beauty) was a potent and disempowering force. Not only in the French colonies of which Fanon wrote, but everywhere in the world in which Europeans had been the colonizers and White supremacy prevailed, social norms pushed colonized women to emphasize their assimilation into Whiteness as a means of being beautiful.

My generation can recall the many advertisements for hair straighteners and skin whiteners aimed at African American women (and where hair was concerned, at Jewish women as well). Fanon (1967) commented that colorism was often embodied by darker-skinned women seeking intimate relationships with White men as a means of decolorizing themselves: "It is because the Negress feels inferior that she aspires to win admittance to the white world" (p. 60), implied through a relationship with a White man.

Fanon's title for his book refers to the now well-studied phenomenon of divided self that has come to be known to be a common survival strategy among members of marginalized and subordinated groups. This sense of wearing a mask in order to code-switch between one's own culture and that of the colonizer is a phenomenon that is frequently a source of emotional suffering for members of marginalized and subordinated groups. The emotional energy expended, the manner in which a person's core and authentic sense of selfhood must be continuously cast aside in favor of an enactment of that which is socially acceptable, unthreatening to the dominant culture or colonizer or even protective against violent enactments by the colonizer or oppressor, carries a heavy emotional cost; to mask is traumatizing.

The White mask that Fanon describes is a form of exposing one's belly so as to convey submission and the absence of threat. It is also a parasite on the soul of the colonized person, a source of trauma for which the suffering person blames themselves, buying into the falsehood that putting on a mask is a choice they have made rather than something necessary for some kind of survival in situations in which they are trapped, literally or figuratively. The mask is a double-edged sword, one that is a source of trauma, for the person and often intergenerationally both up and down the years. This is because, as Fanon pointed out, the self-protective act of mimicking the oppressor contains within it the seeds of self-hatred, as the hatred, fear, and rejection that the oppressor expresses toward authentic manifestations of the target group are inherent components of the White mask.

Fanon specifically used the examples of racism and anti-Semitism, the latter social pathology being the original European Christian racism and thus well known to him due to his time as a student in France, to argue that these forms of oppression (and by inference, any and all structural and systemic forms of oppression, no matter what their basis) are essentially similar in that they deny humanity to the marginalized and subordinated group. When humanity is socially constructed as belonging only to the colonizer (in the cases analyzed by Fanon, White-skinned and non-Jewish French people), then those outside the group at the top of the social hierarchy are socially constructed, at times specifically so, as other than human or subhuman, as a species of animal that can be killed with impunity, its body mined for its gold or stuffed and placed in a natural history museum (as was the case with Saartjie Baartman, the woman labeled the "Hottentot Venus," who was enslaved, displayed as a curiosity, and after her death, subjected to taxidermy and further display).

A DHCR practice recognizes that survival practices such as these add to the collective and historical burdens of trauma suffered by those marginalized by some form of melanic phenotype supremacy when they are also experiencing the pains of trauma exposure to the structural forms of that pathology in present time. Whether or not a person knows their culture's heritage of masking to survive, the resonances of those masks echo throughout the cultures of, as Fanon (1967) would say, the wretched of the earth. DHCR practice understands that the experience of being born other, being defined as less than human from the first moment of existence, is the source of the trauma. Colonized, marginalized, and subjugated populations with higher rates of trauma-related distress are not manifesting some kind of underlying predisposition to distress. They are living with the threads of social toxicity that wormed their way into the fabric of White supremacist cultures that surround them long before their births. Fanon's work delves into the ways in which one act of devaluation of a marginalized and subordinated group spreads harm to others, creating an intellectual precursor to DHCR models of trauma healing in which the harmed community creates harm for the individual, and healing the individual heals the traumatized community.

Fanon also presciently commented on the ways in which the psychotherapist is infected and colonized with the viruses of supremacy. He describes an encounter with a woman manifesting the early stages of cognitive decline and observes himself changing his language to an infantilizing tone. Honestly confronting himself, he writes, "The fact that I talk down to this poor woman of 73; the fact that I condescend to her in my quest for a diagnosis, are symptoms of a dereliction in my relations with other people" (1972, p. 33).

With this statement Fanon pithily summarizes one of the continuing challenges for decolonial trauma healers. How can we maintain a posture of respect, of collaboration, of equity and humility, when we have been trained so insistently to observe suffering people through the eyes of a pathologizing taxonomy and nomenclature? As he then goes on to confess, he has been trained to see the other, anyone marginalized, as "scum" (1972, p. 110).

While the training of modern-day trauma healers is likely to be more politically correct and careful in its use of language, the aversive and nonconscious biases with which all humans are afflicted lead us to nonconsciously perceive some of the suffering trauma survivors who seek our care in similarly pejorative ways and to enact those biases in how we deal with those "scum."

Fanon was influenced by and refers to Adler's work in *Black Skin, White Masks* (1967). While he was also influenced by more mainstream psychoanalytic and psychodynamic thinkers, not surprising due to his having trained as a psychiatrist in France, Fanon draws the clear link between Adler's constructs of inferiority and the internalized racism and colonization of whose effects he writes.

ALBERT MEMMI AND THE DAMAGE DONE TO THE OPPRESSOR

Yet another weathered paperback has traveled with me across the years and miles from that radical psychology class in 1972: Albert Memmi's *The Colonizer and the Colonized* (1957). As, over time, I have attempted to explicate the ways in which systemic forms of oppression are damaging psychically to the oppressor as well those who are the targets of social pathologies and thus to dismantle false hierarchies of victimhood, I have often returned to Memmi's analysis of the ways in which the system of oppression, not those who enact it, is the ultimate social pathology and source of distress.

Memmi was neither a psychotherapist nor a psychologist. His life spanned the century from 1920 to 2020; he was born a Mizrachi (Arab) French-Italian Jew in Tunisia and became a writer, first of novels and then of social theory about the effects of social subjugation and oppression on subjugated groups. Where his work has informed the paradigm of a broader decolonial psychotherapy for me is in his identification of the colonizer as a different kind of victim of the colonial experience.

Memmi had a unique standpoint; Tunisia was a French colony at the time of his birth, and he was a member of a Jewish community that had been historically tolerated by Muslim rulers and included people like himself of mixed Mizrachi and European heritage. It was a community that, for its social survival, had sought to identify with the (mostly Catholic and historically virulently anti-Semitic) French colonizers rather than the colonized Muslims who were the indigenous peoples of Tunisia. He lived in liminal intersectional identities within the overlaps between his divergent social realms for his entire life. Under the rule of Vichy France, he was interned in a Tunisian camp for Jews. Although he had been active in the struggles for Tunisian independence, he was nonetheless expelled from his homeland by the new revolutionary government both for being a Jew and for being Europeanized. A quote from his diary (Memmi, 1955–1956/2017) illustrates this experience of intersectionality and liminality: "La multiplicité des personages qui sont en moi m'étonne toujours" (the multiplicity of people within myself continuously astonishes me (p. 12))—a lovely, pained, poetic description of intersectional identity penned in the late 1950s.

Because one of the challenges for a DHCR trauma healer is to remain open to the suffering of members of the dominant culture, those who operate and appear to benefit from structural forms of oppression, Memmi's work is especially informative. Acknowledging the damages done to the oppressor is not, he notes, a failure to see the damages of oppression (Memmi, 1965). Instead, it is to see the dangerous nature of a system of oppression—in his example, of colonization—on all of its members, the colonizer and the colonized alike. DHCR trauma healing work is not about inducing pain in people with colonizer identities in the strands of their intersectionalities; it is about holding space for the pain of moral injury, of guilt and shame, so that room is made in that traumatized person's heart for compassion and connection to the pain of the colonized.

Memmi also tells a painful truth. Continuing to knowingly participate in and derive benefit from structural oppression (e.g., in Christian European colonized nations to benefit from White privilege) is something that the DHCR healer must, at some point, turn the suffering person's attention toward. This is because it matters not to the degree of moral injury one suffers nor how liberal one is in one's stated views toward and treatment of the oppressed. Conscious and knowing collusion with systemic oppression is ongoing trauma. DHCR healing with this suffering person necessitates inviting a particular kind of critical consciousness, the consciousness of how one can disengage from and work to dismantle those systems that have appeared to be the source of privilege.

Thus, in the DHCR practice model, in order to decolonize our epistemic frameworks, it is an ethical imperative for trauma healers to identify ways in which we benefit from and uphold structural inequities. This is not to induce guilt nor shame. It is to create the space in which to actively explore how to own our participation in structural oppression, and then own the struggles of ending those social pathologies, learning not to make them the problem of the marginalized and subordinated traumatized humans who suffer obvious and direct harms. This creates an understanding of the process of decolonizing the self that allows the DHCR healer to hold space, as described earlier in this book, Memmi noted that to be a person of good will counts for nothing when one continues to unmindfully participate in and allow themselves to benefit from the colonizing/oppressive system. I will share my own explorations of how I benefit from White skin privilege at various points later in this volume as an example of how a DHCR trauma healing practice can operationalize Memmi's observations.

Memmi also explicates the powerful role of social class as a tool of the colonizer used to make solidarity between different marginalized groups seem a near impossibility. He noted that a poor or working-class member of the colonizing society who shares phenotype supremacy with the ruling class is fed the illusion that it is possible to rise to a position of more power in the social hierarchy due to having phenotype privilege. In this manner, Memmi noted, these groups can be exploited by the elite as tools to maintain the social order and taught to feel aggrieved and angry when a member of a marginalized and subordinated group appears to take on privileges—education, wealth, political power—that were meant to be reserved for the phenotype-privileged group. Such persons know that they are outsiders, playing the part of how a White person should speak and act should they overcome barriers to reach some kind of professional success. One White friend and colleague of mine, who grew up in extreme poverty, has spoken with me about how difficult it is for her to embrace her many professional accomplishments for fear that her roots will be unmasked and thus herself expelled from her professional world as some kind of charlatan who does not belong there (J. Henning, personal communication, various dates 2018–2024).

Or as Lyndon Johnson, no stranger to the wounds of growing up in abject poverty, once said about the social control function of White supremacy, "If you can convince the lowest white man he's better than the best colored man, he won't notice you're picking his pocket" (Moyers, 1988). The fragile nature of the colonizer's social standing is the model for the brittle and temporary nature of privilege for most members of such groups, whose intersectional identities often contain a variety of target group memberships. Frantic efforts at concealment of those marginalized identities, frequently manifesting as self-hatred and disconnection from important internal sources of power and capacity, are often part of the trauma of being of the dominant culture. For a DHCR trauma healer this dynamic, so clearly explicated and embodied by Memmi's own life (as well as, to some degree, my own), points to the core importance of understanding social class as a phenomenon that can be weaponized through the social pathologies of classism and phenotype supremacy. A DHCR healer must be skilled in exploring the suffering engendered by marginalization and devaluation of a person's class status, seeing that internalized classism as a source of behaviors with which the suffering person struggles.

Memmi additionally describes the phenomenon of identification with the oppressor from a decolonial rather than intrapsychic epistemic framework, using the experiences of his own Jewish community in Tunisia as the example. The Jews of Tunisia had been historically oppressed by the Indigenous people of Tunisia, Arab and Berber Muslims. Some of the Jews of Tunisia had themselves been Arab and Berber Muslims, some of whom, like Memmi's own parents, married European Jews.

The arrival of the French colonizers, despite the anti-Semitism endemic to French society, offered the Jews of Tunis an apparently less oppressive ruler, with whom the community and its members frequently attempted to identify by assimilating in language, dress, and social customs, becoming Francophiles. This narrative echoes Fanon's concept of the "white mask" worn by colonized people of Black African descent: a false self taken on as protective camouflage, yet one that, like a mask, can be stripped off at any moment.

For a DHCR trauma healer the phenomena of passing and masking as survival skills, whereby a member of a marginalized and subordinated community intentionally obscures their group membership so as to escape notice from the colonizer, all while knowing that danger can emerge should the mask slip, is illuminated in Memmi's discussion of his own liminal group's experiences. As noted at various points both earlier in this volume and as we proceed with these ideas later in the book, it can sometimes be difficult for a DHCR trauma healer to recruit within themselves compassion for the suffering of the person who appears to have been doing their utmost to distance themselves from their own marginalized and subordinated group's suffering through assimilation. It can be even more difficult to hold the healing space for the person who, trying to survive, seems to have protected themselves, if only for a moment, by colluding with the suffering of those even more marginalized and subordinated in the social hierarchy.

These manifestations of internal colonization, which commonly lead to experiences of betrayal trauma, alienation, and isolation, may seem morally difficult to defend. They are moral injuries that have required a betrayal of self, a failure to form a coalition with other marginalized and subordinated people against structural forms of oppression and social pathologies. And yet, such trajectories are painfully common among members of marginalized and subordinated groups whose intersectional identities hold false promises that, should one assimilate enough, mask enough, punish one's own group enough, that one will be fully and unconditionally taken into the fold of the colonizer. Memmi's work, because it is so personal in nature and so eloquent in its description of the pain of living in apparently conflictual intersectional identities, is foundational for DHCR healers who are struggling to grasp the complexities of these kinds of liminal identities and to be able to clearly see the price paid in suffering by those appearing to benefit from structural oppression.

IGNACIO MARTÍN-BARÓ AND LIBERATION PSYCHOLOGY

The social psychologist, Jesuit priest, and martyr Ignacio Martín-Baró is generally recognized as the primary initial explicator of liberation psychology, which he derived from liberation theology. Murdered, along with five of his Jesuit colleagues and their Indigenous housekeeper, by U.S.-trained and U.S.-supported government forces for his alignment with the peasant revolt against the dictatorial government of El Salvador, Martín-Baró's work integrated liberation theology, Paulo Freire's liberation *Pedagogy of the Oppressed* (1972), and social science of a sort easily recognizable to psychologists trained in the logical positivist empiricism of U.S. and U.S.-influenced research psychology.

Martín-Baró moved critical psychology from the realm of the theoretical into that of the practical, exploring how an analysis of the social conditions of oppression leads to collaborations between professionals and oppressed people with the goal of liberation, equivalent to healing. In the past decade, students of liberation psychology have become more active in making his work, and the theory and praxis of liberation psychology, available to a wider audience (Comas-Díaz, 2020; Comas-Díaz & Jacobsen, 2024; Comas-Díaz & Torres-Rivera, 2020). While liberation psychology has always been foundational to DHCR practice, which would not exist in its absence, the healing applications of this work have become more accessible with the contributions of Comas-Díaz and other healers, which I discuss later in this chapter.

Martín-Baró expanded upon Freire's notions regarding learning from oppressed people in his own work and elucidated the construct that the promotion of conscientization, critical consciousness—that is, the fact that one is not to blame for one's sufferings—is a powerful decolonial and potentially healing step for individuals who have experienced and are suffering emotionally from the effects of systemic oppression.

In this approach, the healer engages in a dialectical process with the suffering person, encouraging curiosity about the question of who and what benefits from the acts that caused harm to that sufferer, a literacy of the suffering process that becomes liberatory for both the person suffering, who is more accurately read, and the healer, whose lenses become more finely tuned (Freire & Macedo, 1987). The goal is to elicit the suffering person's critical consciousness regarding the power dynamics that have been disempowering and dangerous, but to do so in a manner where the healer neither leads nor makes pronouncements but rather empowers the suffering person's own capacity to think critically about what has occurred.

In practice, with a DHCR trauma healer, this might look like the following. This material combines the stories of several different individuals, thus disguising all identifiers of the various contributing parties. Sylvio, the person seeking healing, was a lighter-skinned person of mixed Zapotec and Spanish ancestry, who came to the United States undocumented and was the beneficiary of a blanket amnesty in the 1990s that allowed him to be a legal resident after 2 decades of daily worry about "La Migra." His family were farmers in Oaxaca State. He worked in the restaurant industry, first washing dishes and then, demonstrating his skills in the kitchen, rising to the level of sous-chef. He was a natal man and heterosexual; raised Catholic, he was now a member of an evangelical Spanish church. He lived with his partner of many years and was the father of two children. Efrain, the healer, had not only been born in the United States; he told friends that "before Texas was America, my family was there." Both of his parents had bachelor's degrees, and Efrain had a master's degree. A natal, heterosexual man, he had been raised nominally Catholic and defined himself in adulthood as Buddhist. He grew up entirely bilingual.

So it would appear on the surface that the DHCR paradigm would see these two as a good fit for therapy. But what about the power dynamics? Efrain had never been poor and never worried about being deported (despite being stopped regularly enough by Border Patrol in South Texas that he always traveled with his passport on his person); he never worked in a job where being burned and cut were simply by-products of the working conditions. He had an advanced degree; Sylvio had dropped out after primary school because his family could not afford school fees. How many differences of power are here in this short description of their differences?

To do DHCR trauma healing work with Sylvio, whose official trauma had been to suffer a severe burn injury at work which had activated layers of other trauma experiences, Efrain needed to address, early in the healing work, the ways in which there are these power dynamic differences that are built into their intersectional identities. He needed to explore with Sylvio what it means to be in therapy at all, as this kind of healing is a colonizer phenomenon, not part of Sylvio's Indigenous culture. Efrain also needed to explore unspoken assumptions.

So he started their work by inviting Sylvio to set some of the ground rules, collaborating with the suffering person rather than imposing those rules on him. "So we usually meet for about 50 minutes at a time, one time a week," Efrain said. "That's not how we have to do it. If this were set up the way you wanted to do it, what would that be?" Sylvio replied, "Uh, well, you're the expert, so I shouldn't tell you." "Sylvio, I am a kind of expert, and you are another kind. Seriously, if you decided how we worked together, what would that look like?" And so on; Efrain invited Sylvio to collaboratively dismantle the Eurocentric colonial rules of how the healing process will take place. Over time they would explore deeper issues of power between them.

The DHCR healer, knowing the vulnerability inherent in more marginalized identities present in the sufferer, starts with what appears to be on the surface: how many minutes, how often; do we use honorifics, formal address, or first names; do we sit in the office or walk together on the bike path; all of these structural, apparently superficial, aspects of a healing practice empower the suffering person's skill in thinking about power dynamics, in experiencing their own voice in balancing these dynamics. It took 6 months of 2-hour-long weekly meetings before Sylvio asked, "So what do you think about me being an illegal?" and Efrain said, "You know, hermano, the White guys didn't ask our people where to put their borders, did they? So no, it doesn't make any difference to me, speaking just for myself as another Mexican who happened to be born in El Norte."

In this response Efrain demonstrated critical consciousness about the Christian European colonization process, one whereby various Christian European nations traded off the rights to control the people and resources in tracts of land without the consent of those already living there (Jones, 2023). That critical consciousness is embedded in a DHCR paradigm of trauma healing. Without it, Efrain is just another Spanish-speaking therapist to whom Sylvio, the client, is assigned by the agency without thought to what their very similar and very different intersectionalities might mean, without attention to whether or not the healer has the necessary critical consciousness to do decolonial work.

Although many of the constructs of liberation psychology focus more directly on collective actions than on individual healing, a number of constructs that are central to research or action projects also appear to be central to a DHCR healing practice. One of these is *vivencio,* lived experience (Burton & Guzzo, 2020). In the usual, colonized models of working with trauma-exposed suffering people, the lived experiences of the sufferer are not given weight anywhere near equal to that accorded to the expertise and training of the healer. An emphasis on the lived experiences of the suffering person means that if they say, "This doesn't work for me," the healer listens rather than pushing back, is curious rather than interpreting that response as defensive. The lived experiences of the suffering person in the healing relationship are foundational to a DHCR practice.

The critical recovery of history (Fals-Borda & Rahman, 1991) is another liberation psychology research value that is central to DHCR trauma healing. If the DHCR healer locates the source of distress somewhere within a social pathology, doing so requires critical recovery of history: What stories have been told, both personal and cultural? Which have been silenced, which distorted, so that the suffering person is unable to know that their story has a place in a larger story, that they do not stand alone in their pain? The #MeToo movement, which was started by BIPOC women, is an example of a collective critical recovery of history—in this instance, the history and pervasiveness of sexual assaults in the lives of modern women at a time in the mainstream cultural narrative that proclaimed things to have changed.

As Comas-Díaz (2020) wrote, "Liberation clinicians believe that the purpose of psychotherapy is to change people, so that they can change the world" (p. 170). This could be the motto of a DHCR healing practice, reflecting a similar construct from the Talmud that says that if you save one life, you save the entire world. Both Comas-Díaz and the Talmud demonstrate systems thinking about the place of the individual rather than separating the individual—in this case, a suffering, trauma-exposed person—from their social realities. Consequently, one can, from a liberation psychology standpoint, work with a person and still be working collectively and in community, using the focus on raising consciousness with regard to social pathologies and unsilencing the true stories of the past, whether one's own past or that of one of the components of the suffering person's intersectional identities, as a way of integrating individual and community.

Comas-Díaz adds one interesting, unique, and, I found, essential message to what constitutes the practice of a liberation healing modality—to live well, "Buen Vivir." As the poet Ross Gay (2022) has commented, it is not only permissible but necessary for the survival of systemically oppressed people to find joy, and to find it everywhere and anywhere in life through the paradoxical door, which is consistent with DHCR healing practice, of inviting sorrow in. He writes, "Rather than quarantining ourselves or running from sorrow, rather than warring with sorrow, we lay down our swords and invite sorrow in" (p. 4). Make space for human response rather than pathologizing it.

Thus, a goal of a DHCR healing practice is not symptom reduction nor merely the addition of the working through of the existential meanings of the trauma at the individual, cultural, and historical levels. It is also that the suffering person find ways in which to live well, to be, in Gay's words, incited to joy. Joy, after all, is one of the first things that colonization attempts to steal from the colonized: our songs, our dances, our art, all demonized. Sneaking around the colonizer, appropriating the colonizer's metaphors so as to express joy, is the necessary work of survival. Thriving, living the good life, a life of joy, is a goal for DHCR practice that has its roots directly in liberation healing paradigms.

CRITICAL PSYCHOLOGY: AN OVERARCHING FOUNDATIONAL EPISTEMOLOGY FOR DHCR PRACTICE

Critical psychology (Fox & Prilleltensky, 1997) is a term describing a growing group of theories that operate from the perspective of critical analysis of the dominant culture through various antioppression, decolonial, and intersectional lenses. As such, critical psychologies challenge much that is taken for granted regarding methods and practices in the social and behavioral sciences. The critical psychologies are interested in unjust and unequal dynamics of power and privilege, although in these instances the emphasis is less on gender and more on other aspects of identities and social locations.

Some of the theories that come within this definition include liberation psychology (Duran, 2007; Duran et al., 1998; Martín-Baró, 1994), intersectional feminist, mujerista, and womanist psychologies (Brown, 2009; Greene, 1990, 1992, 2000, 2007), and multicultural psychology (Comas-Díaz, 2006, 2010; Comas-Díaz & Jacobsen, 2001), all of which are located epistemologically and methodologically at the margins of mainstream psychology and critique those professional cultures' assumptions about health, distress, normalcy, and the nature of the therapist-client relationship. Many critical psychology theorists have either themselves been members of colonized cultures or have been directly informed by the experiences of those so colonized. Thus, a critical psychology perspective will always be foundational to DHCR trauma healing practice.

Values of Critical Psychology

Critical psychology emphasizes knowing through a diversity of epistemologies and methodologies, including those not valued by the colonized world of academia. These include story, song, film, spoken word and other poetry, and personal narratives of trauma exposure and healing. In a DHCR paradigm reflecting the insights of critical psychology, these sources are treated as valuable, not anecdotal evidence to be swept to the side.

The Practitioner as Self-Aware and Self-Reflexive

Audre Lorde (1984b) expressed the value of the critical psychology practitioner being self-aware and self-reflexive, writing that each of us must "reach down inside yourself and touch that terror and loathing that lives there. See whose face it wears" (p. 1). Thus, critical psychology points to the necessity of holding a "qualitative stance" (Kidder & Fine, 1987) on the experience of others; such a stance, they write, requires the professional, researcher or healer alike, to be "propelled by a desire to know what is unknown, to unravel surprises, to be alarmed and jostled in our own thinking" (p. 37).

Critical psychologists have proposed a number of methodologies for offering both emotional healing and social justice to survivors of trauma; we will explore this material in most of the later chapters of this volume dedicated to the question of what makes for a DHCR healing practice. Many of these methodologies derive from the liberation struggles that have identified the systemic traumas experienced by colonized people, as well as from torture survivors and other traumas that result from overt abuses of governmental and institutional power. Some of these methodologies reflect modalities that emerge from non-Western healing traditions integrated with those of the dominant culture of the mental health professions.

Syncretism: The Integration of Indigenous Healing Strategies Into 21st-Century Treatment

Syncretism is what is often implied in other writing on decolonizing trauma healing, as that work refers to Indigenous methods from parts of the world colonized by Europeans. These colonized cultures have always had healing strategies that have been found helpful for suffering persons. Many of these approaches are spiritual, invoking the divine or spirits to assist the emotionally wounded person. Others reflect types of medical epistemologies, such as those of Asian medicine and acupuncture, which diverge sharply from those of Western allopathic practice. These healing modalities, which have been colonized and appropriated under the rubric of complementary and alternative medicine reflect an evidence base of having helped suffering, trauma-exposed humans over very long periods of time. Openness to the integration of these approaches into treatment is consistent with a critical psychological perspective of valuing knowledge from a variety of sources, not only those approved by dominant cultural authorities. A thorough and nuanced discussion of a range of

Indigenous healing strategies that have clear application to work with trauma survivors can be found in Comas-Díaz (2012) and Comas-Díaz & Torres-Rivera (2020). A DHCR trauma healer is open to learning about and integrating these Indigenous and syncretic healing modalities.

Critical and liberation psychologists have also emphasized attention to the social, moral, and political implications of their work, which is an ethic informing a decolonial trauma healing stance. They insist that a healer abandon a stance of moral neutrality with regard to social pathologies and structural and systemic forms of oppression. Similar to an ethics code, critical psychology has a set of values that are foundational to DHCR trauma healing work.

Included in this value set is the idea that a healer identifies as problematic the radical individualism of Global North, Europeanized dominant cultures, which stresses individual happiness and values it over community and relational well-being as if the two are separate from one another. In DHCR trauma healing work, the continuing oppression of a suffering person's community affects their own healing, and their healing affects that of their community. Such radical individualism is also at odds with the goal of solidarity, allyship, and equal collaboration between a DHCR trauma healer and the suffering person. Individualistic paradigms for life are conceived of as risk factors for suffering, increasing as they do the distances and voids between humans and their communities.

Critical psychology attempts to expose the degree and pervasiveness of inequality and disparity of treatment and the ways in which the dominant culture attempts to obscure those realities. One dominant strategy for accomplishing this is via the creation of tokens—members of oppressed, marginalized, and subordinated groups who are permitted to succeed due to extraordinary talent, special access, or evidence of willingness to serve the oppressor (e.g., U.S. Supreme Court Justice Clarence Thomas) and who are then pointed to as examples of what any marginalized and subordinated person can do if they only exert sufficient effort. This individualistic narrative makes invisible the systemic nature of oppression and disparity of opportunity.

Within the context of emotional suffering this framework functions to make invisible the ways in which systems of oppression, the social pathologies, are the sources of suffering not simply for the person but also because they create cascading barrages of vulnerability-inducing experiences that exacerbate suffering, as we explored in all of the earlier chapters of this book, and will explore in greater depth as we go along, about how the gender binary creates unsafe spaces for people who do not conform to it.

Disparities in access to resources, including healing care, then aggravate the experience of suffering by making healing space either completely unavailable or less available in some way based on a person's economic status and social identities. Members of oppressed, marginalized, and subordinated groups are thus further oppressed when experiencing suffering due to unequal availability of necessary treatment. Institutional betrayals play into these forms of oppression and inequality. For example, when a combat veteran is denied care for trauma-related symptoms by a government that has pledged to care for that veteran yet has chronically underfunded veterans' services, healing options are open only to veterans who have means to purchase care on the open market. But for veterans who are too economically disadvantaged to purchase such care, unacknowledged and unhealed suffering engendered by trauma exposure has had the consequence of the prison system becoming the largest treatment facility for veterans suffering from encounters with trauma.

Critical and liberation psychologies trace the effects of systemic oppression through the life cycle of these individuals via the social pathologies of classism. Poverty creates systemic barriers to obtaining postsecondary education; in the militaristic social pathologies that inform U.S. culture, joining the military is offered as a better job opportunity for poor and disenfranchised young adults whose educational opportunities did not prepare them for academic or vocational success.

The military does not offer training for life in the civilian world; it creates opportunities for various kinds of trauma exposure, be they direct combat or flying drones from a windowless room somewhere in Nevada and watching people die because they were the ones pulling the triggers on those drones many thousands of miles from the death they have inflicted. Members of the military live in a culture that both valorizes what they do and simultaneously punishes anyone who manifests posttraumatic distress through marginalization that leads to premature separation from service and sometimes other than honorable discharges from the military due to the service member's employment of problematic posttrauma coping strategies, such as overuse of a substance. This last leads to denial of access to care designated for veterans, as the other than honorably discharged veteran has been defined as unworthy of care. Even with an honorable discharge a suffering veteran faces a years-long wait for care within the underfunded veterans' care system.

In these times of abandonment, during which the veteran has no skills that are useful in the civilian world, acting out of distress from trauma exposure may ensue in the form of abuse of substances, escalation of use of violence as a problem-solving strategy, and entry into the role of criminal. These are all institutional betrayals, which critical psychology describes as a built-in component of structural forms of systemic oppression and inequality. A DHCR trauma healer attends, then, not only to the obvious wounds—combat and moral injury—but also to the betrayal, to the abandonment, to the destruction, not simply the loss, of a person's just world hypothesis that are often normative in these narratives.

Critical psychology asks healers to hold ourselves to account. As the saying goes, "If you're not part of the solution, you're part of the problem." Critical psychology differentiates between the benign intentions of the social and behavioral sciences as expressed in the preambles to their various ethics codes and the actual consequences of taking stances that passively uphold the oppressive social status quo. The dilemma, as experienced by critical psychologists, is whether to use the master's tools to remodel or even bring down the master's house, to rephrase the words of poet Audre Lorde, or to depart entirely from the norms of dominant disciplinary culture to explore new forms of interventions that may lead to more fundamental, less superficial change. This is the dilemma of the DHCR trauma healer: Do we try to adapt what is already here, or do we take our stand in solidarity with those suffering from exposure to trauma and become the guardians at the gate, stating which healing modalities are liberatory and acceptable to us and which are assimilationist and potentially dangerous to people already harmed by social pathologies?

Critical psychology calls particular attention to the ways in which systems of inequality are rationalized through individualistic values so that justice is distorted to become the equivalent of receiving what one deserves due to one's individual qualities. Socially constructing human suffering as one form of evidence of systemic social injustice, of the traumagenic presence of social pathologies rather than simply as miswired biology or irrational thinking, breaks through the trance of unknowing inherent in the individualist emphasis of psychotherapy as generally practiced. DHCR trauma healing is not individualistic, although healers work with individual suffering people.

Questions of self-determination and participation are relevant to designing systems of care for suffering people in that they challenge the notion that designated experts will know better than those who suffer how to develop holistic models for healing that are congruent with clients' own values and goals. From the critical psychological perspective it is grossly insufficient and yet entirely telling when systems of mental health care delivery act as if it is a meaningful change to rename clients as "consumers." A consumer, eh? In other words, a purchaser of good and services in a capitalist economy. To the degree that access to care for wounded souls is being drawn into the maw of corporations, this supposedly progressive renaming seems more like a portent of corporate overlords than the empowerment of suffering people. This latest trend has emerged in many of the mental health settings to which the most disenfranchised, marginalized, and subordinated of suffering people are sent for their care. Suffering people are not fooled; their awareness of their disempowerment, by whatever name their role in the trauma factory is being called this year, has not been dulled.

Consumers are not citizens or true participants. "Consumer" is a role in a culture where everything is for sale, and thus that which is being sold must be attractive to those purchasing it. There is an illusion of choice but no real power. The consumer role lacks moral agency and creates an illusion rather than a reality of participation. Citizens, conversely, are potentially the moral agents of their culture and society and can potentially be in an empowered and active position in which real change is within reach. Critical psychology perspectives query how healing can be offered to suffering people in ways that are genuinely collaborative. Critical psychology has explored how not to reenact the disempowerment of systemic oppression in the healing relationship or in any system of which that healing relationship is a part. DHCR trauma healing is thus profoundly informed by the epistemic stances of critical psychology.

CARL ROGERS: CENTERING THE PERSON

One might be surprised to find Carl Rogers in the collection of sources of a DHCR trauma healing methodology. Rogers came from the mainstream of psychology. At the time of his death he was still in the mainstream. His work has not been vanished from the canon. Yet Rogers was, in his own way, quietly revolutionary, and his ideas about the healing process are among those in the foundation of the structure of a DHCR practice.

Rogers's own intersectional identities had many elements of the dominant culture and few of the marginalized and subordinated in them. But he was gifted with an unusual capacity for openheartedness, for feeling with and standing side by side with people in pain. He pushed first to call his work "client-centered" and, by the middle of his career, influenced by his encounters with healers such as Barry Stevens, a woman who had never been formally trained and whom Rogers brought into his world as his coequal and teacher, "person-centered." Rogers was thus the first theorist to say that healers are working with humans—persons—and that those humans needed to be centered in the work and thinking of the healer.

As I wrote in an earlier work,

> Rogers's work can best be described as revolutionary, given his time and place. He moved the field of psychotherapy from a view of our clients as ill patients who required our expert ministrations to seeing them as whole persons in states

of incongruence, possessed of innate capacities for growth and change. His view of the therapist's role was equally important to his subversion of psychotherapy's then-dominant psychoanalytic paradigm. The notion that a therapist not only could, but ought to, step out from behind the faux neutrality of the psychoanalytic frame and be genuinely present in the relationship is the basis for all of the work I have done as a writer, theoretician, and practitioner of psychotherapy. I am not alone in having been shaped by Rogers's insights; the many generations of psychologists of my acquaintance who, like myself, began our doctoral education sitting in triad practices learning to demonstrate empathic active listening are his inheritors. (Brown, 2007, p. 1)

Rogers did not intend to address social pathologies. He was not wedded, however, to locating pathology in suffering people, and he deemphasized pathology even in his foundational work studying audio recordings of sessions with psychiatrically incarcerated people. He was genuinely interested in figuring out how to disrupt imbalances of power in the healing process, although much of his own life and his intersectional identities, as well as the time of the world and social contexts in which he lived, put limits on the degree to which he seemed willing or able to be more revolutionary. He was, at the end of his life, concerned with politics on a societal scale, specifically with some of the U.S. social movements of the late 1960s and with international conflict; he did not see structural and systemic oppression.

What he did, and what is foundational to DHCR trauma healing practice, was to emphasize the essential and necessary skill in the healer of listening to the suffering person and then not deciding for that person what they meant by what they said or what they dreamed. Equally foundational were his conditions for therapy: warmth, empathy, and unconditional positive regard.

While these three conditions, in today's world, sound naive and idealistic, the data of years of psychotherapy research show us that Rogers was right, and his inheritors, in the world of evidence-based psychotherapy and relationship variable research, are equally right. What matters most of all is the nature of the relationship and the suffering person's experience of being heard, seen, and felt clearly (Norcross & Cooper, 2021; Norcross & Wampold, 2019a). Rogers, by being a researcher who listened to what healers and suffering people did in their exchanges with one another, created a foundation for DHCR healing work by pushing past the authority-claiming epistemics of every other mainstream healing modality to the simple truths. While he was unable to see the next layer of truths, about systemic forms of oppression, social pathologies, and the dangers of power imbalances, he opened a door through which DHCR healers could walk. Or at the very least, he opened that door for me.

FEMINIST (WOMANIST, AND MUJERISTA) PSYCHOLOGY: CRITIQUING PATRIARCHAL SYSTEMS OF OPPRESSION

Feminist psychology as a formal discipline emerged toward the end of the 1960s, coinciding with the second wave of feminism in the United States, and reflected the concerns raised by that movement regarding both the formal academic and community understandings of gender. While first-wave U.S. feminism had largely concerned itself with women's right to vote and to participate at all levels of civil society, second-wave feminism had two sets of interests. The first was to ensure that women had equal access and opportunity in all aspects of life. The second, and the one informing this chapter, was to make visible women's normative experiences so as to destigmatize and depathologize these experiences of oppression that happened frequently, mostly to women, and mostly without acknowledgment by dominant cultural authorities.

Feminist psychology initially defined itself as a psychology of women, acting as a corrective for the problem of androcentrism, for example, that almost all of academic psychology had studied only men and had founded its assertions about women and girls on minimal data that were frequently distorted by deeply embedded strains of sexism and misogyny in dominant cultural thought. This androcentric bias was pervasive in psychology's first century.

The field of study renamed itself as feminist psychology during the decade of the 1980s in response to the growing understanding that its adherents were not simply studying women but were more broadly studying gender and power from the standpoint of feminist political analysis. It became increasingly apparent in the field of feminist psychology that simply collecting data about women's experiences in an apolitical and decontextualized manner was not the intended goal of those conducting its research and developing its scholarship. The field now refers to itself as intersectional feminist psychology, with two subvariants, womanist psychology, which is an integration of feminist and Afrocentric psychologies, and mujerista psychology, which derives from the experiences and knowledge of Latinx feminist theorists.

Feminist psychology derives its analysis of information via an intensive interrogation of standpoints that are usually marginal to academic disciplines, such as those of Euro-American women, people of color, lesbian, gay, and bisexual people, transgender and gender-variant people, poor people, people with disabilities, people of minority religious and spiritual orientations, immigrants and refugees. As such, it is a model informed by feminist political philosophy and thought, observing human experience through an analysis of how power and powerlessness are distributed and experienced in various cultural and social contexts. Inherent in feminist psychology's current understanding of human behavior is that although social hierarchies attach power and power-lessness to certain positions and roles within those hierarchies, those ascriptions are not essential but rather constructed socially.

Thus, for instance, the early documented data regarding Euro-American women's struggles with achievement did not reflect anything inherent in being female that would serve as a barrier; rather, the data reflected systemic factors that assigned powerlessness to women in those settings where achievement behaviors might be expressed (Unger, 1989).

Because of this amalgam of science with a defined and acknowledged politics of power and powerlessness, feminist psychology has long eschewed the construct of scholarly or research objectivity or neutrality, encouraging its practitioners to engage in rigorous transparency about the standpoints that inform their research questions, the manner in which they gather data, and their interpretations of what is found. Feminist psychology is interested in supporting the integrity of research via an informed utilization of the scientific method of inquiry, while making transparent the standpoints that inform interpretations of data. Feminist epistemologies in psychology have, however, embraced a broader perspective as to what constitutes scientific methods of inquiry and consequently equally privilege qualitative and quantitative modes of inquiry and both statistical and heuristic forms of data analysis. Feminist psychology proposes that while this dynamic of the researcher's standpoint universally affects interpretation of outcomes in psychology and other behavioral sciences, it is largely within feminist and other forms of critical psychology that there is a norm of transparency regarding the effects of researcher and scholar standpoint on the meaning given to observed facts and phenomena.

As a consequence of this stance on how knowledge is generated and authorized, feminist psychology has had a core and long-standing interest in understanding and authorizing experiences of marginalized and subordinated individuals. An expectable result of this interest in such experience has been that much of the initial work in certain fields of trauma psychology, particularly the study of persons targeted by interpersonal violence and betrayal, has been conducted by feminist psychologists and other feminist behavioral scientists. Trauma, as Judith Herman noted, is itself a stigmatized, marginalized, and subordinated topic (1992). Trauma survivors, no matter what the source of their distress, have frequently been marginalized, subordinated, and silenced; the modern version of fear of the evil eye has prevailed in the form of shutting out any narratives of trauma survivors that disrupt just-world narratives or in any way challenge the glorification of war, which has been one of humanity's most persistent sources of trauma exposure.

DEPATHOLOGIZING POSTTRAUMATIC RESPONSES: A FEMINIST PERSPECTIVE

Feminist healers were among the first critical psychologists to take on the dominant diagnostic systems, beginning with critiquing how responses to interpersonal trauma were labeled and pathologized. Feminist psychological research in trauma was not only interested, initially, in describing the experiences of individuals who had been targets of traumatic stressors. An additional and continuing thread has been to depathologize those persons and shift the locus of responsibility for being a target of interpersonal violence from target to aggressor. This refocusing from a pathology of victims to a pathology of perpetrators, and from describing victims' psychological distress as having been causative of their trauma rather than an effect of the trauma, has constituted a second central contribution of feminism and feminist psychology to trauma psychology. As such, this reframing of the problem from trauma-exposed suffering person to the social pathology at the root of the distress has many roots in intersectional feminist theory and is consequently a main foundation for the DHCR practice paradigm.

Combating Victim-Blaming

What little work had been done on the experiences of victims of interpersonal trauma prior to the contributions of feminism and feminist psychology had been victim-blaming. The theme of such work was to search for the dynamics within the victim that had led the perpetrator to violate her, a classic tactic of social pathologies whose correctness is upheld by social norms that see suffering for violation of the social pathology as a deserved and reasonable outcome.

Articles such as the now infamous "The Wifebeater's Wife" (Snell et al., 1964), a classic of prefeminist woman-blaming in which the authors, all psychiatrists, discuss what in the battered woman is causing her husband to beat her, exemplify this trend in the prefeminist scholarship on targets of interpersonal violence trauma. One can also see this stance in the commentaries even in later volumes of Kaplan and Sadock's authoritative *Comprehensive Handbook of Psychiatry* (1985), in which girls sexually abused as children were described as seductive and contributory to their abuse. Before feminist psychology, the victims of interpersonal violence trauma often were analyzed for the personal flaws that led them to experience trauma.

Present in this pervasive blame ascribed to women who had been targeted by intimate partners or family members was the social pathology of misogyny, in which women's experiences of trauma were defined as inherent to normal female experience. The construct of normative feminine masochism, as promulgated by Deutsch (1944), informed the construction of women who had been violated physically or sexually as not simply pathological but actively complicit in or deserving of their victimization.

Feminist Trauma Healing

Feminist therapy, as it was called at its inception, emerged from feminist psychology as a means of translating research findings on women's experience into healing models that would embody the feminist politic of empowerment. A review of its development demonstrates that much of the theory for this model emerged from work with survivors of trauma, particularly trauma engendered by social pathologies of patriarchy, misogyny, and toxic masculinity.

Some of the foundational constructs of trauma healing thus emerged from feminist practice. One, which we shall discuss and deconstruct at length in all of the chapters that follow, is that of the three-phase model, those phases being stabilization/containment, trauma processing, and reconnection/meaning making (Harvey, 1996; Herman, 1992). Empowering the suffering person is another principle of DHCR practice first encountered in intersectional feminist work (Brown, 2009).

Most importantly, and like critical and liberation psychologies, intersectional feminist psychology focuses on the presence and toxic effects of structural and systemic forms of oppression as the locus of the problem, not on the suffering person. Feminist practice has always had its eye on these larger systems of oppression and could be conceptualized as the first wide-scale application of a decolonial model of practice (Brown, 2021), as its goals have always been the decolonization of the healing practice, the suffering person, and the healer from the toxic effects of patriarchy and, more recently, other phenotype supremacies. Feminist trauma healers were among the first to state unequivocally that trauma is an intended consequence of social pathologies and structural forms of oppression (Brown, 1994). Not simply because this author is a theorist of intersectional feminist therapy but simply because the precepts of this model align so closely with the DHCR trauma healing model, which is in fact an extension of my own previous thinking, intersectional feminist theory is another foundation on which DHCR work stands.

SPECIFIC INDIGENOUS HEALING PARADIGMS

Comas-Díaz (2006, 2020; Comas-Díaz & Jacobsen, 2024) has described the integration of Latino/a cultural and spiritual traditions into the healing process. She notes that all persons from Latin America have been affected by colonization, directly or indirectly, and that many of the cultural healing practices deriving from Latin American societies have been strategies for resilience in the face of persistent colonization trauma. We will discuss some of the specific healing methodologies that she presents in the various chapters later in this book that address what makes a healing modality consistent with the DHCR paradigm.

The Indigenous peoples of North America are an ethnically and culturally diverse group, with different languages, spiritual beliefs, and healing traditions. No one tradition is necessarily relevant or helpful to a person who comes from a different nation's traditions. Thus the use of sweat lodges, smudging with smoke from sage, sweet grass, or tobacco, Warrior Way ceremonies, and other Indigenous trauma interventions that have emerged into the consciousness of dominant culture are not ubiquitous within Native American societies but reflect the traditions of specific groups. A DHCR framework for trauma healing begins with understanding the healing methodologies of the culture of a particular suffering person, without assuming that these are in any way attractive to the suffering person. If and when a suffering trauma-exposed person whose intersectional identities include an Indigenous heritage that is meaningful to them, a DHCR model invites the healer to team with the suffering person and their chosen Indigenous healers and healing practices.

An enormous risk at this juncture is of the appropriation of an Indigenous healing methodology, thus thrusting a trauma reenactment of colonization into the healing space. It is nearly impossible to turn around in the world of trauma healing in the early 21st century and fail to encounter a mindfulness- or yoga-based intervention for a variety of forms of distress, including the suffering of trauma exposure. The fact that mindfulness is a watered-down version of the millennia-old practice of Vipassana meditation from the Buddhist tradition is not necessarily obscured, but equally not necessarily highlighted, by many psychologists who now include mindfulness-based interventions among their collection of evidence-based treatments. The fact that yoga is a Hindu spiritual and movement healing practice, not a neutral series of poses, or that it can somehow be reinvented as "trauma-informed" by persons who primary intersectional identities are those of the nations that colonized the Hindu world, is also often lost.

CONCLUSION

In this review of the family of healing theories and modalities on which I believe a decolonial, humble, culturally responsive trauma healing practice to be built, I have emphasized a number of themes.

Trauma healing is ever more rapidly becoming mainstreamed within the larger disciplines of the social and behavioral sciences, which makes the project of decolonizing trauma healing and rendering it humble and culturally responsive even more urgent than in years past. It is now possible for doctoral students in clinical psychology to study in programs where they receive training in evidence-based treatments for trauma, get supervision from trauma-informed faculty in the treatment of trauma survivors, and obtain internships and post-doctoral residencies in facilities with a focus on treating trauma survivors. A clinical or social scientist can build a tenurable research program around the application of various evidence-based practices that were not originally designed to treat trauma but are now being utilized with trauma survivors. The slogan of "trauma-informed care" is slowly and, one hopes, inexorably moving into integrated practice of health care. Decolonial, humble, and culturally responsive practice is not showing up in these places.

The inclusion of trauma within the canon of the healing professions could be a positive move. It risks, however, another layer of colonization. Yet in this progress toward integration into the mainstream of psychology, it remains important for trauma psychologists to remain cognizant of the roots of the discipline in the work of activists from social justice movements who were willing to name trauma where they saw it and to press for attention to the needs of trauma survivors. Feminist and critical social movements and the psychologists who have been affiliated with and informed by those movements are the foundation stones of trauma psychology. Understanding, valuing, and integrating feminist and critical perspectives into one's work strengthens whatever a trauma psychologist does, no matter what their theoretical orientation is.

5 DECOLONIAL UNDERSTANDINGS OF THE TRAUMAGENIC EFFECTS OF SOCIAL PATHOLOGIES

To do liberation psychology requires, first, to liberate psychology.

—Ignacio Martín-Baró,
Toward a Psychology of Liberation (1994, p. 9)

Trauma robs the victim of a sense of power and control over her own life; therefore, the guiding principle of recovery is to restore power and control to the survivor. She must be the author and arbiter of her own recovery. . . . Many benevolent and well-intentioned attempts to assist the survivor founder because this fundamental principle of empowerment is not observed. No intervention that takes power away from the survivor can possibly foster her recovery, no matter how much it appears to be in her immediate best interest.

—Judith Lewis Herman,
Trauma and Recovery (1992, pp. 159–160)

https://doi.org/10.1037/0000421-006
Decolonizing Trauma Healing: Toward a Humble, Culturally Responsive Practice,
by L. S. Brown

RESPONSIVE, NOT REACTIVE, DECOLONIAL WORK: THE HEALING PARADIGM

Colonizers are not simply a case of "Meet the new boss/same as the old boss" (Townshend, 1971), as the rock group The Who famously sang in their satire on political revolutions, titled (quite presciently given the various, mostly regressive, right-wing revolutions that have followed in the intervening half century) "Won't Get Fooled Again." It's not simply replacing one cultural paradigm with another as if they are interchangeable cogs in the machinery of society.

Decolonizing healing work requires decoupling that work from Christian Eurocentric colonizer paradigms of reality. But how to do this? One way is not to engage in acts of physical or psychological violence. This is because to violently revolt against colonization is, in my opinion, simply to reenact its norms and strategies, and in the world, dictatorships often have followed the overthrow of colonial rule, following the theme of The Who's song. I know that there is a fair amount of decolonial writing, including some of Fanon's (1967, 1972) work, that calls for violent revolution as a necessary decolonial strategy. But violence creates trauma for all involved and consequently cannot be a component of decolonizing healing methodologies.

Therefore, decolonizing trauma healing is not creating a new boss. Simply overthrowing the old ways of treating trauma is not what I mean by the construct of doing decolonial, humble, culturally responsive (DHCR) trauma healing. Simply not doing as has been routinely done previously or throwing out what has been done before and supplanting it with a new set of rules would create a form of trauma healing constrained by an entirely fresh collection of problematic notions about what counts as a trauma and what matters for healing. This is not what DHCR stands for.

The challenge of whether it is possible to decolonize trauma healing necessitates exploration of some more philosophical matters that I see as foundational to developing a trauma healing stance and praxis, honoring what is good in the old and yet which can be generative of the new and the decolonial. DHCR trauma healing is syncretic, an integration of all that might heal, no matter its source.

A colonizing power uses its more advanced weapons technology to take over a territory. It then burrows deeply into the culture and people who are Indigenous to the land that the colonizing power has occupied. That power subjugates not only the peoples and their leadership structures but also the institutions, languages, and belief systems of the colonized. Cultural genocide ensues even if actual genocide has not, although historically one has frequently accompanied the other. Ultimately the effects are similar.

Colonization in which lands and peoples are conquered also appropriates the foods, the argot, and the healing practices of the colonized and then announces to all who will listen that the entire colonized entity, with all of its material and human resources, has been discovered by the colonizer, the Christian European doctrine of discovery under which colonizers divvied up the non-Christian European world (Jones, 2023). Colonization of a place exploits, marginalizes, rapes, and murders the people who are inconveniently living on the colonized land, access to and control of which is asserted as its own by the colonizing power. That colonial power enslaves the people living on the conquered land, should they survive the barrage of technologically more advanced weaponry. Colonization sells Indigenous people to other colonizers so as to raise capital for further exploitation of resources and defines the humans dwelling on the conquered land as other than human so as to conveniently rationalize what is being done, feeding the social pathologies that rationalize these murderous behaviors.

The epistemic through-line from the notion that the Indigenous people of North America are not human to the establishment of the patterrollers, the first organized police force in the United States, whose entire job it was to hunt down enslaved Africans who were trying to escape, to the "no humans involved" label applied by some law enforcement personnel today to the killing of one Black, Indigenous, or person of color (BIPOC) person by another is also the trauma through-line of the Western Hemisphere. The social pathologies of White supremacy in its various forms are the strands of that rope.

Notice some parallels between what is generally understood as colonialism of lands and peoples to the colonization of the planets of emotional trauma and to the experiences of traumatized humans who have been targeted by social pathologies at work. The lands of the walking wounded, of people harmed by various exposures to trauma, the big traumas that are easier to see, the smaller paper cuts of the systemic oppression of daily life, are lands in which real or emotional violations, betrayals, and appropriations have been enacted on the bodies and psyches of trauma-exposed humans. Whether or not a person has experienced formal colonization arising from membership in an Indigenous or enslaved group is immaterial in this model, which presupposes some kind of colonization experience happening to all traumatized humans. Exposure to trauma created by social pathologies resembles all too closely in its biopsychosocial/existential-spiritual effects the experiences of people who were physically conquered, colonized, enslaved. Thus, we can expand the DHCR paradigm to people who are not among the officially colonized but are otherwise colonized and subjugated.

Trauma healing that is decolonial, humble and culturally responsive will of necessity allow a healer to notice that this suffering person sitting with them has had an experience of colonization of some kind, even very subtle and apparently invisible kinds. DHCR trauma healing must entail liberation from those less obvious forms of colonization of the self, every bit as much as it leads to the surcease of the distress for which that trauma exposure has been the catalyst.

MEDICALIZATION AS COLONIZATION: SOME MORE WORDS ON THIS TOPIC

The suffering of trauma-exposed people has been colonized over the past 150 years by the official mental health professions, invaded by the health professions—first medicine, then psychology. As discussed in all of the prior chapters in this book, this has led to the misattribution of the problem to the suffering human and to a tendency to avoid staring down social pathologies. The powers that the government gives to medical and mental health professionals make all of us with a license implicitly complicit with this continuing colonizing effort—a dilemma for which, as of this time, I do not see a clear solution. The question lingers, nonetheless: If the DHCR trauma healer is licensed by a state that also incarcerates people, pays law enforcement that sometimes terrorizes and sometimes murders some people, and in various ways upholds the ethics of individualism that are at the core of the Christian European colonization of this continent, how does a DHCR trauma healer attend to being loyal to the healing process when and if it comes into conflict with the law?

A logical consequence of trauma healing being colonized by licensed professions is the creation of an otherizing mentality. A suffering person is reduced to a case with a particular diagnosis, a case who is not us, who is an other. The narratives of a culture imbued with the toxicity of social pathologies then portray this kind of suffering human as potentially dangerous, definitely ill, possibly violent, or perhaps entertaining if their story makes for good drama on a streaming service. How often is the story of the antagonist in the script of some filmed drama that of a combat or law enforcement veteran who is struggling with the psychic wounds of trauma or of a woman sexually abused as a child or being savagely beaten by a husband or boyfriend who is now some kind of private avenger of the wrongs done to others? As a consumer of popular culture, I can say with certitude that this is increasingly common. Trauma makes for good drama and is rarely portrayed in ways that do not otherize, pathologize, or exoticize the trauma-exposed character. People who've experienced trauma consequently learn to see themselves reflected back in popular media as damaged rather than as having a human response to something that overwhelmed their neurobiology in one or many ways.

Through this same medium, social pathologies are also hidden, very occasionally hinted at, even more occasionally made foreground by creators from marginalized, subordinated, and socially aware communities (everything coming out of Shonda Rhimes's production company Shondaland is, for example, replete with commentary on social pathologies). For the most part social pathologies' continuing contributions to the suffering of a trauma-exposed person are barely alluded to in most storylines.

Because not only the health care professions but popular culture have been infected with the toxins of social pathologies and their distorted perspectives on what people suffering from trauma exposure are like and what heals them, the DHCR trauma healer will need to keep those contexts in mind. It's not part of the usual intake process to find out what media a person is consuming or what music they listen to, yet such questions acknowledge two DHCR practices. The first is to attend carefully to the intricacies of the person's social context, including those the person chooses to bring themselves into contact with, such as their preferred shows, movies, or video games. The second is to begin to demonstrate our interest in sources of joy in a suffering person's life because, as noted in Chapter 4 when I referred to the work of Comas-Díaz, joy is necessary for liberation. Joy, and the capacity to live a life that is good in the suffering person's eyes are components of the liberation psychotherapy underpinnings of DHCR trauma healing.

Asking such questions is also an avenue for bringing awareness of the presence and continuous effects of social pathologies into the foreground in a way that gently teases them out of the substrate of the person's own life. So a DHCR healer might inquire, "Hmm, do you notice how the show/podcast/ Instagram thread that you watch portrays people who share your identities? And what are the messages?" We take care to never imply that someone's enjoyment in the media they consume is a problem, because it is not, all the while integrating the social pathologies communicated by such media into the healing narrative of how a person was harmed and into how they might be liberated into healing partly through the development of critical consciousness about that media.

The DHCR model of trauma healing continuously interrogates and challenges assumptions about suffering people that arise from the pathologizing treatment of our trauma responses. The DHCR paradigm inquires, at each step of the healing process, into the influence of social pathologies, on how we and the suffering people we work with might be seduced into the colonizing narratives of the medical model. These colonizing influences can be difficult to detect, in part because so many suffering people have soothed themselves with knowing that they are not crazy but simply have posttraumatic stress disorder (PTSD).

There is irony here. In the early years of my therapy practice in the 1980s I would open whatever edition of the *Diagnostic and Statistical Manual of Mental*

Disorders (*DSM*) was sitting on my office bookshelf and have a suffering person read the definition of PTSD as validation that what they were experiencing was so common that, look, here it is in the book of diagnoses. I did not then consider that I was offering a toxic soothing experience, toxic because it taught people that they indeed suffered from a mental illness, albeit one that meant that they were not simply indefinably nuts because horrifying images, smells, and sounds kept intruding into their waking consciousness in ways that made it hard to live in their worlds.

I have found it useful, in developing a decolonial stance, to analyze the methodologies of colonizers. In the next section of this chapter, I will explore some of what I think of as typical colonial dicta conveyed to colonized people as best practices for surviving and appearing to thrive, for seducing the colonizer into believing that they have done a good thing by colonizing you. The French called this piece of the paradigm the "mission civilisatrice," the civilizing mission that was an alleged end goal excusing the horrors perpetrated on Indigenous peoples of North America and North and West Africa, the notion of the colonizer believing they did a good thing for you by colonizing you. In the world of trauma, this shows up as, "It's an evidence-based treatment; you're going to feel worse until you get better, but trust me, this will help you."

These best practices preached to the colonized—and frequently incorporated into cultural norms for colonized groups as means of protecting the community from attention or reprisal (and thus, over time, appearing to be norms native to the colonized culture rather than the cultural artifacts of oppression, as I first referred to them in 1992)—operate for the ultimate and sole benefit of structural social pathologies and those upholding them. Even when these coping strategies appear protective of the marginalized and subordinated traumatized person and/or their culture, such protection is typically transient, illusory, and entirely contingent on the colonized person maintaining their allegiance to the rules of the social pathology, never letting the mask slip.

WE WILL SURVIVE

Assimilation

A colonizing power typically offers a few so-called privileges to a select number of the colonized as a means of dividing while conquering. This strategy requires members of the colonized culture to assimilate into the culture of the dominant as the price paid for being temporarily given protection, which may look like privilege, in exchange for maintenance of assimilated practices and abandoning or hiding Indigenous ways of being. Handing out protection and the illusion of privilege to those, often few, who assimilate as fully as they are allowed to do so then functions as a false narrative about the value of colonization to the colonized—the adoption of a better religion, a more civilized language and style of dress. Assimilation preaches a false message promising that some of the colonized can become safe, made respectable, if they only assimilate thoroughly enough. The fragility of this position is always obscured in the narrative of assimilation, and its risks are hidden or denied by both the colonizing social pathologies and those who are most forcefully upholding assimilation, often rejecting or othering members of their own culture who resist assimilation.

An Assimilation Story

In Poland in the 1600s there were assimilated people of my repeatedly exiled and colonized culture, the Jews of Eastern Europe, who were often referred to as court Jews. They were members of an otherwise despised and endangered group but were singled out and encouraged to assimilate. As the prize for shaving their payot, the side curls worn by observant Jewish men then and now, and taking off their tallit katan, the fringed garment that can be seen even today dangling over the waistbands of observant Jewish men, these assimilated men were given positions at the courts of the Polish nobility as managers of the nobles' estates, which were worked by serfs and peasants who, unlike Jews, tended not to be literate.

The court Jews were held up, directly or indirectly, to their unassimilated brethren as an example of two things: (1) that a well-behaved, assimilated member of the oppressed group would be tolerated by those who usually put Jews in terrible danger just so long as that person did not advocate for the well-being of the rest of the group (should a court Jew advocate for his Jewish community, he was at risk of being stripped of his job and the illusions of protection that came with it); and (2) that it would remarkably easy for such a person to fall from grace, from court to the grave, when it suited the political aims of the oppressors.

The court Jews were put in the position of being the human face of the nobility in dealings with their serfs. They collected the rents and brought the news of new taxes, while the nobility played in Paris or Baden-Baden or Saint Petersburg. When serfs rebelled, as was the case during the Cossack rebellions of the mid-17th century, the court Jews, and then all other Jews, were the targets of pogroms of murder and rape while the Catholic nobility were safely away from the fray—which could then be blamed on the poor management of the Cossacks and serfs by the Jews.

These select few, highly assimilated pets among the colonized demonstrated their fealty to the colonizer through a process that in nature would be called a form of protective mimicry. They took on Polish names—in the English-speaking version of this, Gittel became Gertrude, Cohen became Cole. They accepted new gods, converting, or at least pretending to convert, to religions of their colonizers. They eschewed their own ways of marking the passage of time for the Gregorian calendar of the oppressor, so that there came to be "the calendar" (Gregorian) and "the Jewish calendar" (the one their ancestors had lived by for centuries, and which their descendants still follow where holidays are concerned). They changed their dress to copy the outfits worn by the nobility they served.

Assimilation is the symbol of acquiescence given in exchange for false promises of protection from the worst depredations of a colonizer. That promise is the ultimate lie, as my culture learned repeatedly. Jews were invited to Poland by its king, offering a place of refuge after the terrible massacres of Jews that had occurred in the Rhine Valley during the crusades in the first centuries of the second millennium of the Common Era. By the time the Nazis marched into Poland in 1939, Jews had spent most of that second millennium assimilating or not, dealing with the broken promises of protection, and experiencing individual and intergenerational trauma.

Most Jews in Poland, which in 1939 had the world's largest Jewish population, had not assimilated. Those who had assimilated, who had followed in the footsteps of the court Jews, died equally fighting for the liberation of the Warsaw Ghetto, or herded into the ravine at Babyn Yar to be gunned down by the thousands, or sent to the gas chambers of Treblinka, where my great-grandfather—unassimilated and unwilling to join his children in America—perished.

I am telling this story from my culture because although this story exists in many other cultures—think, for a moment, of the boarding schools into which the Indigenous children of Canada and the United States were forced, or schools for Deaf children, who were punished for speaking their native language, ASL, or the lynching of African American servicemen returning from World War II in uniform, a garment they believed might protect them, or the adoption by Hawaiian royalty of Victorian era garments and Christian beliefs—I don't want to appropriate the stories of other colonized people to make my point. That's why the through-line story I will tell in this book about social pathologies is going to focus on the ones arising from the lived experiences of one of my cultures. Because Jews have had liminal intersectional identities for two millennia, we are also a good example of what it means to be in the position of subjugated, but not clearly so, and able to subjugate, but not entirely; in other words, we have been both colonizer and colonized, pale of skin but not White (Brodkin, 1998) for much of the last 2,000 years.

Jews have been using assimilation as a strategy for dealing with colonization for more than a millennium now, all over the Christian and Muslim worlds in which we live in exile from our Indigenous homeland. We began to do it the minute we landed on the shores of the United States and Canada, or in South Africa, which was kinder to Jews than to its own Indigenous African peoples, or Argentina, or . . . fill in the blank. I was raised to believe that a little surface-level assimilation was a good thing, so long as, at the core, being a Jew was still present. After all, what kind of nice Jewish girl has a name like mine? And like my ancestors who suffered in and fled from Poland, it is turning out that assimilation is no protection from the reemergence of the social pathology of anti-Semitism, even in the place to which my grandparents fled for safety. Assimilation tells a lie: Give up something about yourself and we, the upholders of the social pathology, will keep you safe—but only so long as it's convenient for us. Anne Frank's diary is a poignant illustration of just this point, and of the impermanence of privilege when it is tied to assimilation (Brown, 2023).

When we take this analogy to other people who are suffering from exposure to the traumas of social pathologies, we encounter the notion of the high-functioning trauma survivor, supposedly assimilated into the culture of normal. "Look, she's been raped, but she's still going to school every day" and is consequently appearing to assimilate to the world of not-traumatized people. Such statements are microaggressions, saying that yes, trauma engendered by systemic misogyny and toxic masculinity has invaded this person's body and psyche, but she is performing the part of the unaffected person: "You're doing so well for having been raped a year ago." Valorizing the assimilation of a suffering person to the society of those not yet traumatized and lauding their performance of nonsuffering creates an untenable trap. Should they disclose that they are indeed still suffering, they risk the loss of the rewards of their assimilation, the praise given for doing so well.

But if the assimilated trauma-affected person believes they must double down on their performance of being fine, the cost is frequently the employment of strategies for soothing their neurobiology that then themselves become problems—using substances, food, or overwork until their use can no longer be sustained. It is often the case that the explosion of a life that occurs when whatever strategy has kept the performance going is no longer working leads to terrible shame. When a person has been deeply invested in being assimilated into the world of the not yet trauma-affected, their own responses are perplexing and terrifying to them: "I thought I was doing so well."

Unfortunately, this emergence of evidence of pain through the cloak of assimilation can become a kind of confirmation that this wound is indeed a thing that can destroy the suffering trauma-affected human. Lewis B. Puller Jr. was just such a person. A man whose intersectional identities were soaked in privilege, growing up as a White-skinned, natal man from a famous military family, able-bodied until he went to Vietnam, his combat trauma, which included loss of limbs, was something that he proclaimed in his memoir to have healed from (Puller, 2000). He was not healed; he shot himself not long after publication, his performance collapsing under the weight of what was considerable pain and loss, particularly the loss of his underlying beliefs in the just world.

Another Assimilation Story

I have also seen this dynamic up close and personal, when I had the honor to work on the project of seeking compensation for the enormous number of young women athletes who had been repeatedly sexually assaulted under the guise of treatment by a person with a medical license, who I do not name because that person does not deserve such notice. Most of those he violated were gymnasts, and the culture and governing organizations of their sport were the colonizing entities functioning to enable this sexual predator to continue in his actions. He was allowed to continue to inflict harm even well after all of the organizations involved had been made aware that he was sexually assaulting almost every young woman who was sent to him for care.

The very few young women who protested at what was being done or who reported this man's actions to his employer or to the sports federation, the women who refused to assimilate to the culture of silence and minimization and the protection racket run on behalf of the rapist, were typically marginalized and subordinated, made unwelcome in the sport, and eased out of the precincts of the elite athletes heading to Olympic glory. Those who kept silent forced themselves to continue to assimilate to the culture of gymnastics, which enabled many forms of abuse of girls and young women. They continued to be sexually assaulted and to suffer severe and long-lasting psychological pain arising from the trauma of the assaults. Eventually they also experienced the trauma and pain of realizing how they had been betrayed by the colonizing organizations.

Some of them were briefly rewarded for their assimilation. These rewards took the form of scholarships and inclusion on elite teams. When, one by one, these young women's distress became such that they were unable to perform either the role of the high-functioning, one apparently unaffected by trauma, or the role of an elite gymnast, they were cast off, no longer of use to the colonizers. Simone Biles's courageous description of her own violations at the hands of this man, and then having to withdraw from certain activities during the 2022 Olympics because they were trauma triggers, tells the story of these twin traumas—sexual violation and institutional and organization betrayal that required assimilation as the price of admission—better than I ever could (Macur, 2021).

When I met with some of these women I was impressed with the degree to which each of them had had to unknow, dissociate from the danger they were in during their so-called treatments with the predator, a phenomenon I will discuss at greater length in Chapter 9, in Marisol's Story about getting closer-to-safety. I was also a witness to the pain that each of these women carried for the utter destruction of the fabric of their lives arising from the toxic combination of the effects of rogue capitalism (the gymnastics organizations and the university employing the perpetrator all benefited financially through the sales of swag and media sponsorships, some of which used the names and pictures of the violated women), systemic misogyny in the form of never believing anything that any violated girl reported to these organizations, and the perpetrator's extreme expression of toxic masculinity in the form of his sense of entitlement to digitally rape hundreds of young women, some of them hundreds of times.

Just as so many of these young women were convinced that their silence and assimilation into the official culture of elite gymnastics would somehow balance out the repeated violations to which they were subjected by yielding scholarships or membership on the Olympic squad or a sports apparel company's endorsement, with the attached income, so assimilated colonized people of all kinds in all times and places have been at first entranced and tricked by narratives of the colonizer into believing that they have chosen their psychic immolation voluntarily, that by accepting colonization they have been civilized, made better than they were before they were colonized.

Eventually assimilation reveals its price—witnessing the betrayal of their own people and cultures, standing at the edge of the territories in which the destruction of the souls and spirits of their extended families and civilizations is perpetrated. For the gymnasts who kept silent there was the pain of watching friends' suffering while feeling trapped in their own silence by their reasonable desires to reap the rewards of having dedicated a life to their sport, a life filled with pain other than the rapes, and by knowing, through the examples made of those who spoke up, of how easy it was to be exiled.

The double price of telling the truth about the cost of assimilation, when one of those who can no longer tolerate the shortness of the leash around their psychic neck speaks out and throws off the disguise of being high-functioning and thus not suffering, can also be very high, because it entails exposing institutional betrayal as well. Many of the young women with whom I spoke struggled with the sense that they had betrayed themselves or their peers, seeing themselves through a lens of shame, blaming themselves for not having had sufficient courage or integrity to speak up—and these young women were children, some as young as 6 when they began to be digitally raped. It was their 6-, 8-, and 13-year-old selves they were angry at.

Psychic colonization by social pathologies, embedded in all sexual violations, but particularly those perpetrated on children, leads to such self-recrimination in sexually victimized people. Silence by a child is coded by the social pathology of misogyny as evidence that the trauma was not that bad or, by the social pathology of rugged individualism, of the child's own weakness of character or, as psychoanalysis proposed once Freud turned on and betrayed his earliest analysands, was evidence that the child desired such a violation but had never really been violated. Silence by a violated adult is frequently taken in the legal system as evidence that no trauma happened. Yet when no words can be spoken, the body speaks of fear, of broken attachments, of the need to freeze to survive, through the neurobiology of trauma. A move into a dorsal vagal response of shutdown and numbness means that verbal silence is among the typical human responses to trauma and violation, even while the body is yelling loudly at anyone who knows how to listen. Assimilation is a form of silencing. A DHCR trauma healer attends to the forms of assimilation that a suffering person might have, or may still be using, and not pathologize them but rather see them as the marks of the predator that is a social pathology.

Passing: Deep Assimilation

Sometimes retaining one's identity while tweaking aspects of its expression, which is what constitutes assimilation, does not suffice to distract the predatory system of a social pathology. And so some people pass, utilizing aspects of phenotype or behavior that allow them to precariously engage in a form of chameleonlike social mimicry in a deeper and potentially more dangerous way than is the case with assimilation—and less frequently fully successful. Passing is a fragile, and sometimes dangerous, strategy.

Passing comes at an even higher emotional and relational price than simple assimilation. A passing person must cut all ties with others whose presence or knowledge of the person's intersectional identities might endanger their newly acquired status as a member of a nonmarginalized group. In *The Sweeter the Juice*, Haizlip (1995) tells the story of the branches of her family, one side of which was passing for White, cutting off ties from those whose African heritage was too visible and imposing rules about who members of the White branch could marry so as not to risk the birth of a child with more typically African phenotype. Today, in the age of at-home genetic testing, these stories are told in the results that arrive telling a White man, who has all of his life proclaimed racist views, that two of his great-grandparents had been born enslaved—African—and that he has an entire family tree populated by people who have always been phenotypically of African descent and who identified in that way.

Passing was enabled by the social pathology of racism, which assigned invariant phenotypic characteristics of all people of African descent, and by the social pathology of the enslavement and rape of African women by European slavers, which led to children with a genetic mixture that could, within only a few generations, lead to people who appeared entirely European. Although the pathology of slavery defined those children as Black and enslaved, a raped child of a raped child of a raped child might look more like the rapist's White-skinned children than her own African grandparents.

Lighter-skinned people of African descent whose genes for lighter skin arose from rapes by slavers, living in postslavery regions of the Western Hemisphere, frequently passed for being of European descent or Turkish, which was perceived as close enough to European during the period in which the Ottoman Empire overlapped with the era of European colonization. Defining oneself as Spanish so as to explain one's slightly darker than Northern European phenotypic presentation would allow passing. It meant cutting oneself off from family, moving to a distant city where no one could identify you, and being constantly on guard for the possibility that your one drop of African ancestry might be exposed.

In these stories lies terrible pain. These are grown children who could not speak to their mother, grandparents forbidden access to grandchildren. Passing hurts the passing person because it is a betrayal trauma committed on oneself by oneself, in the name of survival. It hurts the people they pass to or, in passing, are cut off from. Betrayal traumas are ultimately about the price paid to survive social pathologies.

Colonial models of the world assume that social pathologies and structural hierarchies of systemic oppression are the natural order of things, normal. So too do colonial models of trauma and its treatment construct a normal life narrative of some mythical place where social pathologies are not continuously at work and trauma is rare. This discourse of the normal and natural, so embedded in current understandings of trauma, is difficult to resist because, after all, who wants to be abnormal or unnatural? Passing is one way to appear to be a member of the normal tribe.

Some women have passed for men. Billy Tipton, the renowned saxophone player, was one. She was not trans. She was a woman, known as a woman to her female romantic partners, who passed for male until her death, when the undertaker discovered her vulva. Even her female partners insisted publicly that she was a man, just a slightly different kind of man; so powerful was the narrative of passing that she had to adopt children in order to enter and succeed in her chosen profession. In today's parlance, she might be socially constructed as trans, but she only ever changed her social presentation to be male and only for the purposes of her work.

James Barry, born Margaret, passed for male in the late 18th and early 19th centuries in order to be able to practice as a physician at a time when the profession was barred to women. Her natal sex became known only after her death. Was she trans, or was she a woman with a burning desire to do that which was not allowed to natal women of her era—to be a physician, with all the power and privilege that entailed? We cannot know. Passing women socially identified as men in order to escape what the social pathologies of patriarchy prescribed for or denied to women. The social pathology of patriarchy proclaims it natural for natal women to be subjugated and even owned by natal men; passing as a man freed a woman from that subjugation and ownership.

Passing was the most common camouflage technique for queer people living in a world where exposure as being other than heterosexual had serious, sometimes life-threatening, consequences. Gay men from before the liberation era of the 1970s have written memoirs in which they describe how they and their friends would practice behaving in as manly a manner as possible, sometimes joining in hate speech about more effeminate men, and even doing so in the company of other gay men, using derogatory terms such as *queen*, as in, "She's just an old queen." (Of note, drag queens, who outside of their performances may present in a typically masculine manner, reappropriated that self-hating term as a source of pride; no small wonder that drag queens as a group are a target of a new wave of antiqueer legislative actions in some parts of the United States in 2023.)

Gay men who married women and had affairs with men they truly loved left wives assuming, thanks to misogyny, that they must be lacking in some manner because of the absence of sexual energy from their relationships. Or, like Leonard Bernstein, they would marry women with the explicit understanding that they were gay and would continue to have relationships with men. Lesbians would dress and behave in a hyperfeminine manner, practicing not only passing but the phenomenon, described below, of submission and the appearance of compliance. Or they would enter into heterosexual marriages with men and, by giving birth, prove themselves to be toeing the heterosexist line until they could no longer stand the charade.

My vacation home in a lesbian village was built by one such woman. She abandoned the love of her life, her college sweetheart, to marry a man so that she could safely be a teacher without risk of discovery as a lesbian at a time when being one would absolutely disqualify her for teaching everywhere in the United States. Her sweetheart, with whom she kept in touch, was her children's "Aunty," their original relationship well hidden from all. In her 40s this woman finally realized that life was short. She left her husband and lived with her sweetheart until her sweetheart's untimely and early death, no longer attempting to pass. She had enough years to repair the damage done by her self-exposure as lesbian late in life, being able to remain friends with her ex-husband and having grown children, who, when they learned the truth, were relieved to know that "picking up on weird energy" was not all in their heads. It made it easier for her daughter to come out as lesbian to her mother a few years later.

I learned this story when I bought the home after the death of the college sweetheart, a lovely little place which was a carefully planned expression of their love. Stories like this one are not unusual for lesbians and gay men who came of age before the 1980s (Cassingham & O'Neill, 1993), although this still occurs in the lives of people raised in social contexts where the price of being anything but heterosexual remain as high as it was everywhere in the United States before the gay liberation movement.

Sometimes gay men and lesbians would marry one another with the full knowledge of their shared queerness so as to provide a shield under which each could pursue the romantic and intimate relationships that were expressions of authentic self, living always in fear of exposure or blackmail. While this has become less common in the Global North, where queer people have found havens of openness and even allyship from powerful heterosexual people, the fear that the clock could be turned back to a time when passing was the only way to be safe is never absent, even in the most apparently safe of places. This segues us into another common entry in the catalogue of social pathology best practices.

SUBMISSION AND THE APPEARANCE OF COMPLIANCE

The 21st-century groom is usually not buying the 21st-century bride in exchange for a goat or the keys to a kingdom. Nonetheless the implicit message in a typical heterosexual marriage ritual is that one natal male owner has passed control of a wholly owned natal female body to another owner. Until very recently in the United States, there was no such thing as marital rape, since this ownership principle extended to the sold woman no longer having the right to refuse sexual contact. If you were born a woman, you were born into colonization, some of it physical, some of it psychological.

This ownership principle in U.S. law stemmed from a legal construct active until very recently in Blackstone's English law, which has informed the legal systems of most places previously colonized by the British Empire, by which a married woman was considered a femme couverte. The doctrine of femme couverte, a woman covered by a man, states that a woman, once married, had no separate legal existence or personal rights. She was legally subsumed into her husband. It persisted in the United States well past the middle of the 20th century, until nearly 200 years after the United States had proclaimed its independence.

The colonization of the intellectual space of the modern world by patriarchy has also been pervasive despite the entirely archaic notions of what people born female or male are able to do, notions that, as noted at many points both earlier in this volume and as we continue our explorations of decolonial thinking, might have begun to make sense when it was still believed that when we were hunter-gatherers in small bands that the men hunted and the women gathered. But more recent archaeological discoveries have shown that this version of our prehistory was itself colonized by later misogyny; women indeed hunted and fought, and did not simply wait around the fire for men to bring home the hunted game (Anderson et al., 2023).

Phenotypically genitally male members of species *Homo sapiens* colonized natal females so early and so persistently across the planet that when it emerged that our closest genetic relatives among nonhuman primates, the bonobos, were a female-dominated society, the earliest primatologists to closely observe and publish the truths about the bonobos were greeted with disbelief (Silverstein & Auerbach, 1999). How was it possible that a close primate relative was not patriarchal nor ruled by might instead of relationships? Bonobos are now, after decades of observation, known to be not only a matriarchal society in which older, more experienced bonobo females control what happens in their bands but a society in which the skills of tending, befriending, and being sexual with others are used as a means of resolving conflicts and healing trauma within the band (Silverstein & Auerbach, 1999).

The reality that testosterone naturally created more musculature and bigger bodies for postpubertal natal males, which was useful for some tasks required of early hominids, or that only natal women could become pregnant and nurse infants, which is true for all mammalian species, was transformed into the parent of all social pathologies.

This founding social pathology, patriarchy, took the biological facts affecting our distant hominid ancestors and made up multiple iterations of similar sets of rules used to create dynamics of power, value, and ownership everywhere the human species lives today. In the intellectual spaces colonized by patriarchy, women's brains were (and in some settings still are) socially constructed as less good at science, technology, engineering, and math disciplines, less rational and logical, less capable of learning at all, damaged in their natural feminine capacities by study, in some places still forbidden access to education. Submission and the appearance of compliance became primary coping strategies for those targeted by patriarchy; making oneself small, hiding one's desires and talents, agreeing with misogynist norms that one was not as smart, one's career and life desires should not be taken as seriously, one's attractiveness should be defined only by the man in the woman's life, whoever that man happened to be. (And here we are referring largely to natal women and men, although these patriarchal patterns of relating are sometimes also present when one of the people in question is trans, as assimilation into the coping strategies of the native-born citizens of the dangerous country of gender—for instance, wearing makeup and high-heeled shoes and frilly clothing if one is a trans woman—has often been used by the psychiatric and medical fields as the criteria for the willingness of gatekeepers to open the gate to desired gender-affirming medical care even if this is not the version of womanhood that this person sees when she looks in the mirror.)

The manner in which patriarchy became associated with normalcy, particularly in the precincts of gender, illustrates how social pathologies have taken the power to define normal. So too with people suffering from exposure to trauma, where some people's human responses are deemed wrong because those responses do not fit into the gender box in which this person is presumed to live. DHCR trauma healing practice requires holding tightly to the knowledge that while what we are seeing is pain, confusion, and struggle, this is all the human response, really a normal response, to experiences that undermine feelings of safety and/or disrupt connections with other humans. Trauma is a lot, and it's hard; and the fact is that all of this pain is horrifyingly normal, even banal, when it comes to trauma. The social pathologies, conversely are not normal at all, even though they are often a social or cultural norm.

SUBMITTING AND COMPLYING WITH PERFORMANCE DEMANDS: THE BURDEN PLACED ON TRAUMA SURVIVORS

In the daily world of rogue capitalism, in which most adults are expected to appear regularly at a workplace (or its online equivalent) where they will engage in behaviors that will enrich those who are already rich—called "alienated labor" by Karl Marx (1844, Section XXV)—trauma-exposed people find that they must often pass for normal, submit to or at least appear to comply with the rules of a workplace, so as to be productive members of capitalist societies. Not producing is a stigmatized position to which negative characteristics such as laziness (especially thrown at BIPOC people), bad attitude, or general unworthiness of the protections of society are frequently ascribed. Not only traumatized suffering people but many other people who are struggling with their brains and nervous systems, with how their mitochondria produce (or don't produce) energy, with the varieties of hidden ways that they are typically human that do not make them good producers are similarly stigmatized.

Often, then, these people do their best to submit to the rules of rogue capitalism. They perform their best compliance, "leaving it all at the office" being not a metaphor but a lived experience of having no capacity left after complying with the demands of work. They submit to humiliating attempts to get legally mandated accommodations from their employers, a process that many people have described as worse than just trying to do the job without the accommodation, being faced with questions and statements like, "Why do you really need this?" and "The letter from your health care provider doesn't go into enough detail"—an illegal request under the laws that have tried to cover up the depth of the social pathology of ableism. For trauma-affected suffering people who are experiencing distress in mind, body, spirit, and psyche, for whom some characteristics of a workplace might be retraumatizing or invitations to enter the bad movies called flashbacks, passing for normal by practicing submission and apparent compliance frequently come at a high price.

This particular coping strategy of the colonized requires that one wear a mask in one's dealing with most of the world, because to do otherwise means risking being pushed off the edge of the cliff of normal and terminated from a job due to being insufficiently productive. Being made unemployed, which for some people means risking the loss of a home, health care access, and the relationships and meaning arising from employment, adds a whole new layer of economic trauma to the trauma-exposed person's plate of shit.

IMPOSTER SYNDROME OR SOMEONE LIKE ME COULDN'T POSSIBLY BE DOING WHAT I'M DOING–AND IT'S NOT A SYNDROME, IT'S A PHENOMENON

The last item in the catalogue of social pathology best practices that I'm going to discuss here is a thing that was ironically first identified by two natal women, both feminist therapists working in the American South in the 1970s, a time when gendered narratives of work life and rules about how gender was to be enacted, particularly feminine gender, were in flux. They began to notice how frequently highly accomplished members of marginalized and subordinated groups, most often natal women like themselves, would come into therapy and describe themselves as feeling unable to do precisely the work they were doing, often very well. Clance and Imes (1978) named this "imposter phenomenon," the sense that one is an imposter, fooling everyone else by doing what one really cannot do.

Notice that they did not call it a pathology. These two feminist therapists simply named the experiences of women who were getting the message from their contexts that they were not wanted, that those women were personalizing that feedback as evidence of something wrong with themselves, a belief of which Clance and Imes (1978) did their best to disabuse the people they worked with through consciousness raising, through the message of "You are not the problem, sexism is the problem."

The narrative of imposter is that one is doing, often quite well, what one really should not be able to do by the rules of a social pathology. I remember reading this work (Clance & Imes, 1978) soon after it was published and thinking, "But who is that good of an actor, except maybe Meryl Streep?" and then asking suffering people who came into my office with similar narratives, "So, have you been nominated for an Oscar yet? Because anyone who's as good as you are at pretending to do something that you seem to be doing very well has got to be deserving of one of those gold statues."

My humorous response was also a serious one because it did not attempt to challenge the lived realities of these suffering people, all of whom were terrified that their imposter status would finally be discovered, with resultant punishment at some point. Rather, I was inviting them to see what I now know was their intellectual colonization: People of my genital/melanic/not typical body phenotype cannot, by the rules of a social pathology (typically misogyny and/or White supremacy and their various offshoots) do this thing. I am doing this thing. It is not the rule that is wrong. Therefore I must be faking it.

Today, the construct of imposter phenomenon, which has been pathologized into imposter syndrome, has become thoroughly appropriated and colonized by mainstream cultures as a way of saying, "If you're uncomfortable, you don't belong here," which distracts people from saying, "I'm not the problem. Your exclusionary norms are the problem." Of course, one experiences imposter syndrome, a pathology, or so goes the narrative because, of course, the rules about who really is capable of something—building a rocket, developing a computer language, performing surgery, operating weapons of war—have not changed. When a suffering person says, "I feel like an imposter," believe that this is how they have learned to describe what they are feeling about being where the structural inequalities of the culture say they should not—and then notice that you've just seen a tiny, nearly invisible shard of the deeply buried skeletons of social pathologies that are not really dead in this person but simply underground, working their toxins behind the shield of how culture points to exceptional members of marginalized and subordinated groups, their exceptional status evidence that the social pathology is right.

THE RACKET OF TRAUMA TREATMENT

Trauma healing has become, in less than half a century, a colonized territory where once there was wilderness. It was an island that begged to be attached to the mainland of our professions because we island dwellers thought it would help us to help the suffering people with whom we worked if we became a peninsula on the larger continent of psychotherapy.

This isn't what happened. Instead of a causeway over which we could travel to and from our island, the sea was drained, the declivity filled in, and we were merged. Inclusion led to being thoroughly taken over within the larger colonized intellectual territories of modern psychology and psychiatry. By "colonized intellectual territory" I mean that modern psychology and psychiatry, in their collective attempts to be more scientific than actual science, a modern version of "plus royaliste que le roi," have pushed aside any epistemic frameworks excepting logical positivist empiricism as a means of understanding what might help trauma-exposed humans.

Logical positivist empiricism was, but no longer is, a dominant epistemology in the hard sciences of, for example, physics; sciences among which psychology and other so-called behavioral sciences wish mightily to be included. This desire to be seen as a real science has led to the rebranding of university psychology departments as departments of psychological science or neuroscience— anything but psychology with its connotation of being soft. So this epistemology remains, sadly, the false god at whose altar most research into human suffering worships and offers sacrifices. Modern psychology in the United States, which in most versions of history has its roots in the work of the misogynist and White supremacist natal men G. Stanley Hall and William James in the late 19th and early 20th centuries, was a product of such social pathologies as systemic racism, misogyny, classism, heterosexism, White supremacy, and anti-Semitism, among others, all of which were accepted as truths in the work of these founders. As the decolonial theorists to whom I have referred in earlier chapters have noted, American psychology has become as hegemonic intellectually across the globe as have other aspects of our cultural imperialism. So the colonization of trauma healing by the intellectual rules of American psychology is doubly dangerous to the project of creating a DHCR trauma healing.

Fortunately, so far, psychology does not appear to have too many gatekeepers for our published scholarship of the sort occupying the role of Samuel Alito, the U.S. Supreme Court Associate Justice who, in June 2022, proclaimed that anything not referred to in a Constitution written by natal White male descendants of colonizers and enslavers of African people could not be considered a right today. Evolution in my own field gives me hope for the decolonial project.

But the obeisance to the old ways of knowing persists; it is the rare scholar in our field who asserts the value of other ways of knowing, the many methodologies of qualitative study. The logical positivists are still the bulk of the editors and reviewers of what gets published; scholarship is still colonized. Thus, the gatekeepers, not quite Alito, but similarly archaic in their ways of thinking about what constitutes real knowledge in psychology—peer-reviewed articles published in a journal with a high impact factor—are guarding the gates to those journals against anything that smacks of a departure from the logical positivist empiricist religion.

The social pathologies held as truth by the founders of psychology and related fields, and the biases they embedded in psychological science, dominated the academic centers of our disciplines until well past the middle of the 20th century. These biases are not yet entirely absent. By the mid 1960s, natal women, BIPOC people, and lesbians, gay men, and bisexual people were still extraordinarily rare in psychology, which was then primarily an academic rather than a clinical discipline. Elders among both natal women and BIPOC psychologists, some of whom had both intersectional identities (Denmark, 1995; Lott, 1995; Morris & Espin, 1995), describe the undisguised contempt and disdain with which they were treated when they dared to apply to psychology doctoral programs and the overt discrimination they encountered when attempting to find tenure-track academic positions (Chesler et al., 1995).

Of note, these stories come from people who eventually rose to positions of prominence within the field, narrative arcs not unlike those of Ruth Bader Ginsburg, their contemporary, within the legal discipline. These elders assimilated intellectually, and because they did so brilliantly and persistently, they ultimately could not be ignored, although each tells stories of how they had to perform submission and compliance. They often had to carefully, in writing, start their careers pledging allegiance to the false god of scientific objectivity in their work until they came to positions of such power and authority that they could make visible the influence of the knowledge derived from their lived experiences as members of marginalized and subordinated groups. I have encountered this myself as a lesbian psychologist writing about the experiences of lesbians and other women. I have been accused of bias more times than I can count in the half century since I began my graduate education because I skipped the step of appearing to comply and went straight (no pun intended) to the truth as I saw it, peppering my curriculum vitae with the words *lesbian* and *feminist* from the start.

One might argue that by the time trauma became assimilated into the doctoral disciplines these disciplines had changed and had thrown off the social pathologies of their origins. In order to accept that premise, which I believe to be an illusion with which progressives in our field have soothed ourselves for the last several decades worth of guidelines for working with each and every marginalized and subordinated group, it's of value to explore whether psychology and psychiatry have actually decolonized themselves or whether the formerly excluded, marginalized, and subordinated have simply been assimilated. As one who has been a part of this struggle for the last 5 decades, I sadly believe that assimilation and passing to gain acceptance, not revolution in which there has been a throughgoing deconstruction and reconstruction, is what we accomplished. I say "we," because I was complicit in that strategy, which I am now, with the wisdom of greater age, leaving behind. Let's review, because in order to generate a truly liberatory, decolonial, culturally responsive and humble stance to trauma healing, those of us who have wished to transform our fields must tell some hard truths about where we currently stand.

SO DID WE LIBERATE OURSELVES? TOWARD SOME CRITERIA FOR ANSWERING THAT QUESTION

As the 1960s waned, parallel to the uproar occurring in the larger social context, the wretched of the (psychology and psychiatry) earth began to rise up and write the truths about their lives and about the complicity of doctoral disciplines in colonization and marginalization via having lent their authority to oppression. Robert Guthrie (1976), an African American psychiatrist, turned his lens on the exclusion of Black lived experiences and the toxic effects of systemic racism that were prevalent within the discipline; his aptly titled classic, *Even the Rat Was White*, exposed the depth of racism in his own and related mental health disciplines. Naomi Weisstein (1968) and Phyllis Chesler (1972) shone critical spotlights on systemic misogyny's grip on women, and in 1971 Judith Bardwick published a volume on women's psychology that centered women rather than pathologizing them. Psychologists who identified as gay, lesbian, and bisexual (and not trans, because there were so few trans psychologists out in those early years, and they are still few in 2022), some at risk to their careers, began to make their sexual orientations known within their profession and to write affirmatively about the lives of a group that had been defined as a form of psychopathology until the early 1970s. The harms done by various therapies aimed at turning other-than-heterosexual people into something they were not were documented (Duberman, 2002; Feinberg, 2004; Haldeman, 2002)

The wretched of the earth—poor people, LGBT people, people living with other-than-typical bodies, women who refused to submit and comply—all invaded our respective professions—psychology, law, medicine, engineering, the astronaut corps, and so on. We set up organizations representing our principles of social change and rejection of social pathologies: the Association for Women in Psychology, the Association of Black Psychologists, the National Latinx Psychological Association, the Society of Indian Psychologists, the Association of LGBTQ+ Psychiatrists, the Mental Patients Liberation Front, Psychologists Against Anti-Semitism. We demanded changes in publications manuals. We spent years writing scholarly documents showing why oppressive psychotherapies were a bad idea and proposing models for affirmative treatments. We got ourselves into positions of leadership in our various organizations. We had the illusion of change.

> The master's tools will never dismantle the master's house. (Lorde, 1984a, pp. 110–114)

Burning Down the House: Liberatory and Decolonial Epistemologies

These liberation psychology authors–Fanon, Memmi, Martín-Baró—and all of us who have learned from them, these authors, as those they wrote and worked with, proposed to burn down the structures of a discipline that had become a handy tool of the oppressor. They proposed the plans with which to build, from the ground up and from new materials, a psychology and pedagogy that centered in the lived experiences of those who were the targets of colonization and its attendant social pathologies. I think that had Ignacio Martín-Baró not been murdered, and thus the most prominent voice of liberation psychology not cut down and silenced just as his work was gaining steam, the liberation psychology world might have appeared in our midst sooner and the decolonial project on which I am presently embarked would be well in the past. But he was murdered. His works became difficult for anyone who did not read Spanish to gain access to. The most radical voices were tamped down.

Liberation psychology's proposed courses of action represented a radical departure from various attempts made by well-socialized and colonized psychologists, myself included, who were members of marginalized and subordinated groups to adapt the psychology we already knew and were pushing against to become more inclusive. We saw ourselves as rebels because we were starting a process of speaking truth to power within our disciplines, even if we did so a tad politely and in the absence of an awareness that we were simply trying to become the professional versions of the court Jews of the 17th century. We were so thrilled to be invited into the master's house that we mostly failed to notice how we were being assimilated.

Our rebellion was, in consequence, conducted on the colonizer's terms, and we made no structural changes. We did research using the epistemologies of logical positivism and applied colonized definitions of identities as singular rather than intersectional, as strategies for getting our collective feet in the door. Most of us did not, at first, challenge epistemic systems, nor unpack unitary categories of identity, nor challenge ascriptions of pathology once we removed them from ourselves, although we asked rude questions about why certain classes of human were overrepresented in particular pathologized groups.

And we mostly pled allegiance to our disciplines. Only a brave few threw off the chains of legitimacy (Pope, 2016) and dared to expose the worst sins of psychology and psychiatry. A rebel is, after all, defined in relationship to those against whom they are rebelling, unlike a builder or creator, who is making something new. In this instance I use first-person pronouns because in my early career, and in my first attempts at addressing the topics adjacent to those of this book, I too was still caught in that pattern of trying to find a way to remodel my discipline by building out new rooms. I thought I could remodel the master's house, and I was still trying to be allowed to live in it.

No We Haven't, Not Yet

A liberatory DHCR model of trauma healing is the building of a new house. It begins with the premise that the work of healing wounded souls must orient itself within the lived experiences of those who are colonized, systemically oppressed, marginalized, and subordinated by social pathologies. This work must be decolonized of diagnostic categories or officially approved interventions. This new home I am trying to build for trauma healing must also avoid the error of acting as if only those targeted by colonization are harmed by its social pathologies but rather have a deep, complex, and subtle understanding of how social pathologies wound all but the sociopathic few.

As Albert Memmi (1965) noted very early in the development of a decolonial epistemology of healing, the experiences of the colonizer qua colonizer, of the person privileged by social pathologies and thus totally in the poisonous embrace of lies that have had to be thrust by force upon the colonized, needed to be studied. The lives of colonizers are not centered within a colonizing epistemology by DHCR practice. Rather, they are interrogated from the standpoint of the colonized, asking the question of how the colonizer's lives were differently deformed by colonization than those of the colonized, never accepting colonization or social pathology as a norm that does most people good.

The humor of colonized people might make a good starting point for this kind of research. What does it mean when someone says, "White men can't dance," or "Men are incapable of doing the dishes without being told how," or "Only the goyim drink and beat their wives"? While these sayings are full of error, they are observations about the dominant seen through the lens of the marginalized and subordinated and not always too far from truth.

Decolonial understandings of the traumagenic effects of social pathologies start at the nexus of this sort of observation that all is not well in the mansions of the dominant. A DHCR model of trauma healing is thus not only for those whose oppression we can see but also for those who, believing themselves shielded behind the walls of their colonizing forts, have been traumatized when their illusions of superiority and invulnerability have been shattered.

While Martín-Baró and his colleagues, working in Latin America, focused on the lived experiences of impoverished and colonized persons in that region, their attention to social pathologies as the sources of psychological distress went hand in hand with feminist (Brown, 1994; Kaschak, 1992; Lerman, 1996), Afrocentric, queer, and other critical psychological thinkers from American psychology who had begun to make the epistemic move in the 1990s from simply critiquing academic colonialism and the exclusion of the lived experiences of marginalized and subordinated humans to analysis of how emotional distress among these people had its roots in social pathologies (Fox & Prilleltensky, 1997; Sanchez-Hucles, 1998) and how the epistemic models of the field were themselves flawed by their foundational assumptions. Doing so for trauma itself seems like a natural next step.

AN EPISTEMOLOGY CENTERING THE EXPERIENCES OF SUFFERING HUMANS

Telling the Truth Can Heal

This starting premise of the liberation/decolonial model—a preferential option for the (distressed, colonized, marginalized, and subordinated of the earth) poor—which is a construct at the core of liberation theology and moved with its practitioners into liberation psychology and the various critical psychologies, profoundly informs my model of decolonizing trauma healing. This means that our work is centered in and informed by the voices of those who are marginalized and subordinated, although it is not solely for those at the margins. This centering of previously silenced or pathologized knowledge is not an exclusion of the experiences of those who live in the confusing world of both causing suffering and being caused to suffer. It is simply, and potently, a recentering of the narrative. Did Columbus discover America? Or did Columbus invade the Western Hemisphere, armed with the Christian European doctrine of discovery and . . . the truth becomes the center of the story, and the old story is exposed as a cover-up. This takes us to the decolonial healing methodologies of truth telling.

Truth telling in the healing room includes, but is not limited to, interrogating the ways in which a person or their affinity group and its heritage have been the targets of some form of colonization. It always entails the raising of consciousness about the nature of colonization and systemic oppression (Torres Rivera, 2020) and about the location of the problem in the social pathology, not in the suffering person. What G. Lerner (1994) referred to as the development of feminist consciousness is generalized in the decolonial trauma healing model to this consciousness-raising, and thus truth-affirming, exploration. "You are not the problem. You hold the power to be a solution." These are the core truths of decolonial, humble, culturally responsive trauma healing.

#ColonialMeToo

In my own meandering 4-decade path from trauma treatment to trauma healing, I moved from the colonized and assimilated approach that says, "Look, your suffering is in the *DSM*, it has a name, so it's real and you're not crazy," which I described earlier in this volume as a methodology for validating people's pain in a way that never questioned the notion that it was okay to call some other people crazy, to the edge of where I am now.

This was an epistemic location to which I came, toward the end of my career as a psychotherapist, where I finally learned to more effectively tell the suffering trauma survivors who entered my office that they were not the problem and that whatever name they wanted to call their problem, if they wanted to do that at all, was theirs to give, not mine.

I needed to conceptualize what was happening with them and within them for myself so that I was not too lost in the project of how to proceed as their healer, but I became more emphatic that my categories of analysis were not the right ones; they were simply my own starting hypotheses.

One of my own most frequent utterances was, "You know, I could be full of shit, so if I am, please let me know," said when I would offer up a tentative hypothesis about what I might be hearing (apparently so frequently uttered that one person I worked with would interrupt me after the word *full* and finish my sentence, then laugh at me, thereby decolonizing the entire power dynamic of what we were doing in one fell swoop). Thus, decolonizing trauma healing means witnessing and being willing to offer tentative hypotheses that we identify as ones that are tentative, are fluid, will change as we learn together what the layers of this person's pain might be—and that could be wrong, which we might not know for a while. When I think about the first person whose dissociative ego states I missed and misnamed, and who had the guts to write to me later to tell me precisely what I had missed, I wonder about everyone else whom I did not see clearly, hear fully, because of how colonized my own epistemics of suffering were.

What a decolonial mindset tells suffering people is that their distress cannot be defined by the authors of any powerful dominant-culture book, such as the *DSM*. As DHCR healers we need to convey to these courageous humans that the pain and shame they have been given to hold is not of their making, not evidence of their weakness. They are the canaries in the coal mines of social pathologies that have harmed them. While they have been defined as not normal because of their distress or because of the ways they have enacted that distress, their responses are quite normal because they are those of a traumatized human neurobiology of fear, stress, and attachment. This is the pain that points out the presence of systemic oppression and its depredations in their lives.

Those structural and systemic forms of oppression are pathological. Say it again. And again. Because this is a difficult message for anyone to believe, for any of us who have been raised in the vicinity of the authoritative voices of these social pathologies. Before I knew how to decolonize, but was still trying to be liberatory, I would offer this idea, only not nearly so clearly articulated. "Bear with me," I would say, "You know we therapists are crazy. Just try this idea out, that you are not the problem. Don't take what I'm saying as truth because I said so. But try this on for size."

What I did not realize until much later was that by offering truth telling to suffering people while not insisting that they accept that truth simply because it came from someone with a doctoral degree, I was engaging in a somewhat unintentional decolonial approach to trauma healing. I invite you, my readers, to consider some version of these opening lines in your own work if you are a trauma healer who would like to move toward a more decolonial stance. Begin the relationship by telling truth, unequivocally insisting to yourself and, if they will listen, to that the suffering person that they are not the problem. And while you might at some point offer one of the alphabet soup of things that trauma healers can offer that might reduce suffering, especially after running it through the sieve of Chapters 12 and 13 of whether it meets DHCR criteria, never forget that it is primarily, centrally, and most potently in the healing relationship between humans in which truths are told and truths are witnessed that the surcease of pain can occur.

CENTERING TRAUMA HEALING WORK IN THE DECOLONIAL PARADIGM

It would be impossible for me to write this book with integrity and continue to refer to "trauma treatment," or the "diagnosis" of the distressed emotions and behaviors that follow exposures to trauma. That will be hard to do, and I invite us again, together, to give up that language because to relapse into therapy speak would be to epistemologically reenter the colonized intellectual spaces in which I have spent most of my career, the spaces which I entered when, as an adolescent knowing she would become a clinical psychologist, I first read Sigmund Freud, Carl Rogers, and Fritz Perls. It's a powerful pull to resist. It's a good time to embrace being countercultural as a trauma healer.

Everything about this book is countercultural, so if you want to fit in or get tenure, don't cite me, please! Or do so should you choose, the informed consent to your risk offered herein: to speak truths about social pathologies, about embedded inequities of power, access, resources; to call into question that elusive thing we used to think of as safety before a little speck of protein invaded us—all of that narrative is countercultural.

6 EXPLORING INTERSECTIONAL IDENTITIES IN DHCR TRAUMA HEALING

Despite being an assimilationist stance, it remarkably remains somewhat countercultural to assert that all one needs to do to make trauma healing more accessible is to adapt interventions developed in colonized settings with colonized epistemologies to some stereotyped model of a particular marginalized and subordinated group. Such a strategy, the equivalent of dressing an intervention in an ethnic costume, although first seeing the published light of day in the middle 1990s (S. Sue et al., 2006), continues to hold sway right up through American Psychological Association's latest set of treatment guidelines (APA, 2019) for working with poor people. The adapt strategy assumes homogeneity of a given marginalized group in a way that entirely ignores the effects of intersectionality.

And what a diverse group that is, poor people with extremely varying intersectional identities. Some poor people are psychologists with quarter of a million dollars of student loan debt, a fact not addressed in those guidelines, struggling every month to meet the bills and living on ramen while passing for middle class because of their doctoral degrees. Some poor people are psychologists who have been trauma-exposed, experienced betrayal, become unable

https://doi.org/10.1037/0000421-007
Decolonizing Trauma Healing: Toward a Humble, Culturally Responsive Practice,
by L. S. Brown

to continue to pass for normal and thus expelled from their work, living on disability payments that do not cover rent, much less food. Poverty is different if you live on a farm rather than in a city, if you are an immigrant rather than a person whose family lost all of their money in Bernie Madoff's schemes, different if you have children than if you don't, if you're Black, Indigenous, or a person of color (BIPOC) rather than Euro-American, if you're trans or otherwise genderqueer. Poverty is different if you're neurodivergent and your measured cognitive skills are high but your support needs are even higher and you have to spend every penny you earn on getting those needs met. Adapt as you will, the question of how being on an economic margin interacts with the rest of one's intersectional identities will make it harder to see those other strands clearly at times, for both healer and sufferer. Add trauma to the mix, which is often a door opening onto the path to poverty, in this person's life or in the generations before them, and you can be fairly certain that your adaptation will result in high dropout rates because the inherent assumptions of what you are doing haven't been challenged to become humble or culturally responsive.

This strategy of adapting the thing you're already doing was what I used to call the "Handbook of Psychotherapy With Alien Species" approach, an add-and-stir method in which the clinician was exhorted to adapt standard ways of responding to suffering trauma survivors to the most foreground component of the sufferer's intersectional identity that could be observed when they came into the room. If a pinch of Indigenous healing practices was to be added to the mix for Indigenous people, so much the better; voilà, trauma treatment for diverse/special populations (Marsella et al., 1996).

Twenty-five plus years ago, this was not a bad start, as it was after all the first step in the direction toward much of what I am exploring here. It was a necessary step, one the resistance to which tells me much about its necessity in the longer arc of the decolonial project. That the add-and-stir methodology remains a common and prevalent perspective, and that there remains resistance in some quarters to any adaptation of approaches even in the face of evidence that simply doing that helps a little, troubles me and speaks loudly to how colonized the healing of the pain of trauma continues to be and how assimilated the voices from the margins have become.

I think that something missing completely from the add-and-stir approach is a discussion of how trauma is an experience of disempowerment that closely mirrors and is often perpetrated by a social pathology or a person who subscribes to and enacts its values. Rape—usually of a natal woman, sometimes a trans woman or trans man or a natal man adjudged feminine by the rapist—has been found, in research on trauma, to be among the worst, if not the ultimate, form of trauma when contrasted with, for example, a nonsexual assault. Adapting an intervention for a raped human whose only resemblance to the gold standard treatment is being a natal woman risks missing a lot.

The high-end badness of rape has to do with several factors. First, it is a violent and intrusive abuse of a person's right to bodily autonomy, which constitutes an ultimate form of disempowerment. Next, it is the purest expression of the twin social pathologies born of patriarchy, misogyny and toxic masculinity, enacted on the bodies of anyone with a vulva, be they natal women, trans women, trans men who have not had bottom surgery, or nonbinary people with a vulva, as well as on the bodies of natal men whose gender expression is defined as effeminate. Next, rape is a violation conveying information about where people should exist in patriarchy's hierarchies. Butch (masculine of center) lesbians, who are natal women, are raped so as to teach them a lesson about the error of their sexual orientation and gender expression. Men are raped by other men to assert the position of the rapist in the power and dominance hierarchy. Natal women whose mode of dress is deemed too provocative are raped to teach the lesson that a woman must only dress in ways that no man would be provoked by. The death, in September 2022, of Mahsa Amini, a woman arrested and tortured to death in Iran for the crime of having a lock of hair stray out from under her headscarf, demonstrates the ultimate point of the messaging of rape.

POWER AND DISEMPOWERMENT: THE EXAMPLE OF RAPE

The fact that sexual assault appears to be the ne plus ultra of trauma is due not only to the violation of a person's body. Being badly beaten by a stranger is a violation of a person's body. Being nearly crushed to death in a car accident is a violation of a person's body. These are terrifying experiences, physically and emotionally painful, potentially threatening to life, and they cause distress.

These painful traumas do not, however, communicate rape's message of social pathology. Rape says that the raped person, not the rapist, should feel shame for having somehow violated explicit or implicit norms of the social pathologies of patriarchy's offspring, systemic misogyny, and/or homophobia or trans hatred. The last two are subsets of systemic misogyny; natal men who are raped as adults are more likely to be gay men or trans women, defined by their rapist as having become included in the category of woman and thus appropriate targets for behavior that is usually directed at natal women. All rape is an expression of toxic masculinity. A rapist may be cheered on by other men watching; images of extremely violent rapes, including those leading to the death of the raped person, have become pervasive in online pornography. No shame in being a rapist; huge shame in being raped, because if you were raped, you broke the rules of social pathology.

The disempowerment of being raped is thus not simply the disempowerment of one person's body at the time of the violation. It is a reminder to that person that they are systemically disempowered by the social pathology of misogyny. It is often meant as a cautionary tale to others about adherence to patriarchy's rules. The rules of these social pathologies subjugate all women—natal, nonbinary, or trans—and all femme of center natal men with the threat of being raped. A person can be raped because of having a vulva (which is true for many trans men as well) and also because of being or being perceived to be a feminine person with a penis who is violating the toxic masculinity subcomponent of systemic misogyny. The crime of not having a penis or not living in a gender orientation that is considered right for someone with a penis is punished by rape.

Rape can be used to assert authority when someone is in a subordinate position in a hierarchy of power and authority, such as in a military or quasi-military setting, in which rape and its close cousin, repeated sexual harassment, is a strategy for putting people in their place. Rape is the reminder that women, both natal and trans, and nonbinary people do not have the power to decide who touches their bodies, when, and how, that no does not mean no. The shadow of possible rape is what whispers in the ears of many female-bodied persons of any gender orientation and causes them to walk into a parking garage with car keys pushed through fists, the sharp edges poised to act as a weapon against the possibility of an attack that they know might come, even if it hasn't yet. I turned 71 as I was finishing this section of the book, and while parking garages are less common in my life now than they once were, I still return to my car and enter it with that knife-edge of keys sticking out to be used if needed.

The phrase "the spoils of war" has always meant not just the gold and silver of the conquered but the freedom to rape their women (Brownmiller, 1975). Lose a war, lose possession of the vulvas of your women. If your village, your culture, your country is on the losing side and you have a vulva, you are very likely to be raped, whether you were in Rwanda during the genocide, or in Berlin in 1945 after the Soviets came in at the end of the Second World War, or an Indigenous woman in the wake of U.S. settler colonialism, or an African woman captured and enslaved and shipped to Virginia in 1630.

What a Trauma Represents to You and Your Culture Matters

The infliction of particular kinds of trauma as a colonizing methodology for keeping people in the positions assigned to them by social pathologies consequently contains an extra layer of disempowerment, the toxic brew of two kinds of power grabs living in the psyche of the trauma-exposed and suffering person. Decolonial, humble, culturally responsive (DHCR) trauma healing must always take those additional layers of meaning into account.

There are layers of disempowerment that need to be interrogated, some of which might not even be visible yet to the person who walks in the room in tatters from the official trauma. In a DHCR methodology of trauma healing, we must integrate an exploration of the questions of what this particular experience represents to the person with this unique set of intersectional identities into our paradigms for healing. This is where cultural responsiveness takes the lead.

So we ask ourselves and, when it is the right time, the suffering people with whom we are working the questions responsive to culture—How has this person, with their family, their culture, with all the pieces of their intersectional identities, been and/or continue to be assigned to a lower-status, lower-power position in the social order, an assignment in any way reinforced by the official trauma? How has this person experienced a particular trauma or set of trauma exposures that were further disempowering because of the meanings those traumas had to that person? Healing the official trauma, be it combat or a car accident, or even a sexual assault, is the usual focus of the trauma treatment literature. As I've said, not a bad focus, just a deeply incomplete scope for our work.

This is because in the absence of addressing the interplay between the persistent, systemic forms of social pathology traumas of the nonofficial variety to which the suffering person is exposed on the other side of the door of our office, in failures to understand and listen for cultural and contextual meanings, a trauma healer will place a thin bandage each session on the surface of a wound that is deep and festering. That covering that will then be ripped off on the other side of our door or even used by a predator as a sign that here stands prey. The therapist then wonders why, despite using an evidence-based intervention, the person isn't getting better. What happens outside the door, what happens the rest of the week, counts. That's being culturally responsive: not knowing how to behave with a person with *x* intersectional identities but knowing what that means for how and who they are, both for the wounds with which they walk in our doors and the wounds inflicted when they leave—or even, by us.

FOR EXAMPLE: POWER DYNAMICS OF TRAUMA ON MULTIPLE DIMENSIONS

In the middle of the first round of writing this chapter, I reviewed the transcript of a deposition I gave in a sexual harassment case in which I was the forensic expert for the plaintiff. Aliyah was a heterosexual natal woman[1] from a Middle

---

[1]Case material has been disguised to protect client confidentiality.

Eastern country who came to the United States a decade before I met her with a significant history of all kinds of trauma. These included war—in which she had lost friends and during which, between the ages of 4 and 16, she was exposed to nearly nightly shelling—a highly disruptive natural disaster, violent rape by a stranger, and intimate partner violence. In addition to these Criterion A traumas, the culture in which she grew up was a fiercely and overtly misogynist one in which all natal women were at constant risk of being harassed for not covering their bodies sufficiently and could be thrown in prison for the crime of having their hair show. In the culture in which she grew up, the social pathology of systemic misogyny was accepted and overt, not problematized or made more subtle as it has been in the colonizing Global North.

She told me that she had always believed that the United States was a place where, as a woman, she would be safer and freer. But soon after she arrived here, after more than a decade of applying for admission to the United States, she entered a setting where, for many years, she was the target of sexualized behavior perpetrated by Andrew, a natal male, Euro-American, heterosexual, U.S.-born, native-English-speaking person who had a position that was many links up the food chain from her in the institution's own hierarchy.

The institution had known of Andrew's proclivities for at least a decade before Aliyah came to the school. She was not the first, or second, or tenth woman to have complaints about his sexualized behavior with women in subordinate positions. A reprimand had been placed in his file several years before she came on the scene, but he experienced no other consequences of his actions. The institution sent him on his way to continue his behavior, unmonitored.

He thus continued his career of sexual harassment, almost entirely with immigrant young women of color like Aliyah whose activities in the institution brought them into unavoidable contact with him because of his role. He was able to enact expressions of multiple social pathologies—racism, xenophobia, misogyny, all rolled into one. Aliyah complained about Andrew to many different people in positions of authority, following the institution's rules about what to do. She spent several hours in tears with a staff member whose job it was to intervene on behalf of people with sexual harassment complaints. That person listened to Aliyah and did nothing more.

In my deposition, I spoke of his actions that had been so distressing to the woman I evaluated; many of them were what some people might be consider paper cuts, not knife wounds. He didn't penetratively rape her. Rather, he put her in fear of that happening at some point as the audacity of his violations escalated unchecked. He performed toxic masculinity and systemic misogyny repeatedly, rubbing his erection against her more than once, which factually meets our state's definition of sexual assault but was considered to be not a big deal because no "real rape" occurred (Estrich, 1988), that is, no penetration.

A paper cut. He exposed his clothed erection straining through his pants to her more than once, sitting across from her with his legs spread wide. Another paper cut. He followed her into a physical location into which she had been told he could no longer go and where she had believed herself to be safe, leaving her feeling trapped when she fled. Another paper cut. Nothing happened.

Because there was no "real rape" (Estrich, 1988), the other side had asserted in its pleadings that Andrew's actions, and the school's inactions, were nugatory given her prior history of Criterion A trauma. I disagreed and in my deposition had spoken at length about the power differential between the two of them as an important factor in the degree of trauma she experienced. I also addressed the emotional reality that what Andrew had done represented something that was bigger than the uninformed eye might see, the "putting her in her place" component of sexual harassment.

The power differential between Aliyah and Andrew was the size of a gaping crevasse. Her intersectional identities and his overlapped only at the point of being natal members of their respective sexes whose gender expressions fit within expectations for members of those natal sexes. Andrew identified as heterosexual and Aliyah was perceived as such, although she was asexual, a posttrauma sexuality that she expressed no interest in modifying. Otherwise, in every way that mattered, both individual and systemic, he had more power than she did. He knew that he could act with impunity, given the very minor corrective action that had been taken the first time someone had been persistent in their complaints about him. As with colonizers who have felt that they could commit atrocities on the colonized with impunity (see Hochschild [1998] for a harrowing account of how the Belgian colonizers of the Congo region of Africa lopped off the hands of Indigenous African people or Northrup [1853] for a description of similar acts of torture committed on Black bodies by slavers in the United States, for examples of this), Andrew understood himself to be sufficiently powerfully positioned in the institution's social hierarchy to be protected from any meaningful consequences of his actions and thus would implicitly be enabled to continue his reign of terror. He was correct in those assumptions, just as the slaveholders, including several counted among the earliest presidents of the United States, who imprisoned, raped, and tortured their African captives knew that they would have no consequences for their actions (Hannah-Jones, 2021).

That perceived impunity in the context of an institution willing to look the other way and willing to marginalize women like Aliyah who complained had another consequence that was a trauma of social pathologies at work. The passive, enabling stance of the institution gave Andrew's actions a kind of force as a message about the position of women, and in particular BIPOC and immigrant women, in this institution. They were designated fair game, and Andrew knew it because when he preyed on them, he got to stay, got promotions and raises, and the women would eventually leave.

These subtexts of social pathologies made Andrew's behavior more frightening and distressing to Aliyah because she could sense them, even though she could not articulate them to me. Power differentials and their effects on a person's well-being can be systemic; the shards of their venom can also be found embedded deeply within a person's intersectional identities. The persistence of systemic hierarchies of power and dominance, which infiltrate everyone's sense of who they are and what they may do in the world, can allow someone to accrue power and privilege from the social pathologies that operate for their benefit without ever having to ask.

While these power differentials are socially constructed (e.g., in Saudi Arabia and Iran power accrues to adherents of Islam, while in most parts of Europe, the United States, and Canada it is given to those identified as being adherents or descended from adherents of some Christian faith) and vary from place to place and from time to time, they have the force and feel of being something real and palpable. Persons who have once been colonized (e.g., Irish people colonized by the British) are assimilated into and given membership in a group that is privileged by a social pathology, such as (in the case of Irish people in America) Whiteness. They can then be recruited to join forces with and attempt to become among the oppressors.

ASSIMILATION AS TRAUMA, NOT JUST A COPING MECHANISM

Colonized people are vulnerable to pulls to assimilate, as described in Chapter 5. Colonizing dynamics use the assimilated to inflict further pain on another group for whom assimilation has been made impossible. The trauma of the assimilated colonized then is used to shame them for their "bad" behavior of harming other more vulnerable people at the behest of, and in the attempt to please, the colonizer. The weapon is demonized, the invisible hand holding the weapon colludes in the demonization. To assimilate as a price of inclusion within the group privileged by a social pathology carries a heavy price that trauma healers must learn to detect hiding behind masks of assimilation.

Irish Americans in Boston in the 20th century violently attempted to stop African American children from integrating schools in their neighborhoods. Those Irish Americans had been given White privilege in the century following their flight from their homeland, and the conflict over busing exemplified this strategy of allowing people into the club of one's social pathology to serve as weapons. Irish people were decidedly not defined as White when they first arrived. They were allowed into the club so that the "real" White people of

Boston, those whose families were of English descent and were descended from the first colonizers, could hold their noses and distance themselves from the overt expressions of a racist social pathology that the upper-class White people could disclaim and criticize. This chance for a sort of apparent path out of marginalization (you can join our group now if you take our enemies as yours) is frequently dangled in front of persons for whom some component of their intersectional identity—for example, lower economic class status—renders them lesser members of the colonizing group.

"Poor White trash" and "hillbilly" are stigmatizing terms bestowed by educated, upper- and upper-middle-class White people. Poor White people who have gotten the education to become professionals are plagued by constant fears of being exposed for who they really are (J. Henning, personal communication, various dates). And these same impoverished White people's membership in the category of Whiteness can be weaponized by those higher in the social hierarchy in order to punish BIPOC people who are educated, are "uppity," or "do not know their place," creating distance between the powerful and assigning the blame for what happens next to "those ignorant poor folk." This is how lynching became a spectator sport; weaponize poor White people against educated African Americans and then stand back and moralize over the bad behavior of the unwashed.

This dynamic of being allowed to enter the club of the powerful so long as one is willing to be its violent face functions so as to maintain the fiction that equality might be possible so long as one manifests one characteristic defined as valuable by a social pathology. It exploits the trauma living in the bodies and psyches of the formerly marginalized and subordinated to activate them into a fear response and makes them vulnerable to the lies of systemic hierarchies of oppression. Cui bono? Only those at the top of the food chain, none of whom have their picture in the news looking like bad people for spitting on little African American kids trying to go to school.

Because, as noted repeatedly as we explore decolonizing our narratives, the variables in a person's intersectional identities that are markers of power are typically defined by those at the top of the food chain of power as immutable, natural, or essential to the facet of a person's humanity that is included or marginalized and subordinated, the sheer social and emotional energies exerted by power differentials on humans' neurobiology constitute a colonizing force in people's psyches, long after the actual army with the more technologically advanced weapons has retreated from the field. This can be particularly true when a signifier of value that is central to a culture is disregarded or actively devalued by colonization: the woman healer in an enslaved community who knows how to find the roots that are similar enough to those back home, scoffed at as a witch by colonial narratives; the rebbe whose deep learning of

Jewish texts in yeshiva counts for nothing in a secular world that only sees that he has no degree from a real institution of higher learning—these are forms of traumatization arising from colonization of intersectionalities, taking that which was sacred and turning it into trash. This is also why the changing narratives of who is included and who is not are especially insidious, as they hold out the false promise that sufficient acts of assimilation will lead to inclusion, as differentiated from mere tolerance and a brief respite from being harmed.

Privilege as a Tool of Social Pathologies

Feminist psychology (Brown, 2018) and liberation psychology (Comas-Díaz & Jacobsen, 2024; Comas-Díaz & Torres-Rivera, 2020; Montero et al., 2017; Torres Rivera, 2020), as well as theorists of what Fors (2018) calls the "grammar of power," have commented extensively on the necessity of identifying, attending to, and naming the power dynamics that occur in interpersonal and sociopolitical realms as well as in the healing relationship. These commentators have centered much of this analysis on the manifestations of these power dynamics as they affect the healing relationship itself. Because healers and psychotherapists perceive of ourselves as people of good will, it is common for us, when we have not fully integrated a decolonial healing model, to allow unexamined effects of power differentials to subtly undermine the liberatory intent of a healing connection. One important component of noticing how power functions in subtle and problematic ways in the interpersonal field is the phenomenon of social privilege. Trauma can be missed or minimized when the suffering person's intersectional identities proclaim them to have a full basket of privilege. Resilience and capacity can, conversely, be overlooked or de-emphasized when a suffering person's intersectional identities are primarily marginalized and subordinated ones and their privilege supply seems low.

Privilege is the package of social resources that are handed out along with membership in those groups valued by social pathologies. Each intersectional variable to which privilege is accorded also comes with structural forms of social power attached, which is one manifestation of privilege. This collection of resources accrues automatically to the colonizers themselves through the rules of their social pathologies and may be given, conditionally, to the assimilated among the colonized or to others temporarily assigned a status to which privilege accrues.

An excellent example of the latter was Hiram Revels, the first African American U.S. senator, appointed during Reconstruction. His being seated in the Senate was opposed for two weeks by senators representing states in which enslavement of other human beings had been legal before the Civil War. These former slaveholders, traitors to their country, fought against

Revels being seated because of the privileges that would accrue to him as a U.S. senator, the privilege of being treated as the equal of those Euro-American men. He had those privileges only for his brief time as a U.S. senator, at which point his social position was once again defined by White supremacy back into that of any person of African descent in the Jim Crow era.

A decolonial framework invites trauma healers to not simply believe that a person's intersectional identities are a case of "what you see is what you get" and that therefore you can know what kinds of privilege, or absence thereof, a suffering person might have had. Rather, a DHCR trauma healer needs to bring a more finely tuned eye and ear. The healer acquires a deeper understanding and analysis of the layers of colonization and those costs that may be invisible even to the suffering trauma survivor when they have been living with the package of privilege. This subtle and thorough exploration of privilege as it emerges within intersectionalities will expand healing options, perhaps exponentially. This is a topic I will discuss at length in later chapters, with special attention to integration of the topic of the application of analysis of intersectionalities to the concrete work of trauma healing.

If I return to an article I wrote about my trauma healing work with a real client who gave me permission to write about her story and who chose the name of Ruth for herself (Brown, 1986), I can see what I missed by not having a decolonial, liberatory framework to deepen my feminist, not yet entirely intersectional, paradigm for trauma healing. I did not, for example, thoroughly explore what it meant for her to be Irish American nor to be a natal woman educated in Catholic schools through college, schools that were quite traditional in their constructions of gender. I did not explore her family history in light of those two previously marginalized and subordinated identities as, at the time we worked together, we assumed her Whiteness as equivalent to the Whiteness of people whose ancestors had colonized her own.

I did not know to ask whether, as a descendant of a colonized people, anything had been stirred for her by serving in the military as a nurse in this country's colonial war in Vietnam. What I do know is that, years after our work together finished, she participated in a solidarity seminar of poet-veterans of the war, both American and Vietnamese. Perhaps in that decision on her part was a hint of what we might have uncovered had I reread my Fanon (1967) while we worked together or had I understood then, as I did not until much later, that the Irish were colonized people too. I knew to explore her social class as a factor in how she had ended up in the military; the navy had paid for the private college she could not have otherwise afforded in exchange for her working for the navy as a nurse wherever it sent her.

I did not know yet to consider how her Irish heritage was a facet of her family's social class experience. We mainly looked at her cultural heritage in terms of possible inherited risk for alcohol abuse. I did not explore how the social pathology that denigrated Irish people as drunks might have added shame to the fact of her developing a destructive relationship with alcohol in her attempts to manage the pain that emerged from exposure to the deaths of many young men in her care or the sexual coercion she was subjected to by a man higher in the military hierarchy than she was. We were both seduced by her apparent White-skin privilege not to dig more deeply into the layers of intersectional identity that we knew about and whose contributions to her suffering we were not equipped to analyze or understand.

HOW POWER IS MAINTAINED BY SOCIAL PATHOLOGIES: DANGLING THE PROMISE OF PRIVILEGE

I offered this quote up earlier, and I do here again because it is relevant and important. Lyndon Johnson, a natal Euro-American heterosexual man who grew up in extreme poverty and who accidentally became, for a few years, the most powerful person on the planet, once famously said to his former press secretary, Bill Moyers, "If you can convince the lowest white man he's better than the best colored man, he won't notice you're picking his pocket. Hell, give him somebody to look down on, and he'll empty his pockets for you" (Moyers, 1988). Yes, give someone the seductive promise of privilege and most of us won't think twice about the price we're paying for the possible fulfillment of that promise.

Johnson, who understood the social pathologies of classism and White supremacy from painful lived experience in ways almost no U.S. president since the middle of the 20th century has been able to, and who consequently comprehended the ways in which people whose other intersectional identities place them at the fringes of a dominant group can be manipulated with the promise of privilege, thus summed up how White supremacy dangles White skin privilege as bait in front of, as he put it, "the lowest white man." Moyers (1988) correctly identified Johnson's prescient belief about what has emerged in the United States, at a time when the package of privilege emerging from simply being White is still being dangled in front of people like Johnson's own family but the possibility of achieving the associated privileges has been undermined through the depredations of rogue capitalism: "He [LBJ] thought the opposite of integration was not just segregation but disintegration— a nation unraveling," the phenomenon that has been increasingly visible. The trauma here is one of betrayal: If you are White, you will have privilege. Oops, we White people who are also rich don't want you to have privilege. We will distract you from what we are doing by asserting that your loss of privilege is due to greater equity for previously even more marginalized and subordinated people than you, so that you can go blame them for your troubles—and thus we remain in power.

The extreme pain for the survivors of a hate crime murder, of a lynching or an extrajudicial murder by law enforcement, is not only the grief and pain of those left behind by any violent death but also the pain of disempowerment, the pain that this death was a reminder to community members to stay in their place. It is the closest type of trauma there is to rape. It is information about the absence of privilege. It is information about a persistent social pathology and its willingness to commit damage, up to fatal damage, on the bodies of people who were once defined by White supremacy as only three-fifths of a human being or not even human at all.

These murders are a command—to anyone who has other-than-European ancestry apparent in their phenotypic presentation; to anyone who, because of how their brain works, does not know how to respond to a command to lie down and put one's hands on one's head; to anyone who cannot hear that command—to never, ever assume that one has the power or the right to walk or drive or jog freely or even sleep in one's own home freely with the assumption of safety so long as one is violating no rule on the books. These extrajudicial murders of BIPOC people, of people in confused emotional states, and of Deaf people are, like rape, a message that bodily autonomy is not only not guaranteed but rather guaranteed to be violated in the name of social pathologies. They say, "You do not have the privilege to live without fear." This knowledge and this attention to the cultural meanings of these traumas is the culturally responsive piece of DHCR.

As I will discuss later in this volume, particularly in the two chapters about a woman I am calling Marisol (see Chapter 9 for Marisol's story), the entire construct of safety, while central to trauma healing, is also extremely problematic; the illusion that one is safe is part of the nicely wrapped box of privilege offered even to those members of the dominant group who are lesser in status in some way. These folks whose noses are just inside the tent of the dominant, LBJ's "lowest white man," are given the message that they are better and more deserving of safety than any human whose intersectional identities are defined as marginal and lesser than by social pathologies. Sometimes this message is, "You are safe from consequences if you break the law," a belief that we now know was held by many of the mostly working-class, mostly White, mostly natal men who stormed the U.S. Capitol, a belief that they were operating with the same impunity that their upper-class leader had clearly functioned under, with regard to any and all laws, until that time. We know this because many of them, at their trials, asserted the defense that they were doing what they ought to do as White people, defending their country, that is, the country that the doctrine of discovery gave to White Christian Europeans.

When this mirage of inclusion in privilege is swept away, the loss of that illusion, which is a betrayal, can be traumatic. It has also, through recorded history, been a root from which the forests of social pathologies have grown. Instead of looking to those who have lied to and betrayed them, some of those betrayed externalize the problem to the other, which was clearly the case for many of the January 6 defendants. This kind of blame projected onto marginalized and subordinated groups who are not keeping to their place then frequently metastasizes into a new social pathology authorizing the oppression of the marginalized and subordinated. The pain of betrayal is externalized into blame.

Larry was a natal Euro-American Christian man, heterosexual, a blue-collar work in a relatively well-paid union job, in his early 40s and still relatively able-bodied. He was in a contentious divorce and custody battle. His narrative was: "That bitch went to college and got ideas and when I tried to knock some sense into her she went running to that n-word SOB she works with in her fancy new job. I am not letting my kids be raised by an n-word who thinks he's so good because he's got a master's degree. Fuck her."

The story in the legal documents: Larry, who had never previously been violent, had begun to physically abuse his wife shortly after she received her bachelor's degree and gotten a white-collar job that paid about twice what Larry made. She left when he broke her arm, got a domestic violence restraining order, and filed for divorce. About 6 months after the separation, she had become involved with a coworker who was a dark-skinned South Asian Indian. The custody evaluator had requested something unique to Washington State, a nonparenting mental health evaluation for Larry, in order to arrive at a final set of recommendations about custody.

Larry's violence was not excusable, and he was sort of able to admit to that when talking with me. "But I couldn't help myself, Dr. Brown," he said, face scrunched up hard because he was clearly not going to cry in front of me. "She had it good. I was a good breadwinner. I even babysat the kids when she had an evening class. But then it felt like, I don't know, she thought she was better than me. And it felt like shit to have her make so much money when all she ever had to do was sit on her ass and go to school and then get a job where she sits on her ass. I know, I know, I shouldn't have hit her, but I just got so frustrated . . ." his voice trailed off.

Much of Larry's misery was self-inflicted by his use of violence; his ex-wife had reported that while things had become stressful in the marriage after she started her new job, she had no plans to leave until the violence began. But the roots of his violence were in the complex web of privilege that he thought he had as a White natal man, and the privilege he didn't know he didn't have until he didn't have it, that is, social class privilege, which he could only vaguely comprehend in terms of his ex-wife's new educational and financial status. His racist verbiage about her new partner had its roots in the exposure of his loss of privilege; the new partner was more highly educated, which violated Larry's nonconscious rules about who should have power and status—and access to a sexual relationship with a Euro-American woman.

Larry had grown up very poor; both parents overused alcohol, and neither were able to maintain employment for long. His maternal uncle was, conversely, a college graduate, an engineer at the company where Larry hired on as a mechanic, and Larry's cousins had had the benefits of a middle-class life. His parents had disdained the uncle and his family for thinking they were better than they were, thus hammering home to Larry a common coping strategy for the wounds of classism—the projection of shame and devaluation. As Larry became adolescent he experienced shame when around his cousins, who had the Air Jordans which he craved and which his parents could not afford, and rage at his parents for their inability to give him this life just out of reach. Having a good-enough blue-collar job that had allowed him to support his family comfortably, as well as having as little to do with his parents as possible once he was old enough to leave home, had put a thin veneer over the trauma of poverty. His wife's new degree and new job threw him into a trauma reenactment of his childhood, with her standing in for his uncle and cousins in that dynamic of the wounds of class.

In my evaluation of Larry, I discussed these issues of intersectional identities and loss of the illusion of privilege associated with Whiteness, which I saw at the roots of his abusive behavior. I noted that while I thought he might feel empowered by having some emotion regulation skills beyond those he had previously utilized, such as working overtime, which led to more money and gave him a sense of pride, he would likely remain at some risk of becoming violent again if he was not also offered, either in a didactic or healing setting, some information that would give him more understanding of what it was about his ex-wife's education and her subsequent position that had broken open classism and racism-related trauma for him. It didn't much matter if Larry's paycheck was swollen by overtime work when there was no one to come home to. He also, I recommended, needed space to be able to grieve this loss that internalized social pathologies had been a component of his creating for himself. Finally, I suggested to the evaluator that Larry participate in a series of rupture repair meetings with his ex-wife and their two tween children: "Losing access to his daughters has cemented his view of himself as a loser, which then fuels his rage at his ex-wife. Those young women want nothing to do with him because he was violent, and they feel afraid of him. Getting assistance, not for family reconciliation but for genuine rupture repair capacities, will assist him to metabolize both the trauma that he created for himself and his family and the trauma of the loss of his beliefs about a just world and his place in it."

As is always the case when I prepare this kind of report, I went over it with Larry before handing it in to the custody evaluator. He finally cried because, as he said, he'd never been able to put into words "why I had such a stupid response to her getting her degree. I mean, I wanted her to get that degree, I went to her graduation, I was so proud of her. And I turned that to shit in about a second. I think what you wrote here makes sense of it all to me. Shit, I never even thought about. I screwed up big-time, didn't I? Maybe I should have punched out [he named the CEO of his company, at which point I had to do an on-the-spot risk of violence assessment, to which he responded, "No, I mean, the guy is in Chicago, I'm not going to waste any money flying there to do that"] instead of Lucy. Because she never deserved that. Kinsey and Alicia never deserved a father who did this." I included his response to the report in my final version because it demonstrated, more clearly than anything I could say, where the roots of his self-destructive behavior lay.

RESPONSIVENESS RATHER THAN "COMPETENCE" AND THE DEEPENING OF CAPACITIES

As we move deeper into our exploration of decolonial trauma healing, bringing with us our understanding of the layers of trauma, we can become overwhelmed. Stay with that feeling. Allow yourself to sit, as a healer, in that place of understanding that what our work does for us is that it transforms us, makes us more humble and thus less seduced by the false certainties of evidence-based treatments and formal diagnoses.

What does this mean? That no one can become competent as a DHCR trauma healer, although one can, as noted earlier, master a particular healing strategy. To proclaim competence, as I once foolishly did, is to expose one's assimilation into the dominant narratives of the mental health profession. To move away from competence as a criterion for doing the best possible work of which one is capable is not to invite nihilism, but to offer a vision of moving humbly and progressively to deepening levels of capacities as culturally responsive trauma healers. I used to think that one could get to cultural competence in working with trauma survivors (Brown, 2007), a notion of which this book demonstrates my having disabused myself.

What do I mean by deepening our capacities? Let's begin by asking which capacities. Today there is an entire alphabet soup of interventions that one can offer to suffering trauma survivors. As I will discuss at length in Chapter 12, many of these ways of approaching trauma healing can be empowering, reducing suffering, and increasing joy and aliveness for suffering trauma survivors. They can meet the criteria for being part of a DHCR trauma healing relationship. These are not, however, the capacities of which I speak here.

Holding Space

The first, and most necessary, capacity is that of holding the emotional space for whatever a suffering person brings into our rooms, including material that is difficult for us to witness. This is not meant to imply that a trauma healer is an endlessly deep vessel, containing all pain for another person while somehow remaining impervious to the ways in which that pain soaks into their own psychic pores.

Instead, holding the space requires a radically honest, compassionate, and continuing exploration of our own intersectional identities, of how we bring the colonizer and the colonized both into the room. We have to be able to regulate our own neurobiology as it becomes activated by what we witness or by some aspect of a suffering person's intersectional identities. Holding space means that we become skillful in self-regulation, in being fully alive in the ventral vagal state that promotes connection, so that we can offer wordless biological coregulation, the most basic form of human trauma healing, to the suffering people who are with us in our work. As I wrote in *Cultural Competence in Trauma Therapy*,

> if your ancestors came from Europe or Asia to North America, you are most likely a descendant of immigrants or refugees who arrived here to the chilly welcome that has greeted everyone from the Irish of the 1800s to the Eastern European Jews of the early 1900s to today's South Asian computer engineers and undocumented Guatemalans. Some came as indentured servants, sold into labor. If your family came from South and Central America, your ancestors may have crawled under the barbed wire fence at the border. Some of your ancestors came in steerage, others flew first class on a 747—but all experienced the loss of culture and language that is trauma for some. (Brown, 2008, p. 217)

We are also perpetrators. Some of us are the descendants of slaveholders, of soldiers who shot women and children in this country's genocidal wars against its Indigenous people, of those who imprisoned or tortured others in the countries from which they came. Our ancestors suffered what Shay (1994) calls the moral injury of being trauma perpetrators, and in many cases that was traumatic to them and to the family cultures that they created and of which we are the inheritors. Some of our families served in the governments of Batista's Cuba, Stalin's USSR, Hitler's Germany, South Africa under apartheid. Some of our ancestors have been beaten; some of our ancestors administered those beatings. For some of us, our ancestors include both: many African Americans carry the genes of a slaveholder great-great-grandfather who raped their enslaved great-great-grandmother. And each of us, from our positions of dominance and privilege, can perpetrate oppression on others every day in our current lives without knowing or thinking of it (Vasquez, 2007). Perpetrator and victim consciousness live within our cultures, our families, our psychological realities. They are a component of our constructions of identity.

Substitute colonizer and colonized for perpetrator and victim and consider that a DHCR capacity for holding space is not simply the ability to have empathy for the pain of a suffering trauma survivor. It also means being able to identify our complicity, whether direct or indirect, with a self-compassionate and self-regulating gaze, one that does not shame us for benefiting from a privilege we did not seek, but a gaze that also does not excuse us from being responsible to and for those who are marginalized and subordinated by the privileges that have accrued to us. This is hard work to do. It requires us to have people who hold us up as well.

We hold the space because the conversations about trauma are often shoved into corners or, more recently, required to come with trigger warnings, as if somehow daily life is not a reminder of trauma for some. One of the things packed into the box of privilege is often a kind of fragility (DiAngelo, 2018) that leads people to shy so far away from any knowledge of the truths of the world that to even mention them has come to be perceived as a form of social wrongdoing. A trauma healer expands the space available for the suffering person's healing story, strengthens that space, and holds it even when the winds of our own pain begin to blow against the membranes of that healing space.

We deepen our self-regulation capacities so as to strengthen that membrane. This is also hard work to do and requires us, as trauma healers, to continue in the necessary work of healing ourselves from fragility and from unknowing our participation in structural hierarchies of oppression. It is easy to dissociate while sitting with a human suffering in our presence. That dissociation can masquerade as calm or neutrality. But we are not holding the space while dissociated; we are dysregulated into our own dorsal vagal space, which in turn subtly creates less safety in the relationship for the person seeking our care because we have ceased to be capable of responding, of empathy, of connection from heart to heart, and the other person can sense that absence.

MY OWN RECKONING WITH WHITE-SKIN PRIVILEGE

My own progress from being a "good liberal" to my current state of attempting a decolonial stance is reflected in my narrative about getting to know my own White-skin privilege. I offer this story here not to virtue signal but rather to demonstrate two things. First, it's difficult, at times, for people whose intersectional identities include both the colonizer and the colonized to go deeply into the ways in which we have benefited from social pathologies that also harm us. That would be me, the Jew, a descendant of a woman raped during the Cossack pogroms. An Eastern European Jew whose skin is pale and thus passes for White in a place where the Whiteness of Jews has always been a conditional and impermanent thing (Brodkin, 1998). A lesbian who, without trying, passes for not lesbian. An upper-middle-class person. And in that last part of my intersectionalities sits the story of my White privilege.

Second, this is an example of the process by which DHCR trauma healers can work to deepen their capacities to hold space. In my case, this was necessary for me to fully appreciate the traumas inflicted by systemic racism and White supremacy in the lives of BIPOC people and by the genocidal traumas inflicted upon the Indigenous people on whose stolen lands I have always lived. In facing that head-on and doing the work of my own distress not in relationships with the people seeking my care, I was able to engage in self-care, self-regulation, and an embrace of the complicated reality of who I am.

My grandparents were Eastern European Jews who fled to the United States in the years just before and after the First World War. My more distant ancestors had been persecuted, sometimes violently, for most of a millennium for the sin of their Jewishness. All four of these remarkable people faced anti-Semitism in the United States as well, but it was not of the violent variety that had been our families' fate in the Old Country.

My paternal grandfather's uncle, who had come to the States before the war, advised my great-grandfather to change the family name to Brown, and because the Jews of Russian Poland were frequently pale-skinned and red-haired as was my zayde, my paternal grandfather, not speaking a word of English, equipped with his new name of Hyman Brown, was able to join the carpenter's union immediately upon coming to these shores. The story of how my family benefited from White supremacy and White privilege began at that moment. Zayde was entirely a Jew when he left the jobsite, where he acquired some English. He spoke Yiddish at home. He and Bobe kept kosher, and he tried not to work on Saturday, the Shabbat, helped by union rules about the 40-hour workweek and no mandatory overtime (and his willingness to work overtime on Sunday, which made him friendships among his coworkers who, back in the Old Country, would have happily killed him if drunk on Easter). He regularly attended daily services at the synagogue that he helped to found in the early 1950s, and the family finally spoke English in the house as of the early 1950s when my generation, who knew little Yiddish, arrived on the scene. He passed for White, and his last name was Brown. A thin layer of assimilation, a thin layer of Whiteness.

For many years I disowned the notion that our family had benefited from White privilege or White supremacy. We were Jews, not White people, at least not in the eyes of the real White people, aka Christian White people. We were persecuted, a tolerated minority in the United States, particularly after the horrors of the Holocaust, and we hadn't enslaved anyone or colonized anyone's land, at least so far as our official narrative of being Jewish in American went. We got here after the bad stuff was all over with.

Real White supremacists didn't think we were White (and, as the events in Charlottesville in 2017 and the statements of White supremacists in positions of power are making increasingly clear, never have thought that we were). But because our families arrived after most of the overt horrors against BIPOC people in the Western Hemisphere had passed, and we, being the good social justice liberals that Jewish values trained us to be, were active in civil rights struggles, in getting our schools and neighborhoods integrated, I thought, so my skin is pale, so what? So my last name is Brown, so what?

This accrual of White privilege showed up on both sides of my family of origin. My maternal grandfather, a postal station superintendent by the time I was born, became known for actively hiring African American veterans as mail carriers. Because I lived in the zip code of his substation from the time I was 5 until I left my hometown for graduate school, I had the chance to hear this, not from him but from those carriers themselves when my college-age self asked them if they had known him and heard these stories.

I didn't understand that because he had White skin and had arrived in the United States just in time to be drafted into the military, where he caught and survived the flu of the first Great Pandemic in 1918 while in basic training, thus avoiding combat entirely, he had been able to get that job delivering the mail—another inflection point where White privilege operated to my family's benefit. My maternal grandparents were never middle class; they never owned a home or a car, as did my paternal grandparents. But the family did not go hungry during the Depression. My mother and her younger sister both went to college, at a time when only a tiny minority of White-skinned women did so.

It took decades and a good deal of antiracism work with myself to look at how much my family had benefited from slavery and the colonization and genocide of Indigenous peoples. Zayde could join the carpenter's union with his White skin, remain employed through the Great Depression, and then become a developer of suburban homes after the Second World War, which helped to vault his branch of our family into the middle class within one generation. Both of his children, my father and his younger brother, went to college. Both of them able to use G.I. Bill benefits to help pay for that education and for the down payments on their first homes, a privilege denied veterans of color, even though neither of them ever saw combat.

African American carpenters, born in the city to which my zayde came as an immigrant who only spoke Yiddish, had to mount a massive lawsuit to get admitted to that same carpenter's union. That lawsuit was settled in the late 1960s, well after my zayde and bobe had comfortably retired to their second home in Florida, well after my family had benefited from systemic racism and White supremacy. Like the Irish after the Civil War, Jewish immigrants were just White enough to be Whiter than any person of color as far as the union was concerned. We believed in the promise of acceptance in America, although we never put up a Christmas tree or cooked pork in our homes. We were Jews first, but we believed ourselves to be White.

We benefited from systemic racism and White supremacy, my family and I. We were also sometimes its targets. When my parents moved us into a mostly White Protestant neighborhood when I was five, I was beat up on by slightly older girls who told me that I was a "dirty Jew" and that they would not play with me (sending me home in tears to ask my mother what a Jew was—my first of many lessons in anti-Semitism), but we still could afford to build a house in that neighborhood. We could afford it because I had two college-educated parents whose light-skinned fathers had been employed in jobs that excluded men of color during a time when very few people had jobs at all. I could go to the excellent public schools, elementary and junior high just across the street from our home, relatively free from hassle and free of cost, aside from property taxes, to my parents. Because our last name was Brown, the anti-Semitic, very wealthy White Christian woman, without having met him, sold the lot that had been her English garden to my Jewish father to build my childhood home on, thus we could live in that very privileged neighborhood.

Mind you, once she found out whom she had allowed to move in next door, our neighbor put up a very high fence between her property and the lot now occupied by Jews, but oh well. We were already there, despite her best attempts at having my dad and his brother arrested for violating the blue laws that forbade work on the Christian Sabbath, Sunday. When they talked the police out of arresting them by coming out as Jews, this led to anonymous threatening phone calls, destruction of tools left on the building site, all kinds of interesting although not dangerous harassment, which I was told of when I was deemed old enough to learn about the anti-Semitism that had been the welcome wagon for our family. But White privilege got my father in the door.

I have very pale skin, like my zayde. My last name is Brown. I have a blandly American first and middle name. There were times when I had to come out as a Jew, for example, by missing school on Jewish holy days, which would always create a kerfuffle about my having to make up the work I'd missed, or by refusing to sing Christmas carols all through elementary school, which stance was the occasion for my annual visits to the office of the principal, who would attempt to shame or terrorize me into participating, or later, by missing intramural sports in junior high because I was attending Hebrew school every afternoon, thereby incurring the eternal enmity of my P.E. teacher, who already detested me for being a klutz. Aside from those times, I was just another White face, and we were eventually just another White family, one of two educated, upper-middle-class Jewish families on a White block in a very White, wealthy suburb. I had a free public education where we learned set theory and French in fourth grade and had annual trips to the symphony and art museums, which were among the crown jewels of high culture in my hometown, artifacts built by the robber barons. White privilege equals social capital. I left for college and graduate school equipped with the equivalent of an Ivy League education.

The irony is that because my neighborhood and its junior high were the only ones in the entire school district that were not majority Jewish, my high school of 3,600 students was nearly bereft of the White, non-Jewish peers I had been in school with through the end of ninth grade. The majority of the non-Jewish adolescents were whisked away to various private schools whose ratios of Jews to non-Jewish people more closely resembled that of my grade school and junior high. My high school closed on Jewish holy days rather than leave a smattering of other-than-Jewish students forlornly wandering the halls.

But all of this was made possible because most Eastern European Jews are Whiter than most African Americans, and so even though we were not real White people, we passed for White sufficiently to have just enough White privilege available to us that in two generations our family went from being impoverished refugees fleeing violent anti-Semitism to everyone in my generation being American-born and college-educated, replete with advanced degrees. One of my generation was on *Harvard Law Review* with Obama. One of us is me. One is an award-winning documentary filmmaker. We count a research pathologist, an award-winning short story writer, a successful national park ranger, and a rabbi among the ranks of our generation. None of this would have been likely to happen without our benefiting from White privilege.

My grandparents were able to accrue financial and social capital because White supremacy allowed them and my parents across the thresholds of doors that were slammed shut and locked against African American people born in the United States, people often more highly educated than any of my grandparents, none of whom got past the equivalent of elementary school. Because our skin was White and our last name was Brown, my father was not locked in struggle with our suburb's zoning commission when he submitted the plans for our home, which included innovations of his own design that were new and thus potentially off-code.

A few years later, the most distinguished African American architect in Cleveland spent half a decade fighting with the same zoning commission to build homes for himself and his brother, a physician, on a lot he had bought a few blocks away from where I lived. I recall my parents recounting this story to me as evidence not of our family's White privilege but of the prejudice of the goyim, our Yiddish epithet for White Christians.

The architect's elder daughter was my age, in my grade in school and my intellectual equal—but not placed in the college prep classes that in my school district started in the fourth grade, the classes that came with set theory and French lessons. Racism deemed her probably not college material. We were in Girl Scouts together and friendly, and then her parents, protecting her, pulled her out of the public school system at the end of junior high so that she would not be one of only four Black faces in our enormous high school and so that she could avoid being lumped in with the other kids identified as probably headed to vocational school into whose classes she would have been shunted.

White privilege, I figured out much later, meant my parents never paid a penny for my education. Her parents, to protect her from the effects of systemic racism, which kept African Americans out of our suburb during the time I was growing up, had to literally pay a price to create the educational privileges and equity for their daughter that I took for granted.

All of this and more, I'm sure, is evidence of how my family has benefited from White supremacy and the institution of slavery. I, of course, benefit every moment of every day from the dispossession of the Duwamish people from their homeland here on the shores of what the colonizers named Puget Sound. The place in which I have lived my entire adult life, Seattle, is the bastardized, Anglicized version of the name of one of the leaders of the Duwamish nation when White people invaded this beautiful place and shoved them into one of the prisons for Indigenous people that White Americans called reservations. I get to live here and to see the mountains in their glory every sunny day (and we have more of those than most people think), but the descendants of the Indigenous people do not for the most part get to live where the views are because you have to be at least middle class (and these days, quite wealthy) to have a home with a view.

Through assiduous work of cultural and collective healing, the genocide of culture and language perpetrated on these and other Coast Salish nations is being remediated, slowly and painfully. The wounds are still open and reopened from time to time. I benefit from the genocide and displacement of the Indigenous people of the land on which I sit as I write these words, even though I nor any of my relations were present for those wrongs done. I am present daily to benefit from the wrongs that were done. White privilege. Colonizer privilege. In order to hold space for BIPOC people who come to me in pain seeking healing, I need to have done this work of examining my privilege so that I am engaged, openhearted, regulated, in a ventral vagal state when those folks walk into my room. Every DHCR healer needs to do this work, no matter how crappy it feels. I invite you not to feel guilt nor shame, as those affects get in the way of radical acceptance of the truths that we can be both colonized and colonizer. It's easier for me to attend to the marginalized parts of my intersectional identities; it is necessary for me to attend to those that are immersed in colonization.

Tikkun Olam: Heal the World, and We Are the World

These psychic effects, these unacknowledged benefits, of our personal relationships with social pathologies are often subtle and thus difficult to detect. We, the marginalized, have attempted to assimilate, we have tried to pass, we have thrown away the external markers of our marginalized and subordinated status. We speak American English at home and give our children American-sounding names. We stop cooking the foods of our cultures so that the recipes for kreplach (Jewish pot stickers) die with our grandmothers whose hands shaped them. Or we feel so ashamed of these traces of pain that, like other sources of shame, we push the awareness out of our consciousness, or we accuse those who share our privileged intersectional identities of being too woke if we tell the truth about how we benefit from social pathologies. It can be terrifyingly activating to tell ourselves the truth about how brittle is the ledge of privilege on which we stand. I don't love it; I do love what I get from those truths though. Terrified healers, full of adrenaline from the activation of their sympathetic nervous systems, cannot hold space for their own feelings, much less those of the people coming to them for care. To do decolonial, humble, culturally responsive trauma healing work we must look in the mirror with love and compassion, allowing the shame to dissipate.

Grief

I believe that all of these dynamics, if left uninterrogated, contribute to a residual colonial thread in trauma healing that can make it difficult to hold the space and bear witness when we know that we have benefited, that we are somehow complicit, in that which has wounded the suffering person we are working with. I think that a missing piece in the personal work of the trauma healer whose intersectional identities have given them unasked-for benefits from a social pathology, and the decolonizing step that opens a door for deeper trauma healing for all, is the acknowledgment of our own grief.

The grief of the well-intended colonizer for the harms done without their knowledge but with their complicity when they turned their gaze away from what was being done, the grief of the colonized for having been unable to find their voice in the repressive and silencing milieu that is psychological colonization, the grief of the person who, like most healers and many suffering people, is caught somewhere in the middle of all of this, grief shrouded in guilt and shame, and thus in many cases unavailable for us to name, feel, and move into and thus through. All of this grief, and more, needs to be held and soothed, worked through again and again, as we do decolonial trauma healing practice.

Here's what's important for healers to keep in mind when we start to touch the third rail that is the privilege woven into the fabric of some strand of our own intersectional identities. We cannot know what we did not know. We are not responsible for the sins of our progenitors. We are not responsible for having failed to act when we had no idea that action was called for or for acting out of shame or guilt in ways that only made things worse. We are not to blame for having privilege because that is not something we have sought out.

We are responsible for opening our eyes, for waking up, and for taking action and responsibility once we have awakened to what we did not know before. We must, in consequence, be willing to observe ourselves, our actions, and our models of healing through the eye of compassion if we are ever to make space to grieve for what could have been if we had known, if we had been able to act, before we did know and could act in a decolonial, liberatory way. "Shoulda, woulda, coulda," it is said in 12-step programs. Stop that, say I. Guilt and shame are useful only when one has done wrong and only so long as to propel us to do better. Grief is what we need to heal into open hearts.

Because most trauma healers are people of good will, people with excellent intentions, people with their eyes on justice, the realization that we have participated in social pathologies, even without our knowledge or knowing consent, that we have benefited from those pathologies, that the models of treatment that we have learned in our training are often appropriations of Indigenous and Global South healing methodologies—these realizations can stop us in our tracks and lead to the understandable desire to protect ourselves, to go into a state of dorsal-vagal shutdown and unknowing of the sort that all trauma survivors engage with.

For it is painful, deeply painful if not genuinely traumatic to fully appreciate our own complicity. Read that again, and take that in. It is painful to appreciate our own complicity. It is painful to appreciate the complicity of Western trauma healing disciplines in colonial narratives of pathology. It hurts our hearts to let this in. This knowledge, when we fully inhale it, bores into the depths of our souls and spirits. So of course we want to unknow. Of course we want to be numb or externalize. But hold the space for yourself to know. Grieve. Grieve again. Grieve not alone, not guiltily; grieve in the company of others who are doing this work.

Remaining in a state of unknowing, of dissociating our complicity, just as any traumatized person moves to dissociate from the pain and knowledge of what they have experienced and any decent colonizer moves to dissociate from the pain and knowledge of what they have done, is an excellent way to persist in making trauma treatment a colonizing phenomenon where the goal is symptom reduction. I think that this emphasis on reducing symptoms has emerged as the standard by which treatments are judged, because if a person's symptoms are reduced, then they can become a tool producing value for capitalism. They can fulfill their roles as adults in society; they are less likely to harm themselves with substances so as to manage their distress, or to harm others with violence also so as to manage their distress, and thus they won't cost taxpayers money, either in the form of building prisons or funding disability programs. None of these less likely phenomena are in and of themselves bad outcomes—it is better not to be in pain, not to abuse your body with a substance, not to harm another person, not to be incarcerated.

But none of these outcomes, of symptom reduction and thus the reduction of phenomena that rogue capitalism would prefer not to pay for, address the social pathologies that are at the root of most traumas. Symptom reduction does not speak to the profound existential dilemmas that arise on the heels of trauma, nor does it allow sufficient room for the grief of all parties.

So having spoken about the conceptual framework that guides us, let's talk next about that mirage known as safety. Because that topic is so large, I'm going to need two chapters to cover it. Bear with me. Getting to something that resembles safety is foundational to trauma healing. Decolonial analysis shows us how difficult it is to get to that place.

7 DECOLONIZING THE CONSTRUCTS AND MYTHS OF SAFETY, PART I

One of the core principles of all trauma healing, no matter how the healer approaches the process, is that the first order of business entails collaborating with the trauma-exposed person on the project of creating safety for the trauma-exposed person. This apparently simple starting point implies that the person can develop a sense of safety on multiple dimensions, starting with safety in their physical and psychosocial environments, safety in their body, and safety in their emotionally important relationships. Having sufficiency of each type of safety is foundational to moving forward with processing trauma, which means making room for painful emotions and memories to be present.

Having safety means that, at a neurobiological level, someone is able to achieve and return to a ventral vagal neurobiological state more of the time. While their stress and trauma systems are not dormant, the person who is living in safety spends less and less time in either sympathetic nervous system (SNS) arousal, parasympathetic overfunction, which creates a slowed, sleepy state of being in which the person is floating on the edge of full aliveness, or dorsal-vagal states of freeze, numbness, or dissociation, which are the refuge of the person who is both traumatized and trapped.

https://doi.org/10.1037/0000421-008
Decolonizing Trauma Healing: Toward a Humble, Culturally Responsive Practice, by L. S. Brown

Safety creates the biopsychosocial and existential–spiritual context that a person knows to be safe in their own terms, one in which the suffering person can move toward reducing their internal upheaval sufficiently to engage in the healing process and fully encounter the pain of the trauma, knowing that they have an internal harbor to which they can return. But in a world where there is continuous danger for many people, where many people have never known what safety feels like or would be for them, it is necessary to decolonize the construct of safety and speak truth about what is possible in the realm of safe.

This is because in the social part of the biopsychosocial are the realms of the social pathologies, of chronic traumatic terror, of all the structural and systemic forms of oppression and marginalization. For people who were raised in dangerous families, the last moment of safety in their lives was as they exited the womb. As my colleague Tyson Bailey (2023) has noted, exposure to the trauma for this group of people starts when the healer says hello, given that for these suffering people almost every human being is potentially dangerous. With real danger, both acute and chronic, around us, how do we create safety in our healing practices?

The three-phase model of trauma healing, pioneered by Mary R. Harvey and Judith Lewis Herman in the mid 1990s (Harvey, 1996), deriving from both their own lived experiences as feminist trauma healers as well as from the lived experiences of the people with whom they were working, has stood the test of time. This paradigm holds true no matter what epistemic stance or intervention the healer is taking on how to approach the healing process. The first phase, before all else, is to establish safety. Then process the trauma. Then work through the meaning of what life is like in the aftermath of that work. Reiterate safety. Reiterate it further. Multiple iterations of safety, as knowledge of its absence, of disconnection or danger, emerge in the processing of the trauma material.

An ultimate goal of DHCR trauma healing, of which Herman and Harvey can be considered foundational thinkers, is justice. As Herman has recently written, "the first step towards a better form of justice is simply to ask survivors what would make things as right as possible for them" (2023, p. 24). Confronting social pathologies is a step toward creating that justice.

But what do we do if safety of one or several types, or even any type, is not possible when someone walks in our door because there is not yet justice? How does a DHCR trauma healer proceed when, in the opinion of the suffering person, anything resembling safety is likely unachievable in the foreseeable future no matter the best efforts of all concerned? How then do we proceed? When a person's intersectional identities, placed in the context of multiple social pathologies, mean that safety is an illusion, something brittle and easily shattered, how does healing occur? Because we, and the suffering people with whom we work, live with chronic traumatic terror in the emotional ecosystems created by toxic social pathologies, decolonial, humble, culturally responsive (DHCR) trauma healers must interrogate the entire idea of safety and decolonize its meanings. To ignore the brittleness of safety for so many humans is to do them injustice, which obviates the goals of DHCR trauma healing practice.

For who in this world is actually safe? And whose illusions that their privilege protects them from danger are most likely to be shattered in ways that make their pain, and the fragments of their shattered illusions, difficult to gather in for repair, a challenging task for even the most capable of trauma healers? A decolonial analysis of the construct of safety, which remains at the core of all trauma healing work, is necessary if DHCR trauma healing is to be culturally responsive to all. Recently, a measure for formally assessing a traumatized person's subjective and neurobiological sense of safety, the Neuroception of Psychological Safety Scale, has become available (Morton et al., 2024). It could be, for some healing pairs, a tool for collaborating on tracking the neurobiology of the experience of getting closer to safe.

A metaphor might be in order here. When I received my second dose of the Moderna vaccine against COVID-19 in early February 2021, I walked out of the vaccination center into the cold, clean Seattle air and thought, "I'm going to be safe now. In two weeks, no one can kill me with this virus." I had that illusion until that summer. Little did I know that Delta, Omicron, the BA.1 and BA.2, and endless other variants were about to emerge. I've had six booster shots since then (being old and having had cancer has its advantages in the vaccination department) and will continue to get boosters as new variants emerge. A negative test no longer means that a person is not positive for the virus; it may simply means that their immune system, strengthened by vaccines, has fought it off very quickly, to the point where the exposure would not show up even on a polymerase chain reaction (PCR) test.

But I had, for a few months, the illusion that I was safe to walk around in the world of humans again, to eat in a restaurant. An illusion, indeed. I luckily was not among the vaccinated people who eventually became ill, as has been true for too many people I love. Now my supply of masks of every color and every kind for the various places in which I spend time—the food co-op, the cancer treatment center, an airplane, my dojo—grows. It's a fashion accessory. I know that I am not entirely safe. I am closer to safe than if I hadn't had the shots and didn't wear a mask. I even had a quite intense exposure in the spring of 2023 and came out of it not sick. But the illusion that, fully vaccinated, in the early months of 2021 I was safe from this wily virus, erroneously applying my paradigm about how the polio vaccine had in fact made me safe from that virus, has been a potent message about the illusory nature of safety.

In 2022 the U.S. Supreme Court decided to strip away reproductive rights, after a half century of asserting those rights, from women and from people who do not identify as women but still have a uterus and thus still can become pregnant—pregnant against their will and without their consent, pregnant with a much-wanted child who dies in utero and now cannot be delivered because that will be deemed an abortion, mandating that the mother's life be at risk, or pregnant at a time when the arrival of another child in their life and that of their family will be not merely inconvenient but destructive. In the year since that decision, instances of maternal and fetal/maternal death are expected to skyrocket (Gómez, 2023).

For 50 years all U.S. residents had had the illusion, based in part on lies told at confirmation hearings by several of those who signed on to the stripping away of this right, that they had reproductive choice and bodily autonomy, which is not limited to the right to choose whether or not to remain pregnant. And now, in more than half of the states, that right is gone, the first right ever to be taken away.

Bodily autonomy is a component of safety and reproductive justice, and both of these are being stolen or eroded daily as 2024 comes to an end, with regard to both reproductive and queer rights. One of the men sitting on that U.S. Supreme Court, in a concurring opinion, stated that the decision in the *Dobbs* matter opens the door to stripping away other rights having to do with bodily and emotional autonomy that have been a component of perceived safety for many marginalized and subordinated people. These include as the right to obtain contraception, which in turn affects whether someone can choose to engage in heterosexual activity and decide whether it might result in a pregnancy or the right to engage in consensual sexual activity with a person of one's choice.

Things that were felt to be safely available and that created bodily autonomy, reproductive justice, the rights to seek appropriate care if one was dealing with matters of gender orientation, and equality under the law for people of all sexualities and genders have suddenly been put at risk, made dangerous, choice unattainable or criminalized, allowing anyone to sue a person if they learn that the person has traded personal safety against the notion that such safety endangers society in some manner.

These recent and ongoing events demonstrate clearly that, particularly for marginalized people, but in reality for all humans regardless of perceived privilege, safety is an illusion. It's an illusion with regard to apparently prosaic trauma every bit as much because of how the toxins of social pathologies affect every component of how each traumatized person is dealt with by systems, not only those of structural inequality.

For instance, you're driving down the highway, and a drunk driver veers across the median strip and into your car; when you wake up weeks later in a brain injury rehab unit, you can no longer speak—and speaking has been how you have made your living. What happens next has much to do with your intersectional identities, particularly those having to do with access to resources. If you've got great insurance and money and someone who can act as your caregiver, you might get the rehabilitation you need to speak again. But if you have no insurance and no saved funds, the outcome is going to be different, and the trauma will be flavored by your intersectionalities in marked ways.

You're on a lovely ski vacation and it starts to snow; you ski into a tree, snapping your femur bone, and almost bleed to death because no one knows that you're out there. What happens next has much to do with your intersectional identities.

You have a lovely beach house that's been in your family for generations, and a 100-year storm blows it to splinters, washing away beloved family mementos, something that happened to a person dear to me. The degree to which healing this trauma can take place has in part to do with the intersectional identities of those to whom it has occurred. My dear friend to whom this precise thing happened has financial resources, and 3 years later, her home has been rebuilt, although the grief of the loss of cherished family items persists. Her neighbors, who live on that island full-time and are impoverished, cannot restore their homes and live in continuous trauma.

The essence of trauma can be defined as how the illusion of one's safety vaporizes in an instant. In the lives of marginalized and subordinated people, social pathologies continuously create the emotional and psychosocial equivalents of drunk drivers and invisible trees in the snow and 100-year storms. This is part of the quotidian for people with multiple, targeted, marginalized, and subordinated identities in the world of many swirling storms of enormous social pathologies. How does a trauma healer generate something resembling safety in the midst of these storms so that the work of trauma healing can progress?

ONE SMALL POWERFUL THING WE CAN ALL DO TO GET CLOSER TO SAFE: HOW WE BEGIN

Deborah Luepnitz (1988), pioneering feminist psychoanalytic thinker and family therapist, famously wrote that one must "set the fee as a feminist therapist" (p. 83). She utilized this metaphor to communicate that every single decision that a healer makes conveys a message about what is to come next, sets the stage for the epistemic framework of the healing experience. Each thing we do and say, however apparently banal, communicates whether or not that healer understands the concept that distress arises from political realities, from structural forms of oppression, no matter what the identified trauma might be, and that the healer must hold this framework in the background of their awareness so as not to lose that thread.

The ways in which we as healers talk about the pain, about our relationships, about how healing proceeds, are information that the DHCR healing process is a revolutionary act. We overtly or subtly convey that a healer and a sufferer can choose not be seduced into collusion and instead disrupt structural hierarchies of oppression as they have infiltrated the healing process. It's sometimes simple as, "I know that PTSD is a word that feels right to you. How would you feel about taking the word *disorder* out of the mix and just call it posttraumatic stress?" A simple act, a subversive one.

How might a DHCR trauma healer, seeking to be liberatory, make safety? How do we create spaces in which we do our healing work that are safe enough, closer to safe, as safe as possible? In the middle of the tornado, how do we tell truth and still cocreate, with suffering people, places in which painful experiences and difficult conversations about what it means that safety may be illusory can occur and be held, seen, and heard through a decolonial lens, a lens in which the truths about the tornado enter the healing process at some point?

SHALL WE DANCE? THE SPACE IN WHICH WE WORK

I think that we can start making things safe enough with how we present ourselves. Standard training in the psychotherapy world cautions against therapist transparency and vulnerability. In practice, what this means is that the suffering person is entering our realm—and the office or telehealth screen where we meet is indeed our realm, the space that we, particularly if we are in private practice, have chosen. Even in an institutional work setting, we have perhaps decorated the space and made it more comfortable for ourselves. For us, not for the people entering that space, although we imagine that we have done the latter as well. But tell the truth: this is our place, not yet a shared space.

The place where we practice is the physical manifestation of the power inherent in the role of a healer because we have chosen it. It is not the place chosen by the suffering person even when, in a teletherapy session, that person is sitting in a place that is their own in some way.

The space in which we practice our healing work can be a place of sharp imbalances of power, affected by the toxins of a hierarchy of dominance and subordination generated by the social pathologies of which the healer has not yet become aware. Or we can practice conscientization and create a place of liberatory collaboration toward healing and justice. We can begin by telling the truth about this fact, one that typically goes by the wayside entirely. Set the space as a DHCR healer.

Which path we take with telling the simple truth about the power imbalances soaked into the space is up to us. Do we start with "May I be curious about what it is like for you to come into this office/onto the screen? How is it feeling for you? How hard or easy was it to navigate the interface? And how did that feel for you?" Whether this is a first decolonial act is affected by the degree to which we are responsive in the moment to the feedback from the suffering person about whether or how our space communicates the desire for safety or instead speaks to the not so well-hidden artifacts of the colonized paradigms in which the healer trained. Our healing space—often an office in an anonymous building, sometimes a room in our home, sometimes the place where we get online with a person during a time when meeting face-to-face is not yet safe enough or physically possible for one or both parties—is a physical or metaphorical location where historically the rules have been that suffering people seeking care may generally know only the immediately visible components of a healer's intersectional identities.

It is a place where conversely healers claim the right, even the necessity, to know quite a lot about this suffering soul and who they are, fitting that into the healer's ideas of what will work. We thus sometimes, in the process, commence by violating, albeit inadvertently, the boundaries of this suffering person further. The overpowering that happens is complicated by the healer's insistence that what they are doing is right for that sufferer. This is a reenactment of colonization, not a DHCR model but the model of psychotherapist authority. The parallels, when we tease this out, become more obvious: "I am forcing you to speak the colonizer's language." "I am insisting that we begin our work together by going through this list of questions I have."

I just had this experience myself signing up with a new provider for something mental health-adjacent. I am a veteran of these questionnaires, and I found it so horrifically off-putting and invasive that I almost said, screw it; but this provider has something I want, an easier-to-take form of a medication I am already using, so I filled out the endless online screens. Imagine that I wasn't someone with my degree of privilege and power. Oy. Talk about how to create an absence of safety for suffering traumatized people (a group that this provider's office purports to serve).

But back to place. The place itself creates a power imbalance carrying over from old models of power imbalance that were built into the training of most healers, which we must be intentional about noticing and dissolving, creating a DHCR healing space even when doing so makes all of the voices in our heads telling us what is right to do scream that we are messing things up—messing up the artifacts of social pathologies that began when the founders of modern psychotherapy brought the authoritarian patriarchal norms of their medical, professional worlds into the structures of psychoanalytic, and eventually most psychotherapeutic, office spaces.

Without our being conscious about transforming not only the obvious but also the subtle markers of power and dominance, a place where some kind of power imbalance is baked into the furniture is an operational definition of that which is probably not safe for the person with less power in the exchange.

Remember for a second about what it's like to be in a dentist's office having a cavity drilled and filled, or think about a time when you had to have conscious sedation for a diagnostic procedure that involves a camera going up into your colon or down into your stomach. Feel that sense of powerlessness. Now imagine doing that weekly, or more frequently, at a time when you're already in so much psychic pain that you don't know how you'll get through the next day? That's how the power imbalance built into the physical spaces of many trauma healers can feel—not very safe, eh?

I've certainly had those experiences when I was in the position of the suffering person, knowing in my body that something in the entire gestalt of the space was not quite right, and then having the therapist in question act in ways that were overt confirmation of what my trauma neurobiology was quietly telling me each time I walked into the room. You may have had those experiences yourself, even when the therapist is doing things that are objectively perfectly okay, but which leave you feeling a little bit icky, a little bit more reluctant every week to show up for the session. We can create spaces for DHCR healing that are based in the application of our core principles to the space itself so that there is congruence, which enhances the potential of getting closer to safe for the suffering people we work with.

So how can we begin our connection by rebalancing power from the start, given the unavoidable reality that healers invite trauma-exposed humans into our spaces? As Luepnitz (1988) exhorted, let us do all things as liberatory DHCR healers. All things.

FIRST TOUCH

What would happen if we ceased to focus on having boundaries, being neutral, and all of the other things that people doing our work have been taught forever, all ways of being that tend to increase the power imbalance and make our workplaces feel less safe for many suffering trauma-exposed people because the dynamic is replicating one in which they were harmed? What if instead we practiced a form of radical transparency in which our humility and our openness to deeply knowing the lived experiences of the suffering person were the first things that we offered? What if we immediately created relational dynamics that were free of dominance or coercion? What would happen if we did not pretend to be invisible, if we queried the dictum that we must be neutral and pretend to be blank walls onto which the suffering person could project the movie of their life, a social construction of the healer's role that is painfully dehumanizing to the healer? What if we explored the roots of those rules in the colonization and medicalization of the healing of wounded psyches? How might we decolonize the first touch? "Love is touching souls," sang Joni Mitchell (1971). Healing is a kind of love, a touching of souls. So how do we decolonize the first touch? To know, as Bailey (2023)so eloquently said, that hello is the first touch, and the first risk, for suffering traumatized people.

This language of first touch comes from my practice of aikido, the martial art of peace. There, we learn that the first touch with our training partner is not the physical one that occurs when one person offers their hand and their training partner grasps it. First touch instead happens in the moment when that person touches the energy of their training partner and is touched energetically in return, the two people entering relationship, agreeing to attempt connection for an agreed-upon purpose. First touch is the establishment of a ventral vagal through-line for the work we do together because it requires an open heart from the person who is assigned power, the open heart of the ventral vagal relationship system in our neurobiology.

Trauma healing is touching souls; the construct of vicarious traumatization, proposed a quarter of a century past by Pearlman and Saakvitne (1995), speaks to the transformation of a trauma healer that happens when we allow our souls, our hearts, and our beings to be touched by the suffering people with whom we work. We decolonize trauma healing and liberate it from the faux medical framework into which psychotherapy is increasingly attempting to squeeze itself by interrogating what is not liberatory, what does not fit into a DHCR paradigm, in the standard first touch, and then transforming that. We can now do so informed by science as well as poetry and martial art, integrating the understandings of polyvagal theory into the project of creating something closer to safe in the first touch.

AWAY WITH THEE, INTAKE INTERVIEW!

Generally, the first touch of psychotherapy is an intake interview, which is an assertion of dominance over the suffering person, a colonization reenactment, and at times it feels to the suffering person like a coercive experience: "You must complete this form before I can listen to you!" The intake interview— or worse, the online form with a million boxes—creates a perfect way to ensure that the underlying power dynamics are firmly in place by the time the trauma-exposed person leaves the office for the first time—and sometimes, the last as well, feeling silenced, defeated, made invisible by that form being the first touch.

If it's an actual interview, what often occurs goes something like this: The therapist asks questions, many of which are intensely personal, painful, and intrusive. They require answers at a moment when they are still a total stranger in every way to the suffering person. The trauma-exposed person is expected to give the answers to those questions; therapists even learn interviewing techniques to slyly coerce answers out of people who are not yet ready to share their most shameful experiences, for example, asking "What's the obstacle to you answering this question for me now?" The real answer, "That I don't know you, and I don't trust you, and you can take your list of questions and stuff them," is rarely spoken, and when it is, this goes into the chart as evidence of negativity rather than autonomy and a sense of personal privacy boundaries.

What frequently happens in this variety of first touch is the communication that one must comply with the rules of the psychotherapy game. Refusing to answer—or even more radically, questioning why a particular question is being asked—is rarely coded as evidence of a suffering person's striving for autonomy. Rather, it is more likely to be recorded as that person being resistant, oppositional, defensive, or even worst of all, possibly borderline, all words in therapy-speak that boil down to "bad person, whom I, the therapist, do not want to work with." Take that attitude about this suffering person into the next encounter, if they come back for a second round, and you can count on one hand how many sessions will transpire before the client departs, deemed a failure or still in the precontemplation stage, well in advance of that departure by the therapist, who thereby continues to not notice their complicity in this power dynamic.

The highly compliant person, someone whose traumatized neurobiology has led to a chronic fawning response of overcompliance and fear of loss of relationship, will not be less harmed by the assertion of the therapist's power over them. They will fawn and also be harmed, and the foundation of the work will be firmly seated in a trauma reenactment. This is a first touch that conveys the message: "Let me pin you to the ground and show you who's boss."

Everyone in the typical initial therapeutic exchange expects that the therapist will say little to nothing about themself, although in this day of personal and professional websites, Google searches, interactive commenting and review, and social media profiles where friends of friends settings allow potential clients to send friend requests, there are usually a few more data points readily available about a healer than in the past (unless they have no online presence at all, which I have found to be true for an interestingly large number of therapists). But the old walls protecting healers from being known by the people seeking their care have mostly withstood the test of the internet.

Through this form of first touch the power imbalance is set firmly in place. "I ask the questions, you answer them. You are expected to be vulnerable to me, I allow myself to be protected from you." No amount of cultural competence or even cultural responsivity is going to transform this sort of underlying colonial structure of psychotherapy as generally practiced.

This is how it is frequently practiced. I have the data, having reviewed hundreds of psychotherapy records in my work as a forensic psychologist. This has consequently allowed me to observe this format of first touch in scores of private practices and institutional settings alike. I also encounter people trained in this methodology when they come seeking consultation from me and are shocked to learn that I would like them to consider throwing out their intake questionnaires in favor of a DHCR dialogue with the new suffering person with whom they have started to work and who has deeply confused them. This kind of first touch in the form of an intake questionnaire, interview, checklist, PCL-5 (Weathers et al., 2013), and so on will make it harder to decolonize what follows in the work together because it has set a tone about power dynamics. It will make it much harder to make ourselves, and the spaces in which we work, feel just safe enough for a suffering person to tolerate spending time in. So can we stop doing this, please?

Beginning to Disrupt the Dominance/Submission Power Imbalance

Imagine, instead, that the first touch occurs at the first encounter, which today increasingly happens by some form of electronic communication rather than a phone call (or as one of my friends, born just before the start of this century, teases me, "You mean you actually talk to people on a phone? So last century, Laura!"). But via some means, the suffering person reaches out to a healer, often after long contemplation, frequently acutely in the throes of distress, to ask, "Do you have openings? I need to work with someone who knows about complex trauma and immigrant communities." What if the healer's response was not, "Yes, here's my next opening and my fee schedule, you can make an appointment on my online calendar," but rather offers a connecting response that's not about business: "Thanks so much for taking the risk to make yourself visible to me. This healing process isn't easy, and I know that. Shall we find a time to meet that works for us both, where we can begin to see if we can make a connection?" And "What do you need to know about me before we meet in person for the first time?" First touch, telling the truth that there is risk here, honoring the courage, owning the difficulty, immediately framing this as a joint endeavor through the use of first-person plural pronouns—this might be a way to begin to create something closer to safe in what ensues. The healer offering a willingness to be known, even a little, while still respecting our own privacy boundaries but being translucent, not opaque, the suffering person being seen, heard, with someone's open heart.

Instead of an intake interview or a checklist, ask this: "Tell me your story. Tell me what is important to you, for us to know together, just for now, just to get started. Tell me if we need to explore ways to keep you safe enough from any current present dangers, so that we can together construct a plan for you being safe enough. Tell me what I might be doing now that might be making this place and our encounter feel safer or less safe. Because one of my goals is to make this place, and our relationship, as safe as they can be for you each time that we meet, and I know that whatever makes things safe enough might change from time to time."

This is flipping the script. The suffering person tells the story they want to tell. The healer emphasizes the cocreation of safe-enough spaces. From the beginning, truth is allowed to emerge, and the centrality of getting to safety is foregrounded.

CODE-SWITCHING, PART THE FIRST

This is also, sadly, the point where a DHCR trauma healer must often be bicultural and code-switch for a few minutes, as the rules for healers who have licenses for our work include the requirement to produce a consent form and get the suffering person to sign it. Healers in the United States from 2023 onward are under the bizarre yoke of a well-intended federal law requiring that they give people an estimate of what the cost of the healing process will be and how long it is likely to take. State laws require consent forms to explain about billing to insurance, and if that is happening, the necessity of defining the person's suffering as a pathology in the form of giving a diagnosis.

Feh, as my grandmothers would have said, phooey to all of this, and yet, DHCR trauma healers are working in the realities of the societies in which we live and have to figure out how to engage in some form of civil disobedience. Some of you are already brave enough to practice healing work outside the safe confines of licensure and can ignore this whole section. Most of us are not, myself included.

There is, I think, a way to decolonize this still required bow and curtsy to the medical–industrial complex that controls our right to call ourselves psychologists or social workers or counselors or doctors. That particular workaround is accomplished by engaging in radical transparency about this deviation from your framework and entails collaborating with the person on how to arrive at the name that you will give to the insurance company for their distress.

You will need to make time for this collaborative process, as it requires explicating, in the most healing and empowering manner and nonpedantic way possible, how diagnoses and diagnostic manuals are developed and why they mean nothing to you. Inquire of the suffering person—do they want the whole story, or do they want you to skip to the part where you know for sure that it's all made up but where you have to work within it for now, like we work with so many other made-up rules.

If someone says yes to the whole story, you can share what many critical thinkers have concluded about diagnoses being made-up political instruments. Their roots in the United States began as expressions of White supremacy or were planted in the soil of misogyny, the construction of women as hysterical, unable to differentiate between being sexually abused and having the fantasy in which such abuse is desired. And think for a minute: who in their right mind would come up with this monstrosity, one that only someone who had themselves never been violated as a child could ever even imagine, yet one that was a truth for over a century?

But wait, as the TV commercials say, there's more. There is the insistence in these systems on the gender binary and on people's cheerful compliance with the same. Gender dysphoria, a diagnosis that reifies the notion that one should be content with all aspects of one's natal sex phenotype and the gender roles associated with it, is a colonized way of saying, this person is in pain from trying to squeeze their triangular soul into an oval box, and that box feels so inescapable and grows ever so much tighter as people get older, that this person just wants to die because it hurts too much.

There are the not very dead ghosts of homophobia in the diagnostic machine. There are zombies of ableism, vampires that rise up with the assumption that an oppositional child might never have good reasons for being unwilling to comply with the world around them. The profound outside-in view of suffering, the version that proclaims, about someone's suffering or their behavior, that "this is a problem because it makes us"—by which I mean the groups currently in power/or those not currently marginalized or subordinated—"uncomfortable" to be diagnoses. Yes, there are some people who, because of their neurotype, seem to be in constant battle with everyone and everything; why not be curious about that, rather than inject them with an antipsychotic and label them crazy? The entire diagnostic system is full of the toxins of one social pathology or another; it creates premature cognitive commitment, the false sense of certainty in the clinician of knowing what is wrong that stops openheartedness and curiosity in their tracks.

A DHCR healer isn't required to give this whole history lesson, although we should be prepared, if asked, to do so. We can give people a copy of Paula

Caplan's (of blessed memory) excellent book, *They Say You're Crazy* (1995), which does a great job of covering this material from a scholarly, liberatory standpoint. Or, if the person prefers, we can share the main talking points, which are that diagnoses are made up, that you don't believe in calling distress pathology, and that if the person wants their health insurance to contribute to payment, here's what we have to do together, which is to pick out the least worst name from the latest version of this book.

We can talk about code-switching, how people have to go back and forth between the language of oppressors and the language of their own truths, speaking the decolonial language of truth in our work and the lying language of pathology to the medical-industrial insurance complex. We can tell the truth, that this blatant exposure of our code-switching activities might make the suffering person feel less safe or suspicious of us or wonder whether we are worthy of trust or a lot of things other than collaborated with and depathologized. Because, as someone reasonably asked me, how can they know when we're telling them the truth if we are willing to be disingenuous with a structural form of oppression? What I said was, you can know that I will tell you the truth. Try me. Test me. I am even telling you the truth about me being a little sneaky with the system, and not asking you to keep a secret, which is one of the ways in which dangerous adults behave when they prey on children. Notice, I'll say, how you deal with some version of this struggle in your own life, between integrity and assimilation, between transparency and getting access to resources for yourself and others. We don't defend; we invite engagement.

The healer will offer the time and space that the suffering person wants and needs to express their thoughts and feelings about having to be named as ill, as well as about our willingness to dissemble in our communications with external structures that do not share a decolonial epistemology. Some people come in our doors wanting a diagnosis or even proclaiming that they are *x* psychopathology; it's not our job to disabuse them of that intersectional identity, our job as DHCR trauma healers is to gently open doors for people to see themselves more fully than that imposed identity has allowed.

Some people have a value system that they describe as telling the truth to everyone, all the time, no matter what, and our transparency about code-switching will create difficulties for them in feeling safe enough with us. The time frame for this process of coming to terms with choosing the name or with your stance that the name is a agent of colonization will not be one whose length can be dictated by any imaginary deadline for billing that the healer might have imposed on themselves but rather will be informed by the goal of creating, collaboratively, a closer-to-safe space in the healing room. It won't usually take more than a few months, and insurance companies are fine with bills that are no more than 6 months old. (Agencies are an entire other universe of completely colonized work that I'm not going to be able to address adequately in this book. Let's just say that subversion is much, much harder to pull off in an agency, other than by being very behind on one's paperwork, so sorry.) So let this part of first touch go at the speed it goes when you are able to take your foot off the gas, because it is foundational to creating safe-enough spaces.

EMPOWERED CONSENT: OUR COMMITMENTS TO CREATING SAFE-ENOUGH RELATIONSHIPS

Creating norms for safe enough in the healing space also includes verbal and written commitments by the healer in those required consent forms to not exploit this suffering and vulnerable person in any way. This means no physical touch of any kind, not even a hand over a hand, without consent, unless one is a body worker, in which case there must be very clear delineations of how touch will be offered for healing and absolutely no sexual or sexualized touch.

As I used to say to my students and interns about sexual touch: Not in this lifetime or any other lifetime or any other galaxy, even if the rules say that it's allowable 2 years after ending the work. Never. Not ever. Because if that door is open even a crack in your mind during your work with this suffering person, it will contaminate everything you do going forward, and healing will be corrupted in the service of getting to genital sexual contact.

We must promise to engage in no financial exploitation, which means never casually mentioning your favorite charity. Seriously, not even that. No playing subtly on the suffering person's vulnerabilities to indirectly coerce that person into participating in any aspect of the healing process that intuitively feels wrong to the trauma survivor—which means never saying, "This is the best evidence-based treatment, can you at least give it a try?" when they are telling you that this thing feels wrong, feels unsafe in their body.

This person in front of you is sometimes desperate to please you, in the fawn position of trauma neurobiology, wanting you to not toss them out, aching from broken attachments in their youngest years or from the time after their adult trauma experience, alone and alienated. They are desperate to find something resembling approval, with which they can soothe themselves for a moment. They are profoundly vulnerable. Heck, remember when it was you, dear readers—they are so much more desperate to get those crumbs of human connection, which our bodies intuitively sense to be sources of some kind of soothing, that their capacities to refuse something that they know will only cause more pain are locked up behind a sign inside of them that warns of the risk of lost connection if they say no. That desperation can be turned into an enormous box of something that's not safety if you don't realize that and tread lightly and include the right to refuse anything you ask, anything you suggest, in your consent form—with the exception of, no, you do not get to kill yourself or other people on my watch, and if you are thinking about harming a child, I am allowed to tell you no, do not put yourself in jeopardy by doing that.

IN WHICH MY STUDENT AND I LOOK INTO THE ABYSS TOGETHER AND PLANT A GARDEN

One of the pleasures of my work as a trainer and supervisor of DHCR thera- pists as they grow and develop has been working with one particular person who started with me over a decade ago as a practicum student. I have a vivid recollection of being at an airport boarding gate in Seattle, about to get on the flight, and getting a call from her on my cell. She was, atypically for her, freaked out because the person who had come up next in the clinic waiting list and thus came into her office for the first time the previous hour, had come out to her about his lifelong sexual attraction to children. "I don't know how to work with this," she said, which was also atypical for her, because she dove into the hardest places with people with an open, loving heart.

I did my supervisory due diligence, which was also part of my own com- mitment to protecting children from abuse, whether any law required me to do that or not. No, he had never touched a child. He had been sexually abused himself, and he had promised himself he would never do that to a child. No, he did not watch child pornography because he knew that he would be watching a child being abused. No, he did not masturbate to fantasies of children, or have pictures of children in his home, or even masturbate at all. He had taught himself to avoid places where children might be. He did not feel good about this attraction. He wanted help. He had never told anyone before he told this gifted therapist. He had, as it happened, figured out entirely on his own how to do the things that people convicted of sexually abusing children are taught in treatment.

We were a protodecolonial, intersectional feminist trauma-informed clinic for poor people, staffed by graduate students. Everything that happened there affected my license. I could have gone into risk management mode, but that would have undermined our philosophy as an organization. No child was at risk here.

Let's take a deep breath, I thought. I first affirmed how scary this was for her, because having a client come out with this kind of information is always scary to hear. I validated that she had done a very thorough job of risk assess- ment and that this man was clearly not a present risk to any children, so no report to children's services needed to be made. She could not report the abuse perpetrated on him, as he steadfastly refused to say who and where that had happened, 20 years in the past.

I asked her: Can you notice that what he is asking for is not to be shamed but to be joined in his goal of never hurting a child? This question, and my support for her, got her out of SNS fear arousal, silenced the critical voice in her head telling her she would get in trouble, and took her into her usual deep ventral vagal place of compassion for suffering humans. Why yes, she thought she could do that. Oh, wow, had this freaked her out, and now she could see that this man had come into her training life at our clinic for a good reason. "He is here so that I can deepen my ability to see people clearly. I got distracted by what he told me. And this man is traumatized, and . . ." I finished the sentence: "And the harm done to him is one that puts him in danger still, today, and is a source of terrible shame for him. And consequently, you know what to do, don't you?" My affirmation of her capacities was soothing, and also true. She did know what to do.

This woman still consults with me today, long after she ended her time at the clinic and finished school. This man has continued to work with her this entire time. Together they formed a safety plan for him, one that would keep him and children safe and allow him to never break his promise to the sexually abused child he had been, the promise to never harm another child in any way, including and especially in the way he had been harmed. In other words, we did not do risk prevention in the usual, colonized manner. Instead, we taught him that he deserved to live a life free of the trauma of moral injury, free from incarceration, and with compassion for the child he had been, who had suffered the terrible wound to his soul that the person who abused him had given him to hold.

He felt fully seen as someone who loved his work, which kept him far from children. He grew into a man who came to respect himself for being able, unlike the person who abused him, to distinguish between a desire and the acting out of that desire. He came, at long last, to love the sexually abused child he had been and to have compassion for how that abuse had distorted and corrupted his own sexuality. We did not try to refocus him on age-appropriate sexual partners because, as it turned out, he was both asexual and aromantic in his sexual and affectional orientations, a community of people who had only begun to make themselves known and to name themselves when he first sought care.

Together with this suffering man, his healer, who was held up by me and the rest of the clinic therapists, created a safe-enough space for him in which he could be joined in protecting himself from his wound. That wound has apparently diminished in its intensity over time, supplanted by a deep engagement with a nonsexual desire, the collection and cultivation of orchids. "My babies," he calls them, vulnerable and beautiful beings into which he can pour his intensity and his capacity for care—with no children involved.

AND STILL MORE CHALLENGES: THE VIOLENCE- AND OPPRESSION-FREE ZONE

Creating the safe-enough space also requires declaring the place where you work a violence-free zone. Some suffering people sometimes feel as if the only way to manage their intense feelings is to engage in violence against someone—themselves, the wall, something. The dominant culture models, and even lauds, violence, and many trauma-exposed people were subjected to someone using violence to apparently solve life's problems. Trauma-exposed people are not inherently at risk of behaving violently, a lie told by cultural narratives that stigmatize these suffering people. Safety cannot be unjust, however, and violence is injustice embodied.

What do I mean by a violence- and oppression-free zone? My version, as I explained it to people I worked with, was that, in my office, it was okay to get angry, to yell and scream, to rage, and it was not okay to verbally abuse themselves or anyone else who was in the room. So a person could say, "Laura, I hate you, you're a terrible therapist and this is hurting me," but could not threaten to hit me or call me a name. They could hurl epithets at an absent abuser as much as they wished. They could not threaten themselves nor call themselves a name. Anger is fine, violence is not anger, and this is a place where we do anger and don't do violence.

I would, at some point when it made sense in the healing process, talk about how some of their own suffering had its roots in being a target of microaggressions, daily assaults on their sense of safety, which I had perhaps inflicted on them or they on me or on themselves through internalized representations of trauma. I also spoke about how these ruptures in the relational fabric between us were inevitable because we were two humans talking about very hard things, and that, in this safer space, when one of us engaged in a microaggression, it would create an opportunity for it to be named and for us to repair, with me as the healer in the position of power, taking the lead in initiating the repair process, making the space safer still. Thus, also, the oppression-free zone in which we named the intrusions of social pathologies as they emerged.

I told the people who worked with me that it was okay to imagine behaving violently and to speak those fantasies out loud, after which we would explore whether we needed to make a safety plan so that no one ended up arrested. My rule was that people were free to destroy as much of the tissue in my office as they wished if the urge to destroy something or do harm became too over-whelming, since tissue is meant to end up in the trash.

I usually had six or eight large boxes of tissues stashed on a bookshelf, easy to get to and to destroy as needed. Shredding tissue became a regular feature of the healing work for some people. After the shredding of much tissue, we would together gather up the shreds and put them in the recycle bin, some-times, when this was a repeated experience, doing so as a ritual of letting toxins be transformed in the recycling plant.

No weapons could come into my office, which meant that law enforcement personnel who came to me for healing locked their weapons in their vehicles or left them at home or at work before coming to see me. It's not that I didn't trust them with the tools of their job; it's that there was one rule for everyone. No guns, no knives, no nunchucks, no throwing stars, no tasers, no pepper spray, not through my office door, because each of these things brought the energy of violence into a violence-free zone.

Some survivors of direct violence who carried one of these things with them at all times in order to feel prepared to defend themselves against the next attack felt as if this rule made them less safe, and they were often vocal about how that was the case. So we collaborated on a gradual process of moving away from those self-protective objects. If they drove, locking the item in a glove box and having me meet them at their vehicle and accompany them to my office, was healing time in which we paid attention together to how it felt not to have the instruments of self-protection with them and to have only me there as a protector. If they took public transportation (on which such items were, in fact, illegal), we immediately placed the item into my locked filing cabinet at the beginning of our time together and then explored how it felt that I was making my "no weapons" rule so important. Was this me abusing my power? Or was it something they had not experienced, the use of power to protect?

Few of these suffering people had ever inhabited, even for an hour a week, a violence-free zone. They might have grown up in a family where the adults were dangerous or unable to protect the children from dangerous adults. They might have grown up with incredibly protective parents in terribly violent zones of active social pathologies and thus lost any belief that they could be safe because the bullets were whizzing around daily. In every instance, there was little or no feeling of safety nor any trust in protection that was not some-thing concrete and dangerous that they could hold in their own hands. This was information, as we explored it, about the pain of unsafety in the core of trauma.

I did not ever ask people to stop possessing these tools unless they intended to do harm with them, to themselves or someone else, in which instance we would make safety plans to keep distance between them and the weapon. I did, in each instance, explore whether they had been trained in safe use and by whom, and if not, how to find smart training. I did explore children's possible access to these tools and the importance of having a weapons safe. None of the people who came to me with pepper spray hanging off their key rings or knives in sheaths under their jeans had ever used them, and the presence of the weapon soothed them, understandably. It also told me, as a healer, volumes about the depth of that person's fear, the intensity of their feelings of being trapped and helpless.

GETTING CLOSER TO SAFE, OR SAFE ENOUGH, OR SOMETHING RESEMBLING SAFER

Why is the topic of safety so central to DHCR work, and why such subtle and elaborate attention to what might seem like the far outer reaches of this topic? Because my best teachers, the suffering people who entrusted themselves to my care, inform this entire discussion and taught me all of this. I remind you of the quote about safety emerging from work done by Bethany Brand and her colleagues (2022, p. 142) mentioned in Chapter 3, if you prefer quantitative data such as has emerged from the Treatment of Patients With Dissociative Disorders study regarding work with highly dissociative people that she and her colleagues have been conducting for nearly 2 decades, and on which they report in *Finding Solid Ground: Overcoming Obstacles in Trauma and Treatment*.

Even though I myself had been raised with a heightened awareness of the fragility of safety, my phenotype skin privilege had overcome that knowing by the time I became a therapist. So I had to be reinstructed in the complexity of this dilemma of safety being an alien experience during my earliest work with people who I knew to be survivors of complex childhood trauma. There had been quite a few of those before the time when I was awakened to this experience, suffering people for whom I didn't have the construct yet, and with whom I was less than healing, in my opinion.

These folks had never been safe during their childhoods. They were in danger every minute they were with their families or sometimes their places of worship, or their schools, or their sports teams, wherever the inescapable predators—adults or much older kids—were. Even if there was a place of temporary safety, such as in a classroom where there was a caring teacher or on a hiking trail with no humans around, these children always had to return to the locations of more persistent danger and disconnection—the homes in which they lived with dangerous adults, the youth groups and sports teams and drama clubs where the predators and exploiters ruled.

Not that any child, not matter how loved, is entirely safe, as the parents grieving their small children mowed down in school massacres by a country that loves its guns more than it loves its children are forced to discover. Until that horrific moment of their deaths, until the minutes of terror preceding the end of their lives as they heard shots ringing out, saw classmates or teachers fall bleeding, many of these murdered children had experiences of emotional safety in their families, which feels like being safe. Their classmates who survive don't get to have a just world hypothesis or a belief in safety ever again, nor do the grieving parents left behind.

These suffering people with childhoods from hell who came to me in the early 1980s, before I understood what I was doing, carried in the very marrow of their bones a powerful felt sense that all humans were likely to be unsafe for them at some point, which of course made the process of healing seem nearly impossible. As one person said, "Therapist is the-rapist, don't you know?"

Walking through the door of my office required astonishing courage. Staying in the room, week after week, required even more as they laid themselves open to me, never knowing with certainty when their worst fears would be proven true and I would turn into a source of danger, despite all of my blathering on about safety plans. Deconstructing the terrors evoked by the comments made to many such people by their primary health care provider—"make an appointment with a psychotherapist, here's a referral"—could itself take an entire book.

I soon was schooled by these brave souls into the knowledge that asking these suffering people to visualize their safe place for our trauma work was not a reasonable request. Duh, said the voices of my grandparents inside of me, what took you so long to remember what we told you? For these suffering people, safety was an illusion, a hope that was dangerous to even imagine. For some of them, the very mention of safety by me opened doors to rage, grief, and, frequently, the profound sense that I would never entirely understand them. Because how could I if I would be ignorant, unattuned enough to ask them to imagine something that they knew was both nonexistent and dangerous to imagine.

Several suffering people I had the privilege to work with come powerfully to mind as I reread these words. On the surface, their lives looked like ones of privilege. Behind closed doors, at home, they were always in danger—danger of being raped, of someone attempting to murder them, of being starved, of being locked in a basement for the whole weekend, of being hurt terribly in ways that didn't show under long sleeves and tights. All the people of whom I'm thinking had privilege deep in their obvious intersectional identities: Christian European backgrounds, pale skin, upper-middle- to middle-class status, fathers with advanced degrees and prestigious jobs. When they tried to tell the truth to a teacher or a scout leader, no one ever believed them because of that privilege; White, Christian, upper-middle-class fathers and mothers didn't do these things, that kid sure has an active imagination. Their pain went deep underground, with the help of various substances, of overwork, of overexercise, of restricting food just enough to feel in control, of inflicting cuts and burns on their bodies in places that did not show, taking a cue from the adults who were harming them.

The people in this collective picture of childhood in hell all had explosive reactions to my asking them to think of a safe place, this being before I caught on that I was asking an unwise question. One of them stomped out of the office and sent me a scathing email. One shut down, resulting in a very young ego state emerging, pleading with me not to hurt her. Another said, "Sure, fine, whatever," and then it took me about 6 months to repair the rupture. I was being schooled in how safety is not a real thing in the lives of many traumatized people. I later realized that I was also being schooled in the illusions about safety that my culture had adopted upon our arrival to the United States, where we believed that Jew-hatred would not emerge as it had for two millennia in the Christian, and later, Muslim worlds.

Suggesting safety frequently led to ruptures in relationships that could take many sessions to repair. I paid attention, began to appreciate that if nothing and no one has been safe, that a DHCR trauma healer (or in the case of the younger me, one in early stages of development) has to meet people where they are and find the words for "as close to safe as you can imagine" (often expressed by some suffering people as visualizing oneself on a different planet entirely, one inhabited by no humans whatsoever).

Omnipresent Danger

There are layers to this dilemma of creating spaces that are closer to safe or safe enough in order to do the work of trauma healing. There are plentiful other sources of persistent danger and risk that are not due to horrific and repeated trauma of childhood. These are the dangers created by structural hierarchies of oppression, the social pathologies generating omnipresent forms of risk for walking while Black, urinating while trans, using a parking garage while a woman, violating the rules of structural and systemic oppression.

When a person begins to shed their emotional protective gear, even for an hour a week in your office, the DHCR healer has a moral responsibility to offer collaboration for walking out the door into the social pathologies of everyday life with something protective in place. Part of creating safety in the healing space is attention to developing new and potentially more liberatory and powerful means of self-protection so that a person seeking healing can begin to simply move about in the world without being frozen in terror as they increasingly know, thanks to the trauma healing process, what they feel and how terrified they always are. As I used to say on my consent form, you might feel strong feelings that you have been unable to feel or avoiding. Feeling those feelings can leave a person feeling stripped of their emotional raincoat. A task for a DHCR healer is not mending the raincoat, which was often cobbled together by accident or borrowed from someone else, but rather collaborating on creating one tailor-made for this suffering person, woven out of the strengths emerging from their intersectional identities, custom-built acid-proofing.

In my own work to build a liberatory and decolonial model of trauma practice I have realized how urgent it is that I ignore neither the more overt manifestations of dangers arising from systemic social pathologies nor the effects of the more subtle, daily ways in which those social pathologies create a psychosocial environment for many people in which safety is always relative and easily stolen. It is simple to notice a hate crime. Hate crimes are large, loud, and violent. It is equally essential, for decolonial trauma healing, to notice how people, in their various intersectional identities, are persistently in harm's way and affected in their psyches and bodies by having to continuously cope with lurking dangers. Thus it's equally necessary to not send suffering people out of our healing spaces stripped bare of all that assists them in being safer enough in the quotidian.

Allowing Ourselves to Know That We, Too, Are Not Immune

For those of us whose intersectional identities have provided some kind of temporary protection against the workings of social pathologies, an awakening to the illusory nature of safety is an emotional capacity required for doing DHCR trauma healing work. This is a capacity that can be developed and deepened. DHCR trauma healing work requires of the healer this kind of painful awakening from many slumbers. It demands that we not turn away from, minimize, or make excuses for social pathologies or pretend that we do not ourselves, at times, embody or enact them.

DHCR trauma healing work necessitates developing an eye that can identify trauma created by the swords of Damocles that hang over so many humans, to trust when someone tells us that they experience one of those swords hanging over them even when we are unable to perceive it because our own positionalities place it out of our view.

Instead of diagnosing their distress as psychopathology, our DHCR healing work requires a close and collaborative engagement around the question of which of a person's intersectional identities may have rendered them targets of marginalization, subjugation, or violence by social pathologies. Those are the junctures at which the person knows, or tries not to know, the presence of chronic risk to safety, to connection, to personhood. The privilege of not paying attention awarded to those of us whose intersectional identities came with the false promises of safety and power in the structural hierarchies of oppression is antithetical our doing liberatory DHCR trauma healing.

A bystander who looks away cannot do DHCR work. We must, for the work to be just, be engaged, outraged, allowing ourselves to feel the danger that the suffering people who seek our care feel. And we must allow ourselves to admit to and feel our own absences of safety. We must disabuse ourselves of the lies that came bundled with that privilege, whatever they were, and turn toward, rather than away from, the truth of this suffering person's experiences, toward truths about the world. Thus, no more neutral position of "trauma is trauma is trauma."

I Heard the News Today, Oh Yeah . . .

My African American colleague, a natal man, large of body and very dark-skinned, has been pulled over by police more times than he can count in his almost 7 decades of life, each time wondering if this is the day that he will die by the side of a road, executed by law enforcement for the crime of driving while Black. My friends and I, natal women, nonbinary people born with a vulva, trans folks, and femme-of-center gay men, all of us breathe sighs of relief when we get into our cars and electronically lock all the doors, but only after having looked carefully to insure that there is no one in the backseat, and this after having walked to the car with our keys out to use as a weapon against a potential attacker. Few of the people in my personal circle have been raped— yet or to my knowledge, except one who was, almost daily, as a child, by a parent. The woman who was the 2023 president of the American Psychological Association has been raped (Bryant-Davis, 2005) and has been vocally transparent about that. A dear young relative was raped in her adolescent years. It is likely that, once this book is published, some of you who know me will let me know that you have been raped too. We live in the omnipresent trauma lurking in the social pathology of systemic misogyny in which a rape is always possible.

The news is with us always now. It is replete with stories of the loss of what was thought to be finally safely held by marginalized people: the stripping away of all women's bodily autonomy, the bodily autonomy of natal female nonbinary people born with a vulva, of trans men who have kept the uterus and ovaries with which they were born because they would like to bear a child someday, by the *Dobbs* decision. The news is with us always, in the palms of our hands, the screens of our phones, 24 hours a day. It activates retraumatization for women who had abortions at risk to their lives, at risk of being arrested, before it was made, for a brief half century, legal; women looking down the maw of a terrifying day in their lives that they thought the younger generation to be safe from. The news is in our faces, perpetually. It is a reminder to the friends of the women that died, septic, because they tried to end their pregnancies with a sharp wire jabbed through their cervixes, that those days of being in danger have returned.

The news is always there, now, inescapable. It is the new of trans kids and adolescents living in states proclaiming that they must urinate in the school restrooms of their natal sex, no matter how long they have been living socially in the genders they know themselves to be, which will open them up to bullying and harassment in the hallways of their schools. That they can no longer receive the care that has eased their minds as their sex phenotype is assisted to become congruent with their phenomenological experiences of gender. Think what you may about children who socially transition. Some of these children's parents are fleeing their homes to protect their children's emotional safety, to keep their kids from becoming part of the statistics about high suicide rates in gender-nonconforming adolescents. The news follows us like some of kind of malign spirit. It speaks to us of new laws reminding every gender-nonconforming person that they must live with some level of chronic traumatic terror simply because they wish to empty their bladder. Not safe enough simply to pee.

The news is there in every language, in every medium. It is the life story of a Persian Baha'i refugee who has too many security cameras in his little store because he knows that his brown skin and Farsi accent place him, ironically, at risk of Islamophobic violence from local White supremacist and xenophobic people. His potential persecutors in this Euro-American world do not know that his faith is the one most persecuted by Muslims, and they do not care to distinguish between Farsi and Arabic, knowing only that he is Middle Eastern, thus the other, a legitimate target of their ideological violence. The news recycles the stories of social pathologies being enacted. It tells us the story of another brown-skinned man accosted and beaten nearly to death on the street not far from his store, an attack heard by this man who is living with a chronically activated trauma-response neurobiology, creating the stress leading to the heart condition that threatens his life just as surely as did the government of the Islamic Republic of Iran from which he fled for his life. He is safe in the United States from being judicially murdered for his faith. He is not safe in the United States from the risk of death due to enacted racism and xenophobia. Not safe enough.

The news to which I awoke on October 7th, 2023. The story of something that was supposed to never again happen, a terrible pogrom inflicted in a place that is dear to me. The wave of anti-Semitism that has followed, leading me to ask my non-Jewish friends, for the first time in my life, "Would you hide me if they start coming for the Jews?" The news of the lasting effects of that day, coming from my friends at the desert university where I was scheduled to teach in December 2023, of their friends murdered and taken hostage, of their children called up into the reserves. The news of their latest protests, their pain at how their government is conducting its war in their names.

The working-class, Euro-American, natal male machinist with just enough seniority that he still has a job, a man who left high school for that good factory job, wakes up each morning after a troubled sleep trying not to notice his dread as his coworkers are laid off by the new corporate hedge fund overlords that have bought out the appliance manufacturing plant where he labors. In the news, plants are closing in an industry he's worked in for 30 years. The news says that the new owners are "right-sizing" the workforce. They're closing the places that have voted to unionize.

When he awakens, it is from a troubled sleep interrupted by his wondering, at two in the morning, when he too will be cashing his last paycheck. He suffers, watching old friends made redundant (the more accurate British terminology for the corporate disposal of the working class), nodding in the stupor of opioids. He sees his neighbors mourning the latest overdose death among their adolescent offspring. The trauma of being the castoff, of the social pathology of rogue capitalism, with all of these manifestations, is not something that allows him to ever feel safe again.

Yet because of his intersectional identities, as a natal male, gender-conforming, heterosexual Euro-American, worshiping in a church, living since birth in the state of Indiana, because of all of these nonmarginalized and nonsubordinated intersectional identities that promised him privilege and safety, he is vulnerable to being misled into believing that all of this background terror, all of this loss has nothing to do with corporate billionaires and instead has everything to do with immigrants coming in to take away jobs. He had an illusion of safety, and because it is woven into the fiber of his intersectional identities, the cognitive dissonance generated by being unsafe when his very identity is "I am safe" feels intolerable. The piece of his intersectional identities that is "machinist" did not signal vulnerability to him—nor should it have in a context not affected by the toxins of rogue capitalism.

So his activated SNS exposes the truths living in his body, of social pathologies that he has been taught are protecting him. He has been taught that a real man does not express fear. So his fear is expressed as anger, as xenophobic thoughts and words, making him a potential danger to other, more marginalized and subordinated people in a country where it's too simple to arm oneself with weapons of war; making him a danger to himself, because if he enacts his terror on the body of another person, he might find himself incarcerated, while the hedge fund managers buy another yacht.

How does a liberatory DHCR trauma healer work with someone who has not only had the core of his life ripped away but has also been, and continues to be, lied to about who did the ripping away? How do we hold the space, witness, have compassion for his rage and what sounds like his entitlement, particularly when he identifies with those who have betrayed him—people who share most of his intersectional identities aside from the one that matters here, the one where he has been disempowered and lied to, the identity of his social class? DHCR healing practice invites us to interrogate how we've thought about privilege, to think about the complexities of intersectional identities and not become fixated on what's easy to see, which is usually some kind of phenotype privilege.

8 DECOLONIZING MYTHS OF SAFETY, PART II

We ended the previous chapter with a brief discussion of the problematic nature of the construct of safety when applied to decolonial, humble, culturally responsive (DHCR) trauma healing work. In this chapter I hope to deepen that discussion. We're going to start where one might least expect us to—with the problem of safety for people who appear, because of their visible intersectional identities, their genital sex, and melanic phenotype privileges, to be safe per se and thus in no need of having safety addressed in any detail before moving on to the index traumatic event. Nothing could be further from the truth. The instability of privilege carries within it an inherent knowledge of the absence of safety, even when a person appears to construct their life around a facade of being safe. I invite you to join me in considering the subtle ways in which aspects of intersectionality affect the first step of DHCR healing, the step of getting as close to safe as possible. When we can see the subtle, we are better equipped to respond to that which seems obvious.

How can a DHCR trauma healer, who, based on my 40 years of observing the folks developing this standpoint, is likely to place themselves squarely in the territory of the progressive world, have a truly healing conversation with someone whose very ability to think critically has been devoured by the

https://doi.org/10.1037/0000421-009
Decolonizing Trauma Healing: Toward a Humble, Culturally Responsive Practice,
by L. S. Brown

toxins of social pathologies and who is not a person from a knowable marginalized group, perhaps even someone spouting the lies of a social pathology? How can we neither judge nor blame, nor be distracted by biased words, by the repetition of lies told by charismatic leaders, or by having grown up steeped in potent forms of phenotype privilege that convey a message that you are safe, that whisper, safe so long as you follow the rules and make sure that everyone else is following them?

When we, our lives and our work, have been focused on the experiences of the most vulnerable, marginalized, and subjugated people, it's unsurprising that we can be lacking in compassion for such folks. We say to them (and to one another), "Check your privilege." Our tone when we offer this or similar verbal correction, like a yank on a dog's leash, is usually of contempt, not compassion. We forget that the poison of being plunged into poverty when comfort in one's last years had been promised because of that very conditional admission to privilege, of being betrayed by rogue capitalism that promised you that it was your friend, and stripped of dignity by having the work of your hands replaced by that of a machine—any and all of these can overpower the illusory, faux-safety promised to those with double phenotype privilege. It's often about social class, because many of those traumatized by rogue capitalism happen to be working class, at the mercy of rogue capitalism. Their alleged privilege has become an empty vessel, a bucket with a hole in it that cannot be repaired with the tools they are allowed to have available to them, no matter how skillfully they attempt to solve the problem of this hole, MacGyvering the heck out of it with no solution—so many blame the hole on those who might have just found a bucket without a hole or who have spent generations learning how to weave baskets, sturdier than a bucket and easier to repair. When these folks hear those of us in the decolonial world speak of privilege, they feel invisible, insulted, microaggressed against—traumatized by our narratives, and poised to take revenge somehow.

It is not that these elements of intersectionality, held by those with double phenotype privilege (e.g., White-skinned and natal male), are not ways that make people who look like him less unsafe, in general, than a woman, or a Black, Indigenous, or person of color (BIPOC), or queer person. In general, this person is safer when he walks around in the world. Realistically, such double phenotype intersectionalities shield against some kinds of danger in the quotidian more often than not. If stopped by law enforcement, a person with double phenotype privilege is likely to survive the encounter. When entering a parking garage this person is probably not thinking about being raped. If, as DHCR healers, we pay attention only to what we see on the surface, we can get distracted from looking at the entire intersectional picture, and we are consequently, sometimes rudely, reminded that we ignore the whole of a person's intersectionalities. We are at risk of seeing vulnerabilities and experiences of marginalization and subordination inherent in a given person's intersectionalities at peril both to healing work with this person and to the project of truly trying to blow up the master's house. Which we are trying to do, right?

THE GREAT SAFETY RACKET OF SOCIAL PATHOLOGIES

For genuine decolonial work to proceed, it requires understanding that almost no one who gets to capital-*S* safety and is allowed to stay there. This is the false promise of the entwined venomous snakes of patriarchy and melanic supremacy, that if one is either a member of the group or conditionally admitted to those groups, one will be safe. Not cannon fodder. Not permanently laid off. Both of which happen, repeatedly, to the conditionally admitted, those who are blue-collar or poor, those for whom joining the military seems to be the only path to a college degree, those who are in the closet so as not to be passed over for promotion, those who have changed their names and joined a Unitarian church and moved across the country from their Jewish relatives or the Black side of the family.

A DHCR healer needs to understand and then bring into their work the truth that there can be the states of closer to safe, safer, and safe enough for now. This radical acceptance of the imperfection and impermanence of safety requires an analysis coding that those reciting or enacting the truisms of social pathologies are also likely to be suffering from traumas inflicted by those pathologies— suffering differently, but suffering nonetheless. Betrayal trauma, in many cases, is betrayal of the promise of illusory safety, if only one plays by the rules of the colonizer game.

Simply because the trauma inherent in double phenotype privilege manifests in ways that are sometimes inexplicable or invisible at first to a DHCR healer, and often in ways that are harmful to other vulnerable people (e.g., proving one's manhood through acts of violence against the woman with whom one is in an intimate relationship), does not mean that we cannot see the forces of social pathologies doing harm to these traumatized humans and find ways to creatively engage with those internalized lies.

Levant (1998) has written eloquently of something he called "normative male alexithymia." Alexithymia, the inability to know and put words to what one feels, is also a normative embodied expression of having been exposed to trauma. If it's normative for natal men, humans with the core phenotype privilege of patriarchy, what can a DHCR healer derive from that picture other than the knowledge that this person's body is screaming trauma at the world?

No One Is Unscathed

As Albert Memmi (1965) presciently noted in his analysis of the psychic effects of the Tunisian and Algerian revolutions, no parties in those conflicts escaped psychic wounds. Colonizers, in order to justify their violence against the people, languages, religions, and cultures of the colonized piece of land, developed rationalizations and justifications for their actions, tricks of the mind that they knew, emotionally, to be untrue. They had to tolerate their own loss of integrity, the violation of values they proclaimed to hold dear. They had to practice continuous denial of the pain they were inflicting, to shut down their capacities for empathy. They had to individually and collectively engage in some form of dissociation from the emotions of shame and empathy that would, and sometimes did, break through when the truth of the colonizing process becomes unavoidable.

So the colonizers have symptoms, which are information about being colonizers, the thing that Jonathan Shay (1994), writing about soldiers who served in America's wars in Southeast Asia, later called "moral injury." To be an oppressor one must violate one's own values and integrity, and unless one is that rare sociopath, this is a betrayal of self from which one is never safe. Being safe enough, ironically, involves being able to live in congruence with oneself and one's values, which can sometimes be easier when one has little to lose by telling truths.

Knowing Unsafety Is Inconvenient

Colonized persons of all kinds, both those physically colonized and those whose psychic colonization results from chronic exposure to social pathologies, must also find ways to go about their daily lives. They must do so without having conscious access to the painful knowledge of the danger in which they continuously live, the tenuousness of whatever faux safety they have found for themselves. Knowing cannot intrude into their consciousness too frequently. From the outside, this unknowing may look like passive acquiescence or assimilation, some strategies we discussed in several earlier chapters. Internally, however, the colonized person is simply striving to find safe-enough, somehow, enough of the time.

Sneaky, Sneaky, Sneaky

It is simply not possible to provide a complete list of examples of systemic absence of safety, of persistent presence of impending danger that can strike at any time and without warning, of threats to connection and love, of chronic traumatic terror, of lies and illusions that vanish into the smog of social pathology. That list is too long, and more facets of it are uncovered daily. The dangers inherent in social pathologies are an omnipresent shadow lurking in almost every person's psychic background. This is a phenomenon that should inform the work of all DHCR trauma healers: the sun shines, the seas rise and fall with the tides (even as they rise and warm dangerously with climate change), and social pathologies endanger people in ways too many to list, all of the time, in ways we can perceive, in ways we cannot yet perceive. This all affects our efforts to create a space in which it is safe enough to do our work. Thus a DHCR healer continuously considers what might create that which is other than safe and what might constitute closer to safe, in all of their work with a suffering person and in their own daily life. Closer to safe is not static; ask anyone living in Kyiv on February 1, 2022, or in Kibbutz Nahal Oz on October 6, 2023. Those people were aware that safety was not promised; they had no idea, on those days, just how unsafe they were, nor how much trauma and terror, would enter their lives a mere 24 hours later.

With the rise of social media, the swipe of a finger across a device's screen reveals, in real time, the kind of terrifying news to which I referred in Chapter 7, news of how someone like us has been harmed, of how someone plans to harm us, the objective definitions of Root's (1992) prescient construct of insidious traumatization now ramped up by the 24-hour news cycle. For each one of these overt episodes that makes it onto some media platform there are millions of humans watching these stories and saying some form of "this could have been me," feeling the tentacles of terror reaching into their safe-enough lives.

Insidious traumatization is the not the realization that one's own life or physical safety is at risk but rather the definitely traumatic experience generated when we witness or learn of danger descending on those who resemble us, no matter that the target is a stranger located far away from us in physical space. I hadn't been to a lesbian bar or any kind of queer bar in about 40 years, but the mass hate crime murders at Club Q in 2022 and at Pulse in 2016 filled me with fear and brought me into a state of deep grief. It could have been me. Likewise, I only occasionally step foot inside of a synagogue, since my LGBTQ Jewish group mostly meets in people's homes. The shooting at Tree of Life synagogue in 2018 hovers over me every time I step through similar doors, thousands of miles away from that massacre, past the armed guards that can now be found at the doors of every synagogue in town, every Hillel organization on every college campus. Insidious traumatization: "It could have been me, but instead it was you."

A DHCR trauma healing framework thus operates from the starting point that almost all suffering people seeking our care, even those who do not carry the label of a "trauma survivor" likely have been and continue to be insidiously traumatized, with this being more the case the more intrusive the news becomes via the explosion of outlets for its transmission. This phenomenon contributes to the strongly felt sense experienced by many people that safety is illusory. One may not have a full-blown experience of chronic trauma terror to experience chronic insidious traumatization and the vague sense that one has never stepped over the finish line into the land of safety.

NO LONGER IMPLICIT: BIAS TURNED VIOLENT, AGAIN

Increasingly, overt verbal and material expressions of the social pathologies of fascism, White supremacy, anti-Semitism, misogyny, heterosexism, transphobia, imperialism, and rogue capitalism, among many others, have become part of today's new normal. Words that would get a politician thrown out of office in 2015 are now uttered regularly by those in positions of power who believe they have impunity. The unleashing of hate speech from national leaders and their many followers offers trauma healers more frequent examples of how marginalized and subordinated people cannot count on being safe, if ever we had such an illusion.

When I wrote *Cultural Competence in Trauma Therapy* (2008), I had, like many of my colleagues, naively bought into the notion that overt expressions of bias were fading away, no longer socially acceptable, to be replaced with implicit bias which healers needed to uncover and address within ourselves. As a group, progressives in the social sciences were so very naive; so very seduced by the progressive cultures of which we were a part, so willing to marginalize the hate speakers as about to fade away. We had no idea of the depth and breadth of the hate media universe; we hadn't heard of Steve Bannon or Alex Jones. We didn't know that a thing called Christian nationalism had only gone underground, not gone away. Now it's back, loud and strong and in control of not just a few state legislatures in 2024. We were naive because we read mostly within our own intellectual universes. A result was that few of us knew the importance of delving into this other universe in which hate speech and hate acts are praised and lies are the currency selling guns and nutritional supplements.

Implicit bias is very much still there, and perhaps has gone further underground in the psyches of folks drawn to any sort of DHCR work because the unleashing of overt bias, embodied in the practitioners of explicit social pathologies, has escalated rapidly since the middle of the second decade of this century with no sign of decline in sight—in fact, quite the contrary. Hate speech, trolling on social media, and proclamations posted by current and former holders of powerful positions in the world is increasing exponentially. Power has welcomed hate to its dinner table, on some media outlets every night of the year, and that hate is proclaimed all good, delicious, truthful, while anything battling the forces of that hate has come under increased scrutiny and denigration, in the media, in the halls of legislatures, on the streets.

This foregrounding and embrace of overt bias is occurring not only in the Western world but anywhere that some component of intersectional identities transforms itself into an arm of oppression. India was colonized by the British. Descendants of those colonized people, Narendra Modi and the Baharatiya Janata Party, have created a Hindu-themed fascist social pathology that has infiltrated the intellectual and social realities of India, enabling terrorizing and at times killing of non-Hindus. The colonized become the colonizers; the formerly marginalized and subordinated adopt the tactics of their colonizers to, in turn, terrorize the new other. Myanmar, formerly Burma, also colonized by the British, has engaged in genocidal practices against its Rohingya minority group.

The psychosocial environment across the planet has become more knowably unsafe as political figures in positions of power lead the way in uttering expressions of disdain and devaluation for the lives, bodies, and experiences of marginalized and subordinate groups and persons and the internet exposes us to the 24/7 cycle of that news. More today than in decades since the defeat of Nazi Germany and fascism in Italy, political and religious leaders appear to be exploiting their power in the social order to disinhibit violence and praise its perpetrators. This in turn creates many more opportunities for being insidiously traumatized because of so many more well-publicized enactments of social pathologies, so easily accessible through so many forms of media. As I sometimes say to friends, it's not that things are getting worse. It's that we know more quickly that things are getting worse.

For a DHCR trauma healer, creating something resembling safety in the midst of these realities presents a real challenge. It requires us to declare our healing spaces to be violence- and oppression-free zones, spaces protected by all parties who enter there. As I mentioned in Chapter 7, I was going to spend more time on that topic, and here we are.

HEALERS MUST BE SAFE, TOO

Safe enough also means safe enough for the healer. My consent form said that a person who did or threatened violence to me, my family, or my space would no longer be able to continue to work with me because I would have become unsafe to work with them. They could be angry and yell at me about what a horrible person I was. They could not threaten harm to me, nor could I to them, which meant that all conversations about going to an inpatient setting occurred, with one sadly necessary exception where the safety of a third party was at risk, without involving any external authority.

Safe enough for the DHCR trauma healer means modeling for the suffering trauma survivor that both parties have a right to privacy boundaries, a component of psychic safety, as well. We each get to decide what we will share and how and on what schedule—thus, as described in Chapter 7, there was no intake interview but instead an invitation for the person in distress to tell their story in their own way, at their own pace. I am aware that, for those of you who work in systems that require an intake form be filled out by the end of the first session, this liberatory approach might lead to problems with those above you in your work hierarchy and that my thoughts reflect the privileged setting of an independent healing practice. One person who worked with me, who was both a traumatized person and a member of the staff of the local community mental health factory, and who shared my perspectives, told me that she had allowed herself to be perceived as "very absentminded, I just keep forgetting to get those forms filled in," making sure that her clinical work was at its usual high standard so that her work evaluations always averaged out to okay. She finally realized that, despite her social justice commitment to working in that setting and seeing people as poor as she had been growing up, she didn't feel safe there—not unsafe from the people who brought their pain to her but unsafe from the attitudes and practices of management—and she left.

Safe enough for healers means knowing that they have the right and responsibility to model leaving a relationship that is not being a safe enough place for them. The right and power of a worker to determine their workplace conditions, which rogue capitalism would like to demolish, is not abrogated when that worker is a trauma healer. If we initiate the end of a relationship because we are caring for our own safety, we carefully assess how best to do this; no one size fits all here. We do this in a humble and nonaccusatory manner, with compassion, and with clarity. We might say, "I am not going to work with you any longer. I can't imagine how painful it might feel to you to hear this. I want us to discuss how we will end our relationship within the next [time period] and support your transition to work with another healer." The time period needs to be short enough to keep the healer safe enough, long enough to establish care elsewhere unless you have consulted with a colleague who agrees that you must refer only to an agency, where whoever sees the person has slightly more institutional support than you do if you're in private practice. If you're already in an agency, be clear with your supervisor about your risk assessment and remember that they are paid slightly more than you are to help you figure out a solution. Expect anger. If you feel unsafe physically with this person, have the conversation with someone else in the room and the door open, and be honest about why you're doing things this way. Expect anger for a long time and crappy reviews on therapist review sites (I can tell who writes the negative ones about me, still angry 20 years after I said that there was not enough of me to go around for one of her, and myself too, and everyone else. I'm mostly just glad that this person is still alive).

If the trauma survivor is the one firing you, honor their felt sense that you are not right for them rather than making that awareness into resistance or avoidance or some other pathologizing set of psychic shackles which many of us have used to protect our own egos. Set the first touch, the second touch, the subsequent touches, as a liberatory DHCR trauma healer who creates the norm that we will get as safe as we are able in the time we are together and depart from one another; last touch, when it becomes clear to either party that safety is not possible for one or both of us in this relationship.

PHYSICALLY CLOSER TO SAFE

There are other strategies for creating safe-enough physical spaces for healing. Buildings in which we work must be accessible to those who cannot climb stairs or drive a car. The neighborhoods in which we situate should, when possible, have a mix of people on the streets that will make no one into an easily visible other. The public restrooms in our buildings should include gender-neutral spaces so that no one feels unsafe when they need a bathroom, and part of our ethical responsibilities as DHCR trauma healers is to advocate with a landlord for the creation of such restrooms, which my pre-DHCR trauma training clinic successfully accomplished well before this was a norm. If we work with a therapy animal, we must ensure that it is well-trained and contained in its crate unless and until the trauma survivor invites that four-legged healer to join them. Our furniture should be comfortable for a wide range of bodies and neurobiologies, which means paying attention to what people tell us about their sensory experiences. If someone needs to wear sunglasses and noise-canceling headphones in our office because these make it safer in their brain, be curious as to how they learned to care for that brain so well and see that as a capacity that the two of you can draw upon as part of this healing work.

We should investigate rates of reported sexual assaults and hate crimes in our office neighborhood, using law enforcement data that are now frequently easily available online in larger cities. This will not give a clear or accurate picture of actual rates, as most such crimes are not reported, nonetheless, if we are considering renting office space in an environment with comparatively high rates of either of these kinds of crimes of social pathologies, then we need to stop and consider what that will mean for trauma survivors as they come and go, whether or not their trauma was due to sexual violence or hate.

We also need to inquire of ourselves about how our healing modalities might privilege or exclude people whose abilities, bodies, or intersectionalities do not fit nicely within the protocols that we have been taught to use. Writing as someone who has used eye movement desensitization reprocessing (EMDR) since 1995 and found it helpful to many people, I know that for some people with whom I worked it was painfully dismantling and dysregulating, so with them I did not use it a second time. For some persons on the autism spectrum, an insistence on their identifying what they feel in their body because you are a somatic practitioner of some kind can lead to sensory overload, which is itself a kind of internal trauma of the nervous system. In vivo exposure therapies can worsen distress for some trauma-exposed people when being safe enough, closer to safe, or safer have not been firmly established for that suffering individual.

Our commitment to engaging in DHCR liberatory trauma healing includes doing our best to work in healing spaces that do not privilege particular bodies or persons with specific intersectional identities, nor put such bodies or persons at greater risk of becoming less than safe simply because they must make a physical journey to our office, as is beginning to occur with increasing frequency in some, but not all places, depending on the culture and norms of the place regarding telehealth and in-person services. A liberatory DHCR stance for creating physical environments that are safer, closer to safe, as safe as we can be for now means simply that we commit do our best, which will be an imperfect best, given our humanity, to consciously and mindfully consider all of these factors as we build a space for healing.

THE FOOTPRINTS OF NEVER SAFE ENOUGH: NOT A SYMPTOM OF PATHOLOGY

Both colonizers, who are the creators and perpetrators of social pathologies, and the colonized, those targeted by systemic forms of oppression and danger, find ways to deny the realities of chronic and persistent danger arising from social pathologies so as to maintain the social, political, and interpersonal order. We turn away from what we see and hear being done to others, from what was done to us, from what we have done to others, from what we reenact on ourselves. When the truth breaks through the layers of looking away, covering our ears, doing what we can to not know, we often experience acute and intense distress, both as individual humans and in the body politic. Consequently, most of the time, the truth is dissociated from our individual and collective awareness in one form or another.

This avoidance, denial, or dissociation all express themselves as what are called, in formal diagnostic manuals, the symptoms of numbing, avoidance, or dissociation arising from trauma exposure, expressions of dorsal vagal shutdown of some sort. A decolonial perspective is that these so-called symptoms are not evidence of something wrong in the person. They are information about ways in which social pathologies have wounded a human in the various Venn diagrams of their intersectional identities and about the strategies they have employed in order to get on with their life somehow. When the exposure to the toxins of social pathologies is chronic, a person may need to escalate the strength of the psychic numbing or analgesic substance in order to keep moving.

Because these manifestations of a person's strategy for being able to simply be in the world eventually work less and less well, such that the person cannot avoid the pain or the consequences of however they are unknowing oppression and trauma, a DHCR trauma healer, while seeking to alleviate pain, is not focused on getting rid of symptoms alone, although we are absolutely committed to the reduction of pain. We are equally interested in and curious about what these manifestations of the attempts to unknow tell both the sufferer and the healer about what it is that someone is trying their best not to know about, which often is the degree to which the person is not safe, not even close to safe.

A wise colleague, with whom I disagree about much, once said something very true to me, that most of the distress people brought to her was about their avoidance of the threat-to-life trauma that they had experienced. She believed that simply getting people to tolerate exposure to things reminiscent of that trauma would heal them, "stop avoiding the avoidance," in her words. She was, not surprisingly, a huge fan of prolonged exposure therapy as the only way to go with trauma-exposed people, which was our point of disagreement. I encountered one of her former clients in my forensic work, who said, "I never could tell that therapist the truth, that things were just getting worse every time I did what she suggested. So I shined her on and said I was fine and quit . . . and I haven't been back to therapy since because I'm afraid that another therapist is going to do the same thing." This very caring, committed trauma therapist, a pioneer, had created a trauma reenactment with this suffering person. Yes, in healing trauma we must touch it. But how? Perhaps by taking the advice of an emerging voice in our field, Bailey (2023), whose wise paradigm is that the first touch, that first hello, is exposure and needs to be treated as part of the healing process.

Would that it were that simple: touching that which has been avoided, doing so again and again, when the trauma itself is both pernicious and ubiquitous. This can at times be almost intolerable, which is why addressing the question of how to assist people to a safe enough, closer to safe place in their lives is so foundational to the work of DHCR trauma healing before making any decisions about what is the right way to embark on the remainder of the healing process, of the path to touching the trauma, the speed, the force, the intensity of that touch. We have to make hello closer to safe.

Addressing the elusive nature of safety and telling the truth to ourselves that pure safety is illusory must come first. This process of radical acceptance of the brittle nature of safety, of its changing face, requires sometimes difficult internal work for the DHCR trauma healer. We have to learn how, within ourselves, to find balance between truth about danger and the capacity to create sufficient safety in our lives to have this balance as part of our own lived experience, as something we feel in our bodies and live in our daily existence. Only when we can do that for ourselves can our speaking of this with suffering people ring true, rather than sounding like the recital of a formula someone has read in a book or been taught along the way. We have to do this hard work within ourselves so as to create the safe enough interpersonal, psychosocial space for healing practice that is the necessary prelude to the state of trauma healing in which we face the pain head-on, together with the suffering people who seek our care.

Much of the suffering that people experience is about having to find ways to avoid not simply the knowledge of what happened, but to accomplish a far more difficult task—also avoiding the knowledge of what continues to happen, the never-post nature of the trauma. When, as liberatory DHCR healers, we redefine what is traumatic to include the persistent effects of structural oppression, we open the doors in the healing process to the question of how to encounter what is continuing to happen, looking together with the people in our care to know without allowing the knowing to have the effect of disempowering a person into high levels of aroused distress, deep frozenness, or passive cooperation with social pathologies. DHCR is not about working with posttrauma alone; it is about, as we've discussed throughout this book, the before and the after and the ongoing as well.

Most people aren't in a state of active and high-enough activation of their sympathetic nervous system that it intrudes into their awareness most of the time, despite the looming presence of systemic social pathologies. Most people seem to be in a state of persistent neurobiological numbing, the work either of the dorsal vagus nerve or of a chemical brought into the body by a substance, a food, a dopamine-inducing computer game, or an endorphin-creating episode of extreme exertion taken, at times, past the point of the body's safety. The absence of awareness of chronic absence of safety implies that in order to engage in daily life without collapsing and screaming, marginalized and subordinated persons who are not having a more overt trauma exposure are doing something, or many things, to cope with this chronic state of being unsafe.

SO IF NO ONE IS REALLY SAFE

Then why are we doing this work if trauma is everywhere and unceasing? Because we cannot wait for the world to be healed in order to offer healing to those who suffer from its current state. It is my contention that a DHCR liberatory approach to understanding healing from trauma must start with these propositions—that almost everyone is living in a state of the chronic absence of safety and that almost everyone is engaging in some form of self-protection against knowing that truth unless and until the truth becomes unavoidable.

That's why I invite you, my readers, to enter healing relationships with this thought in mind, and not only for the people who bring their distress to your doors, since this absence of safety is likely true for all of us as well. Healing from trauma can be transformed from symptom reduction, which is the gold standard by which an intervention is considered successful by the medical-industrial complex, to a revolutionary, culturally responsive, and humble acknowledgment that in front of us sits someone who has had to work too hard and will continue to have to work very hard to carry the weight of knowing on their psychic shoulders. A hero—not a collection of symptoms to be eradicated as if they are pests. As the computer programmers say, "A feature, not a bug" of the traumatized human neurobiology.

Symptoms are not the problem to be eradicated, although we absolutely want to offer ways to reduce suffering. A raised consciousness in a mind that cannot sleep for fear of nightmares is doing no one any good. We do want to listen to what those symptoms are saying so as to hear what they're telling us about the life of the person in distress. A DHCR healer does not simply collaborate with suffering people so that they suffer less, although we absolutely do that. We invite them, in addition, to be able to know the truths about their lives without being destroyed by them, to learn how to become fully alive even in the presence of pain and oppression, so that life can be lived without having to constantly engage the cloaking mechanisms, so that life can be lived with moments of joy and connectedness. Not that we insist that people get rid of those skills of not-knowing, frayed as they might be. Rather, our jobs as DHCR trauma healers involve widening the scope of capacities for being able to live in the world while knowing its realities, and cocreating the definitions of what closer to safe, safe enough, or maybe safe sometimes will look like.

It's a bit like living with an undiagnosed but very potent toxic exposure, for example, the pipes that leached lead into the water of Flint, Michigan, causing an epidemic of lead poisoning until the problem was finally detected. In this case, it is chronic trauma exposure to social pathologies ever present in the political, emotional, and interpersonal background. The toxin in this case, social pathology, is there, doing its damage to the health of the body, the life, the culture and soul of the person, but the person being affected by the toxin can ignore its symptoms, or even go for long periods being asymptomatic, only knowing that they are feeling poisoned sometimes, perhaps terminally so, when the something changes sufficiently that a diagnosis is made. They might mask the symptoms of the toxic exposure with something that reduces the pain, lessens the inflammation—in other words, dissociates the evidence of the toxicity just enough to ignore it.

This is typically the manner in which social pathologies seed the nooks and crannies of the larger society with their toxins, with dangerous seeds that seem so small and inconsequential that it's often hard to know that they are there and at work, sending down their roots into the soil of societies and psyches alike. It's sometimes impossible to allow yourself to know that those occult cells, be they cancer, racism, patriarchy, or rogue capitalism, are even present until the tiny cell of the toxin grows into something large, showing you that you are at great risk.

DISTRESS SPEAKS TO US, WHEN WE LISTEN

The person who comes into the office of the healer saying that they haven't been able to sleep well for years and that their physical medicine doctors are certain it's not something in the sleep disorders category is telling me, with their sleeplessness, that they are trying to not let themselves know something. They are suffering and need to sleep well. Were they to sleep, they might know what they are yet unable to know. Safe enough, closer to safe, safer are all absent, and so this person lies awake at night where they can be vigilant, aware, even though this is not how they frame their inability to fall or stay asleep.

This symptom is not the problem. As healers, we want to address it. As DHCR trauma healer asks, What is the painful thing that this brain which will not rest is trying to tell us about? What version of not-safe will become known at a time when safer, closer to safe, or safe enough have not yet been established in this nonsleeper's life?

Intriguing research by Jennifer Freyd and her colleagues (DePrince & Freyd, 2001) studying people who remembered incestuous sexual assault in childhood much later in life, after not having had conscious access to that knowledge well into young adulthood, has found that most of them suffered from an entire diagnostic manual's worth of symptoms, which became increasingly difficult to live with. The struggle between the need not to know that your beloved father raped you most nights of your childhood and your eventual need to know that you were, in fact, raped and that this man will be dangerous to your own daughter manifests as a symptom.

So not being able to sleep well might be information about the dangers of sleep, because that's when bad things happened. Sleeping is also a time when nightmares can emerge; many trauma-exposed people will be intentional about avoiding sleep because they know that with sleep comes the return of the terror of what happened to them. Sleep disturbance is all kinds of information about not-safe in the past and not yet safe enough or closer to safe in the present to be able to know the depth and intensity of unsafe in the past.

If all a healer does is focus on symptom reduction, then the truth will not emerge. The costs of not knowing may become more painful to live with. "Treatment resistant" is the epithet that mainstream mental health hurls at these folks. If a DHCR trauma healer hears these words or sees them in a chart, that should be an enormous, loud message not to be ignored, saying, "Getting as close as possible to safe in the present is the first, second, third, and next order of business; nothing else, nope. Closer to safe, first." DHCR trauma healing thus takes diagnosis of the various manifestations of not-knowing down a very different path, in the direction of asking, What can this person not yet tolerate knowing or feeling?

We must also accept that there will often be multiple layers of answers to this question. There will be an official trauma, and also the microaggressions and insidious traumas, the betrayals, the toxic substances hiding in the emotional food of daily life. We do not get to being safe enough or closer to safe and call it done. We must seek that state over and over again, listening carefully to the messages that the symptoms are shouting at us.

HOW THE PRESENCE AND CONTINUOUS DISSOCIATION OF AMBIENT DANGER MAKES MICROAGGRESSIONS A FORM OF TRAUMA

Microaggressions are not considered trauma in formal diagnostic manuals. Stressors, yes; trauma, no. Yet the data (Nadal, 2018) show that they are often quite traumatic, functioning as they do to punch holes, without warning, in the cloak of psychic protections that a subjugated, marginalized, and targeted person utilizes in order push out of conscious awareness the constant potential danger being pointed at them by systemic social pathologies. If, for instance, you're going around in your life pushing away on behalf of your own functional capacities the embodied knowing that you are a light-skinned BIPOC person who often passes for White, you sometimes get slammed in the emotional face by a microaggression that conveys that you are marked as other.

This kind of micro-xenophobia can appear to be as simple as someone asking you, "Where are you from?" and when you say, "Encino," they do not respond with, "Oh, I have a cousin about your age from there, did you go to *x* high school, maybe you knew them." Rather, they respond with the othering question, the microaggression: "No, where are you really from?" This is a question saying, "You are not really from here because your pheno-type isn't typical for here, you don't belong here, and so you can be socially excluded [which is a form of endangerment] on my whim or harmed."

This kind of microaggression is an intrusive reminder of a situation of con-tinuous threat targeted at some strand of intersectionality, a continuous threat that must be dissociated or ignored if a person is to live up to the world's expectation that they will function as an adult. An interesting and chilling example of this arose in the *New York Times Magazine* column, The Ethicist (Appiah, 2022), in which a physician, who identified as a White ally, wrote about ethical dilemmas arising from a White patient's overt racist and homo-phobic hate speech directed at nursing staff while being treated in the writer's hospital. The physician posed the question of whether it would be ethical to discharge this patient with adequate outpatient care, knowing that keeping that person inpatient longer would be optimal, if the patient, when asked to do so, refused to stop engaging in hate speech directed at the nursing staff. The patient, in fact, did stop saying racist and homophobic things once the consequences of her hate speech were made known to her, but the physician nonetheless was still struggling with the question of what to do should the patient not have realized the risks of her verbal abuse of the nursing staff.

Among the topics that emerged in the comments section were some in which the physician and the affected nursing staff were excoriated for being affected by these words, scolded, with the theme being that these were "only words" and that the physician's and nurses' duty to care for the patient were more important than whether or not they were subjected to hate speech, which is the higher end of the continuum of microaggression and can be construed as a form of verbal abuse and thus violence. The column's author, who is an immigrant from Nigeria as well as a famous university professor and writer on ethics, agreed with this position. It's not known whether the comments in this thread were BIPOC people or not, as none of them identi-fied any component of their intersectionalities in their comments.

Then there were the comments from self-identified BIPOC readers, who highlighted this strand of their intersectionalities and who were utterly at odds with the message that the staff should simply put up with the hate speech because of some notion that was a burden that they had to bear no matter what, given their professional commitments. There were comments from this group of readers about the pernicious effects of this kind of exposure on the health of the targeted nursing staff. Several of these commentators named the hate speech as a form of violence and questioned why anyone, no matter what their profession, should be required to work in a violent workplace. The places where I get my health care all have signs up that take this position, as it happens. Hate speech in my health care systems will lead to termination of care, which makes me feel safer.

The contrast between the theme of putting up with hate speech and the idea that to put up with it is to tolerate being abused is an example of the balancing act that many people with some kind of targeted intersectional identities engage in daily. Does one allow oneself to know that one is in the presence of potential danger? Does one talk oneself out of this knowledge explicitly—"Oh, I'm making too big a deal out of this"—or unconsciously, by becoming numb through some dissociative strategy or another—turning off the news, using a substance, calling upon a talent for dissociation, "forget-ting"? Does one scold members of one's own or other marginalized groups for saying "ouch" when they are harmed because your version of how to unknow danger has been to suck it up and never know that your toe was stepped on until it was so thoroughly broken that you could no longer walk on it?

The more microaggressions to which a person is subjected, or the more egregious and overtly threatening they are, the larger the hole punched in the protective membrane of unknowing—until the hole gets so large that the marginalized and subordinated person painfully knows not only the social pathology that is continuously preying on them but also whatever other trauma their trauma-affected neurobiology has been protecting them from.

FINDING SAFETY IS COMPLICATED

Thus an initial and continuing challenge for a DHCR trauma healer is inviting people into a healing process in the middle of a dangerous paradox. We need to devote time in our work with a suffering person to develop a shared understanding of two apparently incompatible realities. The first is the one explored at length above: that safety is illusory. If we skip that step, then we as DHCR healers will fail the people we work with because we will have not liberated the therapeutic narrative from the lie that if a person only does x, they will finally achieve safety. Our silence will not protect us; assimilation, changing names, lightening skin, surgery to change noses and eyelids, keeping one's head down—none of these things will create complete and unshakable safety.

In my own work with trauma-exposed people I have sometimes shared a poem by Irena Klepfisz, a Jew born in the Warsaw Ghetto under Nazi occupation in 1941, and one of the foremost Yiddish authors of her generation. Because she and her mother were both blonde-haired and blue-eyed, they fell outside of the Nazi stereotype of what a Jewish phenotype consisted of; they looked Aryan. Her father, with a more stereotypically Eastern European Jewish phenotype, died in the early days of the Warsaw Ghetto uprising against the Nazis. Smuggled out of the ghetto before the final mass murder of its inhabitants, she and her mother managed to survive in Nazi-occupied Poland by chance, in part because they were not phenotypically identifiable as Jews and in part because there were Polish Catholics who risked their own lives to keep them safe. Randomness was the thing that allowed for survival. Being born with a particular phenotype, blond hair and blue eyes, that was considered Aryan, not Jewish, a random expression of genetics, saved lives. And then these people who looked "not Jewish" stumbled upon a particular set of non-Jewish people who were willing to risk their own lives to be allies to these Jews in the midst of the terror and devastation of the Nazi regime. I know the name of one such ally, Krysia Pogoda, the grandmother of a young colleague of mine; Pogoda nearly died in a Nazi work camp because she was among those Catholic Poles who hid Jews like Klepfisz and her mother. She was arrested and imprisoned by the Nazis for her decency, and survived to tell her story.

Klepfisz's canonical poem is titled "Bashert" (1982). This is a word in both Hebrew and Yiddish that translates as "meant to be." The lines of the poem offer a powerful commentary, both on the inescapability of a lethal social pathology and on the utter randomness with which those so targeted can become closer to safe, and even survive, or get farther from safety and die. Taken more symbolically and psychologically, Klepfisz is describing the ways in which people targeted by social pathologies in nonlethal settings survive emotionally until being closer to safe is possible.

The two parts of the poem are titled, "These words are dedicated to those who died" and "These words are dedicated to those who survived." The reasons the poet gives for anyone having either fate are remarkably similar and convey the randomness of outcomes for lives in the presence of social pathology, in this case, a very lethal and organized social pathology, the Nazi variant of anti-Semitism, which is a form of White supremacy that predated the Nazis and continues to be promulgated by modern day Nazis and their fellow travelers in the realm of White supremacist hate.

In the second part of the poem, "These words are dedicated to those who survived," the poem turns into a series of contradictory statements that are the best and most powerful illustration I have ever encountered of the random nature by which marginalized and subordinated people who are targeted by social pathologies survive emotionally, not only literally. Survived "because they did not draw attention to themselves and got lost in the shuffle." Survived "because they drew attention to themselves and always got picked." Survived "because they played it safe." Survived "because they took risks." Survived "because they expected the worst and were always prepared." Survived "because they were angry." Survived "because they endured humiliation." Survived "because they looked the other way." *Bashert.*[1]

More powerfully than I can ever do, Klepfisz's words tell us, as DHCR trauma healers, that in order to survive, to move through the world of unsafety, to hold illusions of being possibly safe, maybe safe, traumatized people do all of these contradictory things, usually several of them at the same time. These were her and her mother's lived experiences of survival as Jews in Nazi-occupied Poland. Doing any and all of these things to survive or in the aftermath of trauma exposure are not symptoms of psychopathology. These are resistance to social pathologies, even to evil itself. These are the paths to survival that have worked well enough, or just barely, or not so badly—well enough, even by a hair, that a trauma-exposed suffering human walks into our healing space still alive.

A VERY COMPLICATED AND THOROUGH EXAMPLE: MARISOL

So what does this look like in a person's life, these layers of personal and familial and cultural responding to the absence of safety? In the next chapters we will spend a lot of time with Marisol, someone who, as promised, is an amalgam of many people who have honored me with their stories over the last 5 decades. Her story is many of their stories, the stories to which we, as decolonial and culturally responsive trauma healers, need to open our hearts and to which we want to learn to listen to carefully. We do this that we might hear the multiple harmonies of unknowing danger so that this woman, and those who came before her, were able to keep walking forward long enough for her to walk into a healer's office.

---

[1] From "Bashert" from *Her Birth and Later Years: New and Collected Poems, 1971–2021* © 2022 by Irena Klepfisz. Published by Wesleyan University Press. Used by permission.

9 STORIES OF UNKNOWING AND WHAT FOLLOWS WHEN WE KNOW

Getting Closer to Safe

What do these core ideas, discussed in the two previous chapters, about chronic absence of safety imply for the work of decolonial, humble, culturally responsive (DHCR) trauma healers? First, we must assume that every suffering person has a lifetime of developing and drawing upon personal psychic and behavioral strategies so as to not have consciousness of danger intrude too much into daily life. It stands to reason that one thing that has led them to be sitting with us is that these strategies for not knowing are not working very well any longer, that the strategies are making life harder, that both knowledge and distress are leaking through—or some mixture of all of the above.

STRATEGIES AND MANIFESTATIONS OF UNKNOWING

A person I know well, who is not a client, told me that she had figured out quite late, in her 30s, that she had been horrifically and repeatedly sexually abused in a family child trafficking ring, in which pedophile parents would share children with others in the group. She had figured out that when dissociating into different ego states didn't work to keep her away from the knowledge

https://doi.org/10.1037/0000421-010
Decolonizing Trauma Healing: Toward a Humble, Culturally Responsive Practice,
by L. S. Brown

of what was being done to her from before the onset of autobiographical memory, she poured some alcohol on top of the pile of scary information that had begun poking into and interfering with daily life. And when dissociating and alcohol combined didn't work, she cut herself. When all of that didn't work, she added risky sexual behavior, at which point someone who genuinely loved her said something to the effect of, "Maybe you should talk to somebody, because I can't lose you." She told me, "And then it took me 6 months, because I already knew that therapists weren't to be trusted, because I had been sent to therapists all of those years that the abuse was being done to me and not one of them had a clue. I did DBT [dialectical behavior therapy], and it didn't do a damn thing except make me feel incompetent. You would think that therapists working with folks who need DBT might have thought about maybe there was something going on in the background, like trauma. Like parts, for [insert long string of expletives] sake! It took me 3 years to tell Sharla anything, and that's only because she had at least been curious enough about my pile of problems to ask if maybe something very bad had happened to me. I kept saying no. And then I knew, and I kinda cracked open, which you know, because I kept calling people up, thinking I had gone nuts, and ended up out on short-term disability for most of a year."

Again, this person was not in therapy with me; she was a friend and colleague who had reached out to me in crisis when things began to fall into place even as her unknowing strategies leaked and cracked. Her story was a mirror of those I heard in my office for 4 decades, which is, perhaps, why she gifted me with her truth. Her story is the story of how people will do almost anything not to know, because not knowing has been survival. When social pathologies add their toxicity to whatever trauma is occurring and bind up the experience with one or more strands of that braid of intersectionalities, the necessity of not knowing in order to survive can become more insistent. Trauma has meaning and weight, and intersectional identities and present-day social and political contexts are the locations at which those meanings and weights are often expressed.

Some of these strategies for keeping an awareness of the absence of safety from intruding into daily life occur in response to trauma that has happened, or is currently happening, in the realm of intimate relationships. The collection of distress that we now call complex childhood trauma is replete with unknowing strategies because there is so very much to have to not know. This was certainly true for my friend, who had to unknow being trafficked and stringently obey the directives from her parents to tell no one, as well as deal with threats about who would be killed if she were to tell, all so that she could be a kid in the world, going to school and Scouts and never allowing the criminality of her family system to leak into daytime consciousness.

Not everyone who dissociates into different ego states has early trauma of this sort, but many folks who have this talent called dissociation have come to its use early in life, before it was possible to rationalize or minimize or use a substance or run their body away from the scene of the crimes being perpetrated on them. These are not symptoms of something wrong. They are evidence of valiant and desperate attempts to survive, to resist the death of the soul.

Some of these ways of not knowing can also emerge to deal with early exposure to war, displacement, or actual colonial rule under which one must find a way to live and go forward. These strategies tend to reflect a person's acquisition of language or their having been accompanied in the trauma by someone older with the language to define what is happening in a way that protects everyone's survival. "It's all right, we are having an adventure," says the parent scrambling to stuff food and clothing into a bag and running into the night ahead of an approaching army. When a caregiver is present, regulating the child during the course of a trauma, the child often also internalizes the caregiver's unknowing strategies as part of that coregulation—for how can a loving parent allow themselves to fully feel the horror of the possibility that their beloved child may soon die or that they might be killed and that child left unprotected? The parent cannot allow knowledge of that question while focusing on keeping their child alive and not frightened. A person's unknowing strategies are bound up in their secure-enough attachment to a loving parent and may look and sound like denial. But no one is denying; a parent soothes a child through danger, a child internalizes that soothing, and to know the truth of the terror at some point means reconfiguring their understanding of a parent who was coded as "stoic" and "not willing to talk about what happened before we got here," perhaps disrupting a fragile family system equilibrium. Unknowing has a role to play in the care and feeding of good-enough relationships as well.

Other symptoms of unknowing develop as a means of containing the awareness of chronic risk in a compartmentalized manner, allowing the person to function but at some cost to capacities for going about life. The person feels the risk from the social pathology that is aimed at some or several components of their intersectional identities and then rationalizes the harm and toxicity as distant enough, or their self as protected enough for now, that the ubiquity of that pathology need not matter to them. The neurobiology of trauma is being activated in their body nonetheless, the sympathetic nervous system (SNS) getting ready for action, the polyvagal system preparing for freeze or collapse, and the prefrontal cortex busily sending that information away from consciousness. The person experiences all kinds of bodily distress as a result of living on constant chronic alert, which they are doing their best to ignore. They seek out medical diagnoses for this distress and, after a multitude of tests, are told the bodily distress is psychosomatic. Eventually the danger breaks through and becomes something that overcomes all attempts at rationalization and compartmentalization.

Dissociation of Collective Knowledge of Danger: The Social Pathology of Colonization, Phenotype Supremacy, and the Genocide of the Tutsi People

The terrible story of the genocide committed by the Hutu majority government of Rwanda against its Tutsi citizens in 1994 illustrates collective unknowing as a coping strategy, layered upon the toxins of colonization, and a divide-and-conquer faux phenotype supremacy promulgated by the colonizers to assert control. It is also a story of how political independence from being a colony does not eradicate the toxins of the various social pathologies that colonization injects into the psyches of colonized people.

"We wish to inform you that tomorrow we will be killed with our families." This was a letter from a Tutsi church member to his Hutu pastor, who was indeed among those who murdered the letter writer and his family the next day (Gourevitch, 1998). Although prior to the outbreak of mass violence, the social pathology of anti-Tutsism had been rising to prominence via the leaders of the Hutu power movement, who used radio addresses to call for these killings, many Tutsi who survived described that they simply could not believe—in other words, could not allow themselves to know—that their neighbors, friends, and even relatives would murder, rape, and mutilate them by the hundreds of thousands in a period of around 3 months. This was a collective unknowing of danger, reinforced in some instances by "calming" messages from community leaders.

What occurred in 1994 in Rwanda was entirely an artifact of colonization, first by Germany, then by Belgium, which "won" possession of these colonies after World War I. Without colonization, the genocide of 1994 would not have occurred; it was the European colonizers who created this artificial divide, defining Tutsis and Hutus as two allegedly phenotypically different groups. This in turn became a narrative employed during the genocide to detect whether a person looked Tutsi, not too different from the Nazi notion of what constituted the Aryan phenotype.

Prior to being colonized, the line between these two groups had been blurred, with shared languages and cultural and religious practices, although one group tended to be farmers and the other herders of cattle. The colonizers emphasized alleged differences between the two groups as a means of recruiting cooperation with their brutal colonizing tactics; the Tutsi were chosen to be the "pets," pitting them against the colonially constructed other, the Hutu majority. The colonizers favored Tutsis, defining them as looking and acting "less African."

The colonizers modeled power as dominance to cultures that had previously been more communitarian, encouraging assimilation of European racist tropes by both groups, narratives that persisted even after the former colonies had gained political independence. By 1994, the memories of how two colonized groups of Africans that had previously shared their lands and identities in relative harmony had been artificially defined against one another solely for the benefit of colonization had faded. What remained were the ethnic hatreds that had benefited the colonizing Europeans and led to the deaths of what is now estimated to be between 500,000 and 620,000 people, uncounted numbers of rapes, and the destruction of social order in Rwanda, which has persisted for almost 3 decades. Rwanda is politically free of colonization. It has never been free of the colonization of minds. Tutsi people had to unknow danger to coexist with their Hutu friends and neighbors. Then they were slaughtered.

Parallels to this collective dissociation can be seen in assimilated or colonizer-identified marginalized groups in many other settings in which a social pathology turned lethal, sometimes gradually and sometimes with apparent suddenness. Examples include, among others, the assimilated Jews of Germany between the two world wars who could not believe that they, Germans who happened to worship differently than the majority, would be at risk. They include the civilized tribes of Indigenous people of the U.S. Southeast who believed that the treaties they signed with their colonizers were meaningful until Andrew Jackson decided that White people needed those lands and sent the military to exile them, sent along the Trail of Tears, the forced diaspora to what is now Oklahoma, during which many Indigenous people died of disease and starvation.

These groups practicing collective unknowing of danger included the Huguenot Protestant Christians of 16th-century France, who believed that they had achieved peaceful enough coexistence with the Roman Catholic majority. They held onto this collective belief until the St. Bartholomew's Day massacre in Paris and the mass murders of Protestants that spread throughout much of the rest of France after the leaders of the French Huguenot community in the capital city were murdered.

Unknowing is clearly not an individual phenomenon, although each individual in a culture practicing collective dissociation participates in it differently. The Cassandras in these groups often find themselves marginalized within their own groups, a relational trauma that may be accompanied by guilt and grief if, following their own inner warning signals, they remove themselves from danger, leaving behind many who then suffer and die.

When having been someone who got away because they knew unsafety in the face of collective and cultural denial is part of a person's intersectional identities, their struggles will be different from the person who remained, stayed somehow alive, and now regrets having dismissed the Cassandras. Just as was true for Cassandra in the *Iliad*, the Cassandras of communities at risk are often shunned by the survivors because their suffering—having seen the terrors wrought on their communities from a place of greater safety— is often dismissed: "You didn't have to go through that. You were here in America." A DHCR trauma healer needs to know if a person was the Cassandra of a community that practiced collective unknowing and suffered great harm that might, in some instances, have been avoided or escaped.

We Don't Know Until We Can No Longer Not Know

Let's explore these various ways in which humans avoid knowing that they are in chronic levels of danger. We will see examples in the stories that follow, because the ways in which a specific suffering person worked to unknow the absence of safety before something broke through those strategies affected how they engaged with the healing process. DHCR trauma healing means, at some point, knowing enough about what has wounded you to heal it, which means that the healer has created sufficient safety in the healing relationship, a container in the space between healer and suffering person that is sturdy enough to hold the pain.

One of the ways in which people's capacities to unknow trauma has been pathologized and colonized has been to treat some forms of unknowing as better than others. Dissociation is "primitive"; rationalization and intellectualization are "more developed" (Lingiardi & McWilliams, 2017). Let's disabuse ourselves of that notion, please. All forms of unknowing can be understood as some component of Braun's (1988) BASK paradigm for dissociation: dissociation of one's behavior, of emotion/affect, of sensation/somatic experience, of knowledge of the facts of one's life, or some combination of all four. Dissociation, suppression, denial, rationalization, intellectualization, use of substances or overwork— all are ways for a person to unknow, to manage themselves sufficiently that the pain of trauma does not intrude. This taxonomy of unknowing strategies artificially privileges those that entail the use of the language centers of the prefrontal cortex or involve activities, such as overwork or overexercise, that are culturally valued in the social pathology of rogue capitalism because they are productive.

This made-up hierarchy, a reflection of structural hierarchies of value (somatic = worse, verbal = better), also ignores cultural unknowing strategies discussed in Chapter 8, such as assimilation, which play a role in how trauma is intergenerationally transmitted, with one generation teaching the next how to survive even when the initial danger appears to be long gone. Knowing the heritage of the cultures of a suffering person's intersectional identities is consequently a further component of a DHCR exploration of that suffering person's collection of ways of not knowing. One person can be unknowing in many ways: dissociating their own trauma, using minimization or distancing for dealing with intergeneration trauma, intellectualization about daily microaggressions, alcohol when none of that works, and so on. Rather than treating each way of unknowing as a symptom, DHCR trauma healing gets curious about the functions and interactions of the various way of unknowing.

From a DHCR trauma healing perspective, one way of unknowing cannot be treated as better than another; they are all human responses to the pain of trauma, all ways that humans find to keep the pain at sufficient distance so that they can engage with daily life. When these unknowing methodologies cease to work, either because of an event in a person's life that is the catalyst for knowing or because a healing process has created a space that is close enough to safe for trauma material to float to the surface, many suffering people become, like my friend, unable for a time to be productive and risk losing the components of their intersectionalities that are valued in the capitalist world in which we live. Knowing what could not be known also creates the new identity of knowing that you had been exposed to trauma, an identity that many people reject out of hand because of the contempt that mainstream culture associates with being victimized. This generates a dilemma for the newly awakened suffering person, which we will address at greater length in subsequent chapters where we explore intersectionality in depth.

The stories that follow may also help show how the healer and the sufferer together find their way to whatever represents being closer to safe, the ingredient that is indeed foundational to trauma healing. These stories represent composites from my work and that of colleagues who have consulted with me and are not deidentified versions of any one person's story.

MARISOL'S STORY: RESPONSES TO EARLY CHILDHOOD CHRONIC DANGER

Complex childhood trauma refers to a situation in which a child's caregivers or other trusted persons are dangerous to them, either because of perpetration of abuse or due to chronic neglect, exploitation, or betrayal trauma (Ford & Courtois, 2020). If having been traumatized in this way is excused as a fitting response to some facet of a person's intersectional identities ("You thought you were so smart, you thought you were better than me, I had to beat it out of you") this also complicates the suffering person's relationships with that part of who they are. When the adult inflicting the trauma on the child is, as is too likely to be the case, also living with their own forms of chronic absence of safety, this renders the emotional environment exponentially more complicated for a child attempting to navigate its dangerous waters. It is not necessary that there be clear intergenerational trauma for this layered experience of unsafety to be present, although when a parent figure was personally traumatized or grew up in a historically traumatized culture, it appears that the risk of trauma reenactment on the child are higher.

A liberatory DHCR trauma healer needs to consider that entire matrix of unsafety so as to skillfully explore how a particular suffering person has coped with life until the time they entered the healer's office.

What follows is a story that is the amalgam of at least five peoples' stories and does not share confidential information about any one person. It's the story of someone I'll call Marisol, a heterosexual natal woman whose mother, Paz, was Filipina and whose father, Duncan, was Euro-American of mostly Irish descent. Marisol was in her early 40s when she started therapy in the early years of the 21st century. She had no romantic partner, defined herself as asexual, and lived by herself. Although phenotypically she resembled her mother, thus appearing Asian to the world around her, she identified as White.

Something she remembered during the course of therapy, after her unknowing strategies had begun breaking down, was that she had been raped almost daily from age 4 to 14 by her father. She did not know this when she started therapy. What she did know was that her mother, who grew up in an impoverished home in the slums of Manila near the U.S. military base at Subic Bay, was physically abused by her father. Marisol witnessed the abuse and remembered vividly stepping in as she grew older, attempting to protect her mother and a younger sibling. She also recalled how her father hurled racist epithets at his wife and daughters, repeatedly reminding them how "lucky" they were that he had married Paz after Marisol was born and had brought them all to the United States, albeit under duress from his military command, when he was transferred to a base on the U.S. mainland. Marisol was her mother's emotional caretaker and confidante and also remembered saying to herself frequently, "Marisol, you cannot end up like this."

What layers and layers of danger does a liberatory DHCR trauma healer need to unpack with this suffering person to develop a liberatory and compassionate framework for being with Marisol as she begins to know what she could not handle knowing before walking in our door and spending several years addressing the official problem?

We're going to start with the unknowing strategies utilized by Paz because Marisol absorbed them, but it's absolutely essential that we don't stop there.

Because the world of decolonial healing has focused almost entirely on work with Black, Indigenous, and people of color (BIPOC), where the layers of oppression by social pathologies might be more obvious at first glance, we become trapped in the narrative about who is and is not colonized if we ignore the unknowing strategies that Duncan brought to his daughter's life. So we'll examine those as well.

Pulling Apart Some Strands, or Why Knowing History Is Part of DHCR Work

Paz had a number of very easy to see and hear marginalized intersectional identities. She is an Asian Pacific Islander from a multiply colonized country. She had brown skin, was of shorter stature than average for a woman raised in the United States due both to genetics and diet, and had an accent that made her nonnative-English-language status, and thus her immigration experience, audible. What was not as visible, and yet core to understanding the heritage of unknowing that Paz passed along to her daughter, has to do with cultural strategies for coping with millennia of colonization that have been developed by the residents of the Philippine archipelago.

Paz came from a society whose Indigenous people had experienced waves of colonization and displacement for at least two millennia, with Chinese settlers displacing many of the Indigenous people of the archipelago around the beginning of the first millennium of the Common Era. Before the Spanish conquest and colonization in the 1500s, and before there was a construct of the Philippines as a country, some of its islands had come under the rule of various Indian, Indonesian, and Southeast Asian empires, leaving a mélange of languages and religions behind them.

The name "Philippines" was accorded to the captured territory by conquistadores in honor of the Spanish king, Philip, who had sponsored their colonizing expedition. Paz's family was from the island of Luzon, where the city of Manila was built and made into the Spanish colonial capital. Her family's mother tongue was Tagalog, which is only one of more than 120 languages spoken in the archipelago.

Spanish and U.S. colonization are historically the events closer in time to the present for Paz's culture. They are the ones whose deleterious and long-lasting effects on the mixtures of peoples living in the archipelago are easier to trace. Spain had completely colonized the islands by 1521, during which time Indigenous languages and religions were suppressed and natural and human resources plundered. Spain "lost" the archipelago to the United States in 1898 at the end of the Spanish-American War. A transfer of ownership of a country and its people as spoils of war and a betrayal of a promise to promote the development of an independent Philippines were the results of this agreement between the rulers of two colonizing powers.

There followed a period of colonial rule by the United States, marked by various liberation uprisings, that lasted until wartime occupation by Japan from 1941–1946, a further brutal period of colonization. Then the country became nominally independent but remained a partially owned subsidiary of U.S. rogue capitalism and the U.S. military until the overthrow of Ferdinand Marcos in 1986 and the closing of the last footprint of colonization, the naval base at Subic Bay in 1992.

What did Filipino people, who sometimes refer to themselves as Pinoy/Pinay, do in order to survive these waves of colonization? Of course, the answers vary. Of interest is that a core value of interpersonal relationships in many of the cultures of the archipelago became that of "smooth relations" between people (Protacio Marcellino, 1990, p. 111). The Indigenous people developed a value of not making waves. This does not mean that there were not repeated insurgencies, some of which have lasted into the present day. Some were led by leftist rebels and, more recently, by leaders among the Muslim inhabitants of some of the islands, who resisted the Catholicism that was imposed on the island of Luzon and its neighbors by the Spanish colonizers and have more recently have rebelled against America's hegemony.

But assimilation, in the form of smooth relations, took center stage in Philippine psychology. A value of having lighter skin (meaning some European ancestry, often but not always due to the rape of an Indigenous woman, sometimes due to romantic relationships that were relatively consensual), adopting the speaking of Spanish and then American English, rather than Luzon's Indigenous language of Tagalog or any of the many other Indigenous languages of the archipelago, the adoption of Spanish names, and overt cooperation with the colonizers' ruling apparatuses became a norm. English, not one of the Indigenous languages, has been adopted as the second official language of the country.

The message of the last colonizers, the United States, was that the Philippine nation needed to Americanize, show progress, and collaborate with U.S. policy in the Pacific as the price of being granted independence. This was the betrayal of freedom that had been unconditionally promised when the Philippines passed from a monarchy, Spain, to a democracy, the United States. In consequence, identification with the aggressor/oppressor continued to be a normative national coping strategy, in this case, a post hoc prerequisite imposed for promised independence.

So How Does All of This History Affect Paz? Or Marisol, Who Is Sitting in the Office?

These are the basic outlines of Paz's cultural story of colonization. Her family, which had moved to Manila from a rural village on the island of Luzon in the hopes of improving their economic status, had instead suffered the experience of being marginalized in the big city by their poverty, their darker-hued skin, and their absence of formal education. This made Paz's impregnation by and eventual marriage to a U.S. military member seem at first to be a path by which not only Paz but her entirely family might improve their lot without one of them having to join the Philippine remittance diaspora. Paz's family did not think to exploit Duncan. Rather, their hopes reflected a communitarian ethic, still evident in the ways in which members of the worldwide Philippine diaspora send home much of their earnings from better-paying jobs elsewhere in the world so as to support their extended families at home.

Duncan not only did not help Paz's family but, by moving Paz to the United States and controlling her finances during a time prior to the existence of cell phones and the internet, he cut them off from her and her from them. They lost her as a wage earner contributing to the family's finances through her work as a cleaner at Subic Bay. They lost her as a member of an extended family that supported each other through chronic hard times. She lost them as social support that might have helped her, not to divorce, as this was anathema to the family's Roman Catholic values, but at least to separate from Duncan as his abuse escalated.

After his discharge from the military, Duncan moved the family to his hometown in rural Alabama, a part of the United States where there were no other Pinoys, much less other people of Asian or Pacific Islander heritage. After the family relocated, there began slowly to be an influx of other Asian and Pacific Islanders; they were not Pinoy but rather Vietnamese and South Asian Indian, brown people for whom she was frequently mistakenly identified, but culturally very different from Paz. When she was misidentified by people of European ancestry, this increased her sense of alienation and isolation, as she was invisible as who she was, Pinay.

Before Paz met Duncan, her family had survived centuries of colonization and occupation. They had neurobiologically and epigenetically adapted to those conditions so as to be able to survive. Their bodies had ceased to respond to ambient lower-level daily threats, which meant that their stress response system and hypothalamic–pituitary–adrenal (HPA) axis had been modified in each new generation to be able to keep awareness of ambient threat to the lowest level feasible. Their ambient cortisol levels had acclimated to chronic stress and danger. This neurobiology of chronic lower-level threat allowed activation when an acute threat, for example, a typhoon or a squad of Japanese occupying soldiers, appeared but otherwise maintained a background level of unknowing.

Behaviorally, Marisol's ancestors had learned to be smooth in their relations with the colonizers and occupiers so as to survive until the next day, week, month, and year, all of which became a part of the cultural norms of behavior that were passed along. "Smooth" meant to be placating, to not show anger, minimizing the effects of microaggressions to themselves and laughing about them with the person committing that violation, and at times rationalizing even active violations in the forms of indentured labor and sexual assault of Indigenous women (Protacio Marcellino, 1990).

Living while actively colonized, with the social pathology being overt, in charge, and holding the weapons and the prisons, was the background noise for all of Marisol's maternal ancestors up through her mother, Paz, who was a tween during the Japanese occupation and in her early young adulthood when the Philippines went from a wholly owned possession to a technically independent but unofficially partially occupied territory of the United States. All of this unknowing of ambient threat in the context of having had to survive the dangers of occupation was something that Paz had had to master and practice before she met, was sexually coerced, was impregnated by, and married Duncan, whose own heritage of unknowing we'll explore next.

The marriage of Marisol's parents represented a small-scale version of colonization. Duncan's behaviors reenacted on a microlevel the colonial dynamics of despoiling the resources of the Indigenous nation. Paz cleaned marine barracks on the base. Duncan found her in his barracks and coerced her into intercourse that she did not know she could refuse. Because there was no other physical violence involved, Paz blamed herself for giving in to his verbal threats to have her fired if she refused to submit to him, and Duncan blamed her for seducing him by being a woman he found attractive over whom he could exert physical force.

Paz and Marisol were Duncan's personal spoils of colonization. He abused the BIPOC woman he had married and then sexually abused their BIPOC elder daughter. Because she was his daughter, she was also, within the social pathology of misogyny and rape culture, his possession, to do with as he pleased.

Another Layer of Trauma: Duncan's Story of Seduction by Social Pathologies

Next, let's take a look at Duncan, Marisol's father, who is also the man who raped her most nights from the time she was 4 until she ran away from home when she was 14. We could make him the villain of the story because he in fact did terrible things. But he too came into this story with his own cultural history of colonization.

Because his visible intersectional identities are those of a White natal heterosexual man who, at the outset of therapy, was someone whom Marisol knew had beaten her mother, it might be tempting to ignore his part of the unknowing structural oppression story. That would be an error, and one that

DHCR trauma healers often make because we get distracted by the issue of who has more structural and social power, which is a real issue, and ignore who else here is carrying the toxins of a social pathology.

When Duncan was growing up, his family lived in a trailer park in a semi-rural area in Alabama, which meant that they were almost as impoverished in their own social context as was Paz's family in the Philippines. His own father abandoned the family when Duncan, the eldest of three children born in close succession, was barely 5 years old. His mother, who had given birth to him when she herself was 15 and his father almost 30, worked a series of low-paid jobs. Misogyny blamed Duncan's mother for becoming pregnant while not married, a thing defined as both sin and a cause for shame, paralleling how Duncan later blamed Paz for the pregnancy that resulted from his sexual assault of her. The misogynist culture into which Duncan was born never considered the fact that having been impregnated as a teen by a man twice her age meant that Duncan's mother had been sexually abused, any more than Duncan understood that the narrative of Paz seducing him and trapping him into marriage so she could set herself up financially had no merit and was the cover story for sexual assault.

Duncan's mother and her children were stigmatized in their small town. Although she had been a bright student, she was forced to leave high school and was kicked out of her family's home when her pregnancy was discovered. This stripped her of the possibility of any further educational opportunities, a not unusual punishment meted out to women who became pregnant outside of the approved setting of heterosexual marriage in the era when Duncan was born. Then, as today, the third decade of the 21st century, reproductive choice did not exist for women in Alabama.

Duncan and his two younger siblings never saw a health professional until each of them started school, and then only when some acute illness landed them in the office of a school nurse. The concepts of a reading disability or atypical attention were not present in the school system, nor were school lunches available for children living below a poverty line that had not yet been defined. Duncan was often hungry and angry, and even if had he been well-nourished, he would have struggled with reading and focus in school. Because he was poor and lived in the trailer park with only one parent, at a time before the term "single parent" had come into common use, he was bullied for his family's violation of patriarchal norms. He often heard his mother referred to by adult men in his small town as a whore because she had been made pregnant so young and then had boyfriends whom she did not marry.

Both of Duncan's parents' family backgrounds were Irish and Roman Catholic. His great-great-grandparents, who had been peasants, fled to the United States starting in 1845, during the Great Famine, a famine that lasted from 1845–1852, a famine promoted by the British colonizers of Ireland as part of their effort to depopulate the country of its Indigenous inhabitants in order to make room for British people to settle. The ways in which Britain colonized Ireland (and Scotland, Wales, and Cornwall) were not dissimilar to strategies they had used with the Indigenous peoples of North America. In the case of Ireland, the British introduced diseases that were new to the ecosystem and for which indigenous crops had no immunity, and they displaced people from where they had always lived on spurious grounds. The Clearances, as this had been called a century earlier in colonized Scotland after it lost its independence struggle at the battle of Culloden, leading to similar famines in that piece of the colonized island that was renamed Great Britain.

Duncan's several times great-grandparents arrived after a terrifying journey in steerage, during which people died all around them, only to arrive to a country that responded to them xenophobically. "No Irish need apply" was the slogan that met them. The full privileges of Whiteness were not extended to people of Irish descent living in the United States until shortly before Duncan himself was born, and as a Catholic in the mostly anti-Catholic Southeast, he and his family were treated as suspect by the members of the various Protestant groups that constituted the majority. He knew, not consciously but very clearly, that the privilege deriving from White skin was a tenuous one. He was confronted with the vulnerability of his membership among White people when epithets of "Papist" and worse were thrown his way during fist-fights with Protestant peers. He coped with that absence of safety by adhering even more tightly to the dictates of White supremacy and by consciously adopting racist attitudes and values, doing his best to assimilate into the rest of the White population.

Duncan's immediate ancestors had migrated southward to Alabama where the social pathology of White supremacy taught the lesson Lyndon Johnson's own family knew well. Once in Alabama, Duncan's great-grandparents started the process of assimilation despite pervasive anti-Catholic sentiment that continued to impose a less than fully White identity, taking up the tenets of White supremacy as their own as a defense against knowing their own marginal position, as did Duncan himself as he grew up. The family's need to dissociate the presence of pervasive threat was reduced by its adoption of White supremacy, helped by the fact that the local branch of the Klan was focused on African Americans and the stray Jew in town and less interested in the persecution of people with White skin who were not members of a Protestant religious faith but who had a cross in their place of worship.

During this pretechnological period before the beginning of the Second World War, the genes for atypical attention and difficulties with the capacity to read that were pervasive among many of his forebears—which had been passed to Duncan along with the epigenetics and trauma neurobiology of colonization, refugee trauma, and xenophobia—were not socially problematic. From the mostly rural worlds in Ireland, where his family had farmed, to the mostly rural worlds of Alabama, where his family farmed and ran a forge, if a person could work with their hands, then having less than a 4th-grade education made little difference for a natal man with kinesthetic intelligence.

Duncan's grandfather, who was probably unable to read, found a job in the foundry at the steel mill in nearby Bessemer, which gave the family financial stability for a brief period until he was killed in an industrial accident in the era before unions and worker's compensation entered the picture. Duncan's father dropped out of school in 5th grade after his father died and, too young to work in the steel mill, did a series of odd jobs to try to support his mother and five younger siblings. He had become a father himself only because he impregnated Duncan's much-younger mother, establishing a pattern that Duncan would reenact with Paz.

Affected by the social pathology of toxic masculinity, Duncan's father had internalized the notion that as the man of the house after his father's death he had the right to rule over his mother and younger female siblings. He began to use violence to enforce his will when words failed to persuade. When Duncan was born to a father who had no interest in being a parent and an adolescent mother who had no idea of how to protect herself, much less her child, the strategy of using physical violence to solve the problems of life was already a well-established pattern in this family.

Toxic masculinity also forbade Duncan's father to feel his deep grief over his own father's horrific death, incurred falling into a vat of molten steel. Instead, he developed a powerful defense against knowing that vulnerable, feminine emotion in the form of rage at his father's stupidity for slipping into the molten ore. His rage fueled his physical and verbal expressions of violence against the family members who were unable to avoid showing vulnerable emotions because of their tender ages; children cry when they are hurt and frightened. Acting out the fear and pain allowed Duncan, and his father before him, to not know about those vulnerable, unmasculine emotions within themselves.

When his father pushed intercourse on Duncan's mother, neither knew anything about how to prevent an unwanted pregnancy because such information was illegal in most of the United States before the mid-1960s and not available to people living outside urban centers, where women who had the financial means to have access to gynecologists might be given information about contraception sub rosa.

Three children and 5 years later he enlisted in the marines and disappeared for good from his son's sight. He was not dead; he simply never returned home. During those 5 years, he brought his rage to bear on Duncan's mother for having trapped him with her pregnancy and, importantly for our discussion of the layers of trauma, on Duncan himself, the result of that pregnancy. He regularly beat Duncan so severely that the boy had multiple unset broken bones before his own father left the family behind.

Duncan carried with him almost as many layers of unknowing ambient danger as Paz did. His dangers were up close and personal, in his immediate family and in ancestors who had had to flee their homeland and endure xenophobia but who had suppressed those parts of the family narrative in favor of the unknowing methodology of assimilation, becoming White, and Irish only on St. Patrick's Day when they could blend into the general debauchery.

Duncan needed to unknow that his own father was dangerous because children must bond with their adult caregivers. Once his father had disappeared, he had no safe enough space in which to allow the knowledge of his father's predation on him to become available. In order to move forward, he needed to unknow that he had been abandoned and betrayed. He needed to unknow the precariousness of his position in the larger social order resulting from his social class, religious affiliation, and atypical intellectual abilities. To accomplish this, he did not know any way to block the messages of the social pathology of White supremacy and toxic masculinity that were broadcasting loudly in his psyche, protecting him from the social pathologies that specifically marginalized him—classism, anti-Catholicism, and ableism—this last because of how his brain handled letters and attention.

Duncan carried the legacies of his Irish forbearers' colonial, famine, and refugee trauma at the hands of the colonizing British. His genes and neurobiology descended from his ancestors' trauma responses and adaptations. He had to unknow that White supremacy and toxic masculinity, from which he appeared to draw benefit, were doing him nearly irreparable moral damage. In an identification with the aggressor/oppressor, he, like his father before him, joined the marines and thus was stationed at Subic Bay Naval Base in the Philippines, where he crossed Paz's path one afternoon as she cleaned his barracks.

None of his heritage of trauma excuses his violence, his sexual assault on Paz, or his sexual assaults on his daughter. None of it excuses his racism and misogyny. All of this puts those ways of unknowing trauma, particularly the identification with the oppressor that is a theme of Duncan's unknowing patterns, into context. Looking at Duncan gives a DHCR trauma healer a richer and fuller picture of the legacies of trauma and the various interactive ways of unknowing that Marisol inherited from both parents.

Both the Colonizer and the Colonized Embodied in One Suffering Human

For many DHCR healers it is easier to see the colonization of BIPOC peoples, the wounds of misogynist violence, and to focus solely on those in making attempts to disentangle the webs of dissociation with which people in distress present us. It is far more challenging, and yet more deeply decolonial and disruptive of the narrative of Whiteness, which denies and ignores the variations on the theme of trauma in the diverse heritages of people assigned to this socially constructed category (Helms, 2019), to trace as many strands of the story of what came before as possible, even when what came before is disguised behind current social constructs of who has privilege.

Upon superficial examination, Duncan is privileged: he is Euro-American, assigned White, a heterosexual natal man, and a military veteran, living in a social context that elevates all of these intersectional identities. All of this is fact. It is not, however, the emotional truth that informs how Marisol came by her own dissociative strategies and how fiercely she will protect them as the healing process moves on.

That's a Lot of Colonization and Trauma and Unknowing—But Not That Much

So why is Marisol the suffering person sitting in the healer's office today? Not, as you might think, because she knows of being raped by her father. In fact, her father isn't even a topic. She's not in the office because she was the target of his racism and general misogyny or because of the trauma of watching him beat her mother. She is not in therapy because something overtly terrible has happened to her, at least so far as she tells the healer when arranging the appointment. She has no idea that she has never experienced safety, and it will take considerable unpacking and reknowing the ways she has been unsafe and her heritages of how to manage unsafety, before she and the healer can begin to address the topic of how to get closer to safe, safe enough, safer, maybe even actually safe.

Marisol early on had developed an assimilationist and dissociative coping strategy that had served her very well indeed in the eyes of the world. Sent to Catholic girls' schools by her deeply religious Catholic mother and her father, whose attitude was "Yeah, I'm Catholic but so what," she found nurturance and love from the religious sisters who taught there. In that atmosphere in which all of her peers were, like her, natal girls and where there were few social class issues because the school was attached to a neighborhood parish which subsidized the education of less affluent children, and where everyone wore the same school uniform, Marisol could be safe enough, closer to safe, for many hours every day and focus on what she loved, which was to learn.

She had not inherited her father's family's genes for atypical attention and reading difficulties. Her mother's family, although not literate, apparently had the genes for attention, focus, and excellent reading and math skills, all of which propelled Marisol into an even greater closer to safety status during her school hours, where she was surrounded by religious sisters who were committed to girls' education and by other smart girls for whom learning was the highest form of being. School was heaven.

Spending every waking hour at school to avoid the unpleasantness of the living situations into which a runaway 14-year-old girl is housed. She had no conscious awareness of doing this. A door opened for her to unknow through her natural talents for dissociation, and she walked through it. She was a star student, her class's valedictorian, who went on full academic scholarship to a prestigious Catholic women's college in Los Angeles associated with the religious order that had taught in her childhood schools. There she had, for the first time, a Pinoy community and also, for the first time, a geographic cure for Duncan's depredations.

After acing her LSATs, she went on to a top-tier law school where she served on the editorial board of its law review and graduated magna cum laude. She had a reputation among her peers as a grind because all she did was study; no dating, nothing that would interfere with her highly successful and well-rewarded dissociative coping strategies. Working, going to the gym for an exhausting workout, volunteering at a shelter run by the religious order that had educated her, work some more, lather, rinse, repeat. She was, in the eyes of the world, highly successful, an exemplar of the mythology that, in America, if you work hard enough, you can achieve anything.

In fact, her dissociation was such a powerful strategy for unknowing the danger her father posed to her that it was not until about a year into therapy that the memories of what her father had done began to break through. She had clearly inherited, from both sides of her family, a rich collection of ways of not knowing danger. This basket of unknowing goodies included dissociation, which is used primarily by very young children who are trapped with a dangerous caregiver, as was the specific case for Marisol. It also included overwork, which both of her parents had also utilized and which translated in Marisol's case into, at first, absorption into academics and then the workplace, first in a highly prestigious position as a clerk to a judge on a U.S. district court of appeals immediately upon graduating law school, the ne plus ultra of postgraduation jobs for a new attorney short of a Supreme Court clerkship, and then in her first job as an associate at an equally prestigious law firm where the routine expectation was that she would be at work 90 hours a week and bill for most of those.

She told her healer that she found none of this difficult because all of this overwork meant that when she went to bed she was exhausted and thus could sleep for a few hours. She could only sleep when exhaustion made it impossible not to. The hours and hours that she spent, first at school and then at work, allowed no time for the romantic or sexual relationships in which she had never had any interest. She made partner at her firm 2 years before the rest of her class, to the surprise of no one. She would joke, "I am married to my job," which was not a joke.

The familial unknowing strategies that she absorbed unconsciously from the layers of unknowing each side of her family had adopted over the generations also included rationalization and minimization. Marisol saw both parents use these with regard to her father's violence, as well as the overtly racist things he said to her and Paz. Paz also taught Marisol, through the course of many mother–daughter talks, that she would do best to minimize whatever distress might attempt to poke through the psychic numbing when she encountered systemic racism and misogyny in her daily life as a BIPOC woman. "Pray," her mother would tell Marisol, "pray to Blessed Mother." Over time, Marisol stopped praying, having discarded religion at the side of her road as she completed school. Degree in hand, she prayed to the deity of overwork instead.

Marisol had a toolbox of unknowing strategies that built wide, thick, and nearly impregnable walls against any sense that she, as a BIPOC woman who thought of herself as White, was in chronic danger from misogyny, racism, and xenophobia. She did not know that she had been incestuously abused. While she knew she had been a witness to her father's violence against her mother, she had not allowed herself to know that she had been in danger for most of her life from the adult male closest to her. She was a success story in the narrative of every social pathology. She made six figures a year, had been promoted to partner quickly, was sought after as a speaker at legal conferences, and lived in a great condo with a view of the mountains.

So How Is This a Problem?

Why was she in therapy? she wondered out loud at the very first session. She told her healer, Sile, who happened to be of Irish descent herself, that she had begun to have what she called panic attacks, "for no good reason." She went on: "I don't like taking drugs, they dull the mind. So, okay, there's this thing I've read about, CBT [cognitive behavioral therapy]. It should get rid of this crap quickly, yes? Do you do CBT?" Two days before her first episode of fearful hyperarousal, she had been told by her firm's managing partner that she was going to be appointed as the head of the firm's litigation division within the coming year if all went as it always had gone with her.

"So why am I suddenly panicking?" she asked Sile. "Do I have imposter syndrome? Because I researched that, you know, when I learned that this was panic and not a cardiac condition, and while it would be logical for someone with my background to suffer from that, I've never for a moment felt like an imposter. The nuns taught me how smart I was, and they were right—they were always right! I'm smart, I'm capable, I work harder than any of the other litigators at the firm, I had a great clerkship, and I've had a brilliant career for a couple of decades. I need tools to stop this because it's interfering with my ability to work, and I don't want to take any pills, because I don't want to be out of control." Words, lots of words, rationalizations and intellectualizations, spilling out quickly, with Marisol stopping herself from taking a breath or crying.

The answer to the question of why Marisol was feeling attacked by her own threat response system, with hyperarousal of her SNS and HPA axis and underperformance by her ventral vagal and parasympathetic nervous systems, was initially unclear to Sile, who was at an early stage in adopting a DHCR liberatory paradigm for her healing work and only superficially acquainted with the emerging scholarship on trauma's neurobiology. "I knew about the HPA axis, of course," she said to Marisol later. "But the rest, ah, you led me to learn, for which I am grateful."

Therapy thus focused, at first, on trying out the usual approaches to reducing unexplained experiences of panic. The healer asked Marisol to engage in experiments with herself that often helped panicking people, such as the 5 × 5 breathing exercise, grounding techniques for bringing a person into the present, and very basic mindfulness skills, as well as some exposure therapy. She introduced Marisol to the cognitive–behavioral strategies that the latter had come into the office requesting.

What surprised both of them was that all of these techniques, which should have worked, only seemed to increase the frequency, duration, and severity of the panic attacks. This was the point at which Sile accidentally turned in a DHCR direction. She did not blame Marisol for the failure of what she was offering her. Instead, she said, "Okay, let's ditch those experiments, because we have the data. This isn't helping the person you are right now, and there's no reason to persist. But what about taking a brief medical leave of absence from work? Haven't you earned some flexibility there, given how much extra you've done all these years?"

On hearing these words, Marisol went into a full-blown episode of terror, sobbing and pleading, "Don't make me do that, please, don't make me go home, please, please, let me stay at school." At which point both of them sat up, shocked into a new level of awareness. Marisol went very still; she later described it to Sile as feeling "like I had just gone dead inside. Gone into a black hole inside of myself," which is an excellent way of describing a dive into a dorsal vagal freeze state common to trapped, traumatized, often, although not always, small creatures. Sile said, "School? School? Marisol, I think there might be something going on here that I don't understand yet. And maybe you don't understand yet. But there is something about what we've been trying that's been making you suffer more than I have ever seen you suffer. I think it's maybe somehow linked somehow to what's happening at work. Maybe to what school represented for you?"

Sile demonstrated a basic important skill for decolonizing the process of trauma healing. She did not assume that she knew what was best for this suffering person, and did not immediately make Marisol the problem or frame her as treatment-resistant when the usual first-line strategies for assisting a person's overactive SNS to calm down weren't helpful. She also didn't assume that she knew what she was hearing when Marisol suddenly begged her not to send her home and to let her stay at school.

What Sile did do was to move into what we would identify as a more clearly DHCR and liberatory stance. She went back to a first touch position, one we discussed in Chapter 7 when describing how to begin our DHCR encounters, without having that construct in her own mind. She simply knew, listening to her own gut and remembering her own healing experiences, what she needed to do. She listened very carefully, with her ears, her psyche, and her body, to all of the layers of what had happened when she suggested that Marisol take time off from work.

Together, over the next several sessions, which Sile requested be increased in frequency "just until we figure this out," thus offering more support without stigmatizing what was happening, they noticed what was emerging, with Marisol setting the pace. The entire idea of not going to work had poked a very large hole in some kind of dissociative process, a premature tearing open of some strategy that Marisol had been using for not knowing about some kind of danger. That hole had already been opened up just enough by the impending promotion, a crack, as it were, wide enough for what had been defined as panic attacks to start to occur—experiences that the two of them later recognized as a younger ego state finally believing that Marisol was closer enough to safe to start yelling, via the panic episodes, about what had been done to her decades previously.

Marisol said to Sile, several years later, if someone is the head of litigation at a very prestigious law firm, then people will probably believe and defend that person, "which makes that person pretty safe, and maybe believable when they tell a story like mine." What Marisol and Sile were witnessing was the wearing out of her strategies for dissociating the knowledge of danger past as the changed circumstances of being barely safe enough to know in Marisol's present eroded the barriers to the intrusion of knowing.

Sile never labeled Marisol "workaholic" or in any other way attempted to pathologize the ways in which this woman's entire life seemed to be one continuous cycle of working and exercising to exhaustion. She did notice how emotionally young the suffering person sitting across from her had suddenly become when she, the healer, suggested cutting back on any of that. Sile invited the two of them to radically collaborate, to be curious together, about what was going on.

"I Feel Like My Psyche Is One of Those Hundred-Layer Cakes, Only Not Tasty"

Things emerged in layers, in a meandering line, feeling like, to quote Marisol, "a not tasty hundred-layer cake from which one layer after another was being peeled back with a sharp knife." Marisol described how the news that she was about to be named head of litigation at first filled her with pride and then almost immediately thereafter with an unexpected and surprising dread. "Pride, I get, because I am proud of what I have accomplished in my career. The dread made no sense. But there it was, and then the panic attacks, and here we are."

Sile invited Marisol to feel where in her body she felt the dread and then to sit in and with that bodily experience, a suggestion that took several sessions before Marisol was willing to experiment with it. "I don't feel anything in my body, and I don't want to" was her first, not surprising, response to this too-common intervention in the world of trauma healing. Sile respected this boundary, getting the message that this was an approach too advanced and disempowering to have requested. She instead asked Marisol in what part of her body, if any, she would not feel endangered by feeling a sensation. They landed on Marisol's big toe, which was sore from a recent running injury. That, Marisol said, she could feel because she knew why she was feeling it and that the pain was the result of doing "a good thing."

"I don't know where this is coming from, Sile," she said to her healer a few meetings later. "But I'm having this sudden memory of how I would feel at the end of the day when I had to go home from school, or from the sisters' residence, or wherever I was. This same dread I started feeling when I heard about the promotion, the dread I always felt knowing that I would have to go home. And yeah, my father was an a-hole [Marisol never used full-on profanity until much further into the therapy], and he beat my mother and said horrible things to both of us, but still, dread? And going home, okay, going home, if I'm the head of litigation I'll still be working really long hours, but I'll probably have to go home because I'll have all of these people working for me."

She stopped and gasped, hearing her own use of language: "Have to go home? Not, could go home instead of sleeping on the office couch? Why should that cause dread? What about going home is the cause for dread, because if I'm all of a sudden starting to dread something, then that would explain the panic. But going home is no big deal. It was no big deal when I was a kid, it was just annoying. Even though I apparently dreaded it. Okay, I'm confused, can we stop now and play with the dog?" At which point Roxie, the French bulldog, was invited out of her crate to be petted and to help Marisol's SNS become less activated, which Roxie was always happy to do.

Here the healer and the person in distress, together with the canine cohealer, were able to encounter and give language to some of Marisol's top layers of unknowing the absence of safety or the presence of actual danger. Home was associated with an absence of safety, and it was in fact quite dangerous to her, far more dangerous than she could know. Her SNS was frantically signaling this danger to her, trying hard to break through all of the layers of dissociation, yelling loudly enough that Marisol was finally able to detect what might be the unsafe place that she had been able to successfully stay away from.

The dangerous place was home. It was her own bed. She had, she told Sile with shame-filled affect and downcast eyes, never spent a night of her life, after leaving home for college, in a room with a bed designated for her. She had slept on couches in semipublic places, in the common room of her dorm, and then in the law library, and then in her various offices, going home only in the early light of day to change clothing and return to the only safe places in her life, which were in the category of "not home" and did not include her bed. Aside from the cleaning crews and the other self-described night owls of her world, no one ever knew that this woman had not slept in a bed since she was 18. "I kept telling myself that if I could just get the right mattress and great sheets, I could sleep in my own bed, but that didn't work either. I even sleep on the couch in hotels."

We next encounter the unknowing strategy of minimization. The place, home, that is giving her danger-warning system conniptions, is "no big deal, just annoying." Dread showed up, dread was shoved away, and annoyance substituted for the more accurate emotional data about the danger zone of sexual abuse into which she was going: her bed, at home, at night. This minimization strategy was well learned from her mother, whose response to misogyny, racism, and xenophobia was also well-practiced minimization and dissociation. She had modeled for Marisol all these ways to unknow social pathologies and the accompanying microaggressions that were rained on mother and daughter, both directly through her father and out in the world of their small Alabama town. Paz taught Marisol these strategies as a component of being culturally Pinay and having smooth relations with those enacting the social pathologies on them.

"I'm making too big a deal out of this, maybe I'm wasting both of our time," was the next line of unknowing that Marisol offered to Sile, who had to stop herself from laughing only because she knew that this ludicrous pronounce-ment was a sign that something scary was lurking just around the psychic corner. This use of minimization and self-deprecation mirrored Paz's response to Duncan's abusive behavior. When Marisol, as she grew older, had come to realize that her father's bouts of violence were not normal (albeit quite normative in most patriarchies as means of enforcing covert norms of the social pathologies of misogyny and toxic masculinity) and had told Paz that she didn't have to tolerate the abuse, Paz had said, "Dear, you're making too big a deal out of this. He doesn't break any bones. We have to be grateful that we're not struggling like your titas [aunts] back in Manila. We are lucky that we have a nice home, and you can go to good schools." Marisol traced her decision to become an attorney to that conversation. "Which is why I do my pro bono work for the battered women's shelter, you know? I might make the big bucks off of corporate America, but I can help women like my mom, even though she still won't let me help her."

Sile, who because of her strong identification with her Irish ancestry had some hints about Marisol's father's family's backstory from knowing of her own ancestors' struggles, was noticing how many different unknowing strat-egies Marisol was employing simply to distract everyone, starting with the religious sisters and continuing into Sile's office, from the whole phenomenon Marisol's dread about going home. She also knew herself to be in the presence of a master litigator, someone who had successfully argued cases at the U.S. Supreme Court and who would thus be able to demolish any cognitive chal-lenges to these rationalizations without breaking stride. Sile also noticed how activated this suffering person was becoming, with the front edges of panic once again entering the room.

So she simply noticed out loud what was happening, using a skill developed in Southeast Asia by Buddhist meditators for many millennia, the Vipassana mindfulness practices of observing, describing, and withholding judgment. "Marisol, I notice that you've said several things about the possibility of going home. Do I have your permission to tell you what I think I might be seeing and hearing?" Notice that an important pathway to decolonizing trauma healing is to obtain consent at each step, not simply in the first session when someone signs a consent form. Consent to notice out loud, to let Marisol know that Sile was seeing her, seeing someone who did not wish to see or be seen.

With consent given, Sile continued, slowly. "So . . . I sense that one thing is that being in your home feels like a terrible obligation, something you must do rather than something you could choose to do. May I keep going?" Notice consent again, at every step. "Okay, so, another thing that we are both noticing is that this prospect mysteriously fills you with dread, and you have been telling us that you realize this is not a new feeling. Keep going?" Consent requested again; and if Marisol had said to stop then and there, Sile would have done so. "Okay. So, you've then said that going home is no big deal and that you are perhaps wasting our time exploring this line of inquiry."

"And now a big ask, about you and your emotions. May I?" Marisol sat with that for a beat longer and nodded her head. "Okay, breathing, and let's get Roxie into your lap now"—an offer of coregulation from a safe species, not a human. "May I notice out loud that at our last session, you were in my office, sounding like a very young girl, sobbing and pleading with me not to send you home from school. If you were listening to someone tell you all of this, what would you think?"

In naming both the multiple topmost layers of protection from knowing that she had seen Marisol utilize, as well as what had happened when full knowing briefly intruded, Sile invited Marisol to also simply observe herself. At this point, Sile had no clear idea of what had happened in the lives or the family histories of either of Marisol's parents. She had some guesses, because of her own heritage and because she vaguely knew something about the American occupation of the Philippines. But she didn't know specifics, nothing about the effects of the layers upon layers of interlocking social pathologies that not only informed the traumas embedded in all of Marisol's intersectional identities and thus her two very different cultural heritages of how to dissociate nor of the ultimate results of all of those horrors that culminated in Marisol being raped by the father who had raped her mother, a man whose own mother had been raped by his father, who was, unknown to him, descended from a child born to the rape of his great-great-great-grandmother by a British soldier.

Marisol herself either didn't know or wasn't yet ready to disclose what had happened in her life, aside from her wonderful times at school, her success in her clerkship, and her stresses at work. But Sile had some very strong hunches, thanks to the brief appearance of the young ego state, as well as the power and sheer volume of the danger warning signs that were coming from Marisol's SNS.

Sile, with all of her good hunches (many of which led to fruitful and liberatory DHCR-flavored discussions much farther down the line in their work together, since she had some ideas about good questions to ask), did not substitute her knowledge for that of the suffering person in her office. That would be a step away from closer to safe. She had become informed enough about DHCR and liberatory trauma healing since Marisol had first sought her out to realize that one of the ways in which trauma healing can be an expression of power dominance is when the healer decides to offer their insights to the suffering person without consent. This too-common practice taught to mental health professionals then substitutes for that person's own self-knowledge, violates the suffering person's pace for being able to know, and shuts down the process of their claiming their knowing in their own way, at their own time.

This sort of substitution of knowledge is analogous to the colonizing dynamic by which anthropologists arrive in so-called primitive cultures and make pronouncements about those peoples, which then enter textbooks and are in turn taught as accurate information to members of that same culture, some of whom get into difficulties with teachers when they protest inaccuracies.

Let's Get Closer to Safe

What Sile and Marisol learned together in those first few years of working with one another was that Marisol's closer to safe place had been first school and then her office. When Sile introduced the idea of using eye movement desensitization reprocessing (EMDR) for strengthening Marisol's sense of being closer to safe, she did not ask Marisol to visualize a safe place. Instead, the two of them had a discussion about whether there was anything, anyone, or any place, real or fictional, that would feel safe enough to experiment with, for use as something resembling a safe place for this stage of EMDR. Marisol said, "I'm afraid to ruin my memories of school and the nuns; I'm afraid I'll remember something terrible that I've forgotten because I needed that place to be safe for me. So maybe, let's try my office. In the daytime, with all the lights on, and the door closed and locked, and the curtains drawn. And oh, can I imagine that Roxie is there with me, please?"

The very slow use of the EMDR safe-place protocol was extremely painful for Marisol because it made her strikingly aware of how unsafe she felt in every cell of her being. She could tolerate doing the EMDR exercise for perhaps 5 minutes at a time for the first few months. In between she cycled back into her unknowing strategies, then into slightly longer periods of knowing, followed by struggles to reassert unknowing. Being closer to safe felt dangerous because some part of her knew what was struggling to be known and would be known if more of Marisol felt closer to safe. The irony of the first phase of this three-phase model, which tells us to establish safety first, is that when trauma-exposed people finally make it to closer to safe, that is the moment at which the knowledge of danger starts to intrude more forcefully. In practice, the model is not linear; it is getting a little closer to safety; then, when trauma shows up, processing, resting, getting a little closer to safety; and on to the next ring of the spiral of healing.

Sile used some of this time during which Marisol was in mortal struggle with herself over whether to allow herself to know what she was trying so hard not to know as a period in which she could invite deeper intellectual exploration into family histories of intergenerational trauma. Marisol, an inveterate reader, gobbled up books about the history of the Philippines and about the story of Irish people in America. She was shocked by what she learned, given that all of that truth had been carefully kept out of the history books she had read during her formal education. Then, as the dust of her parents', and grandparents', and ancestors' lives settled in her psyche, she began to see herself and her terrors of knowing what might have been dangerous enough to provoke dread in an entirely new and increasingly compassionate light.

"I always thought of Dad as just this White racist asshole [by then profanity was a regular visitor to the therapy room], and he is that," she said to Sile. "But he's also a ton of other things. He's a lot like some of the death row inmates whose sentences I worked to get commuted when I was in legal clinic at school, except he never killed anyone, at least as far as I know. And Mom, holy wow. Not the passive pushover. She's been doing her best to make something good out of crap. Moldy lemons into chicken adobo."

This move toward compassion for her parents happened just before Marisol remembered her father raping her. Somehow her beginning-to-know self and her getting-closer-to-safe self were unconsciously noticing that her father was a criminal, not entirely dissimilar from the murderers whose lives she had tried to save. The decolonial conversations that Sile invited Marisol to have are very different from the standard genogram, even those with notations for violence and abuse in a family, because they used the framework of how each family culture had been wounded by colonization and how the results, as expressed in her parents' lives, were not unusual for the descendants of colonized people with the collection of traumatized intersectional identities that were all contained in the amazing human named Marisol.

For Marisol, whose interest in decolonial frameworks had extended only to the Indigenous people of North America, the notion that this was a paradigm through which she could begin to make more sense of her life and her distress was appealing. This will not, by the way, be true for everyone with whom we work: sometimes this paradigm will not be of interest to the person we are working with—we follow their lead on this. Marisol was unusually open to this construct. It was also very appealing to her as a new avoidance strategy, focusing on her parents' distress, a distraction that Sile noticed after a few weeks of "OMG, did you know this? Decolonial Jeopardy, let's have the colonization of the Philippines for a million, zillion dollars, please." Being DHCR in our paradigms does not mean that we make the healing process solely about the pain of ancestors. It does mean that we bring that into the picture so that people in distress in our offices can deepen in their compassion for themselves and the ways in which they have come to suffer.

The Truth and Nothing but the Truth Can Make You Closer to Safe

"Sile, it's Marisol," the voicemail message began. "I just had the most horrible dream. Then I woke up and I knew it wasn't a dream. My father . . ." her voice broke off, sobbing. "I need to see you today if I can, please." Nearly 3 years of working on becoming closer to safe, exploring family heritages of trauma, slowly reducing ways of unknowing, and then Marisol sat down with Sile and knew out loud what had been done to her. "I hate this, and it makes sense of everything, and I hate this. Could this be a false memory? No, no, you've never said a word to me about anything like this, I avoid reading about things like this, oh, I avoid reading about things like this, or working on sexual assault cases. Oh. Oh. That asshole. That asshole. I could kill him, no, I won't get on a plane and go home and kill him, I promise I won't, prison sucks, but right now I wish I were more of a criminal like him. He's a criminal, Sile, he's a pervert, and he's my father, and . . ."

Sile sat with the flood of words and pain. She had wisely ensured that there were no other people coming to see her for three hours from the start of this meeting because Marisol needed almost all of that time that day. At the start of the third hour, Sile asked Marisol what they needed to do together to make the best closer to safe plan that they could for Marisol, who was being shaken by her embodied knowledge of how unsafe she had been, for how long, and from whom. "It's not that I worry that you're going to kill yourself, or him either, mind you, it's that I want you to think out loud with me about what you need to do to get through the rest of today, and tonight, and to consider if you want to see me again tomorrow, because that's an option. You have the right to be as close to safe as we can collectively help you to be, remember? So, ideas?"

Sile's offering to collaborate with a person at an acute intrusive crisis point of knowing is profoundly disruptive to the usual strategy of a healer imposing a safety plan. This collaborative methodology holds firmly to the deeply liberatory and empowering stance of a DHCR trauma healing project. It is about truth telling by the healer: "Hi, we can both see that you're in trouble, not in danger. You're in trouble because you are in great distress. You are being plunged into the loss of your unknowing and into the pain of knowledge.

I trust that you can be the one who takes the lead on ideas about how to be closer to safe, even if you've spent the last two hours sobbing and in a very young ego state."

One very effective way to disempower trauma-exposed people is to send them out of the door of the healing space in a very young, intensely suffering ego state simply because it's time for the session to be over. So if you, the healer, have 50 minutes, start this discussion about collaborating on a plan to get the suffering person closer to safe at minute 25, and no later, please.

Marisol's response: "You know, Sile, it's kind of a relief in a bizarre way to know the truth. Maybe not the whole truth yet, but the truth. Because this is the truth, I can feel it, physically, I feel him raping me. So I think that that's a first piece of me feeling closer to safe. When I know what the monster is that I've been trying to close the door on all these years, I know, I know what I'm dealing with. I know I'm not nuts for never sleeping in a bed. Which makes me feel, in a totally bizarre way, less unsafe, so maybe closer to safe. So yes, please, tomorrow, and please, some safer-place EMDR before we go much further. Also, Roxie in my lap for the rest of our time, please. Does she ever do home visits, by the way?" Which last question led to laughter, a healing moment of joy in the midst of pain, the joy that liberation psychology teaches us is necessary for decolonizing the healing of souls.

Notice that Marisol is identifying ways of being closer to safe that she and Sile have spent several years building in such a manner as to make them familiar and feel reliable. They arrived at a safety plan. Then, as Marisol put it, "I appear to be ready to visit the planet of my own truth. The truth, the whole truth, nothing but the truth. Damn it. But maybe this means that someday I get to sleep in my own bed?"

The only path to closer to safe, safe enough, safer, maybe even safety itself, is to first carefully untangle the thickets of unknowing, which have created the ability to not know that danger is nearby. The reason I have told you Marisol's story in such detail is that, in the hands of someone not practicing DHCR work or one of its close cousins, things could have gone differently and potentially destructively. There are too many stories, none of them apocryphal, some of them written and published by suffering people who sought trauma treatment, of ways in which a healer's insistence on the pursuit of knowing and their inattention to the ways in which unknowing created something resembling temporary safety, led to worsened suffering (A. G. Rogers, 1995).

Decolonizing trauma healing means that we do not put the reduction of a symptom ahead of interrogating how that thing we are seeing, that thing from which the person in our healing space may or may not be suffering, is actually the way in which that person has been keeping themselves closer to safe. Depathologizing is decolonizing. It is treating, with all of the respect that it deserves, the person's indigenous-to-self ways of being closer to safe, which may include individual strategies like dissociation, cultural strategies like assimilation, or some combination of all of the above, lessons taught by a person's intersectional identities and the heritages of each strand of that braid.

So, follow the three-phase model. Safety first, second, third, and again as the healing process continues along its spiral. As close to safe as possible. Truth, rather than minimization of the realities of danger. Because when being close enough to safe is available, then people can turn around and look at the monsters.

10 INTERSECTIONALITIES AND TRAUMA

Risk and Capacities in the Face of Social Pathologies and Relational Harm

A NEW LENS, A NEW APPROACH

When I wrote *Cultural Competence in Trauma Therapy* (2008) a decade and a half ago, my thinking about the ways in which people's intersectional identities were expressed was strongly influenced by Hays's (2022) ADDRESSING model, an acronym for some of the most prominent components of intersectionality studied by psychologists. I spent the majority of that book writing about trauma in terms of specific parts of that model—trauma and age, trauma and disability, trauma and gender, and so on. While I attempted to make my clinical examples intersectional ones, I was using a particular box as my starting point.

From the perspective of the lived experiences of suffering people, a healer's attention to the facet of intersectionality that is most prominent in the suffering person's own phenomenology or the strand that has been most painfully targeted, presently or historically, by social pathologies is not necessarily problematic. I haven't had the experience as a healer, nor have many of the healers who consult with me on their work, of having a suffering person say that they need the healer to deal with their trauma within some particular mixture of their intersectionalities (although this seems to be changing a

https://doi.org/10.1037/0000421-011
Decolonizing Trauma Healing: Toward a Humble, Culturally Responsive Practice,
by L. S. Brown

little as a generation of traumatized people who have already thought about intersectionality are entering trauma healing).

For the most part, in my experience and that of my colleagues, people come in the door saying some version of "I hurt, I suffer, help me, please." It's one of the responsibilities of the decolonial trauma healer to bring the intersectional framework to the epistemic table, to be integrated into and shared with the suffering person as makes sense during the healing process.

Thus, I'm centering this chapter on understanding intersectionalities and trauma at individual, historical, cultural, intergenerational, and larger sociopolitical locations. I will tell clinical stories, none of them based on any single person, all representing amalgamations of at least three, usually more, people, because I find these stories the best ways to teach. First, though, I want to delve more deeply into the construct of intersectionality because I increasingly see it, rather than the identification of any particular strand of it, as central to decolonial, humble, culturally responsive (DHCR) trauma healing. It has been the pathological narratives of colonization of peoples, lands, cultures, and the epistemic systems of healing trauma that have tried to break down people and their trauma into component parts. Reintegrating is decolonial. I also find it helpful in working clinically to have an epistemic framework to guide me, and I am hoping that does the same for you, my readers.

OUR OWN NAMES

Intersectionality is a paradigm developed by women, primarily feminists, many of them lesbians, often Jewish or persons of color who were trying to describe their own experiences of identity development and of living in places for which there were neither neat boxes nor colonial names but in which their lived experiences did not quite fit. Intersectionality is, in consequence, a foundationally decolonial construct, deriving from the observations of marginalized people who insisted that no one person has a single strand of identity, even though the dominant cultures of social pathologies prefer to create binary and mutually exclusive boxes that generate competition for resources and lack of trust among and between marginalized groups (Josefowitz Siegel, 1990).

Well before Kimberle Crenshaw's (1989) now famous article in which she proposed the term *intersectionality* as an epistemic framework for naming the reality that there are, in each human, multiple strands of identity, noting that these strands operate not in an additive but rather in an intersectional fashion, critical thinkers and activists in the worlds of Black, Indigenous, and people of color (BIPOC) women's activism, intersectional feminist therapy, liberation psychology, and trauma healing had been describing the same phenomenon without giving it that name. Crenshaw did not appropriate this other work; she built upon it. What is striking is the number of parallels in the intellectual discourse that emerged as proto-decolonial thinkers and healers began to interrogate the notions of singular identities.

Consequently, while I use Crenshaw's term *intersectionality* because it is wonderfully descriptive, and also has become familiar to many decolonial and liberatory thinkers and healers, I want to give credit to those who influenced my own thinking well before I encountered Crenshaw. The earliest of these authors were not in the mental health professions or in the field of trauma. They were activists, poets, and visionaries, writing of their lives in the intersections and on the margins, or what Gloria Anzaldúa named the "borderlands" of identities (Anzaldúa, 1987; Moraga & Anzaldúa, 1981).

Living in the Borderlands on the Banks of the Combahee River

Before Crenshaw, there were African American lesbians and feminists of the Combahee River Collective (1983), among whose founding and early members were Barbara Smith, Beverly Smith, Demita Frazier, Cheryl Clarke, Akasha (Gloria) Hull, Margo Okazawa-Rey, Chirlane McCray, and Audre Lorde. The collective was named after Harriet Tubman's famous Combahee River raid, in which she freed many enslaved Africans. This manifesto was the first work of its kind to fly into my brain; it was an exegesis exploring the inescapable reality that being Black, lesbian, and committed to social change through feminism was an intersectional location that did not arise from scholarly analysis but rather from lived experience, and this was both similar to and quite different from my experiences as a White, Jewish lesbian committed to social change through feminism. Intersectionality and its implications began to affect my thinking well before they rose to conscious awareness, sending me back to the oldest books in my library while writing this chapter, paperbacks from the 1960s through the 1980s.

The Combahee River Collective (1977) wrote: "Black feminists often talk about their feelings of craziness before becoming conscious of the concepts of sexual politics, patriarchal rule, and most importantly, feminism" (p. 1). I would call the "feelings of craziness" evidence of traumas of social pathologies, of personal encounters with violations, of daily exposure to insidious trauma, betrayal, and microaggression. These women knew that they were not in need of a diagnosis, although they did suffer. They saw the way forward as one of political action, while never denying their suffering and that of every woman whose intersectional identities appeared in a Venn diagram with theirs. They also spoke, eloquently and with pain, of the linked destinies of people of all genders belonging to a group targeted for oppression by phenotype supremacies, in this case, White supremacy.

In the early 1980s two groundbreaking anthologies and one challenging, single-authored volume appeared in which the authors spoke of their lived experiences in the intersections and at the margins. These are works that have also had a profound and continuing impact on my own thinking, deeper perhaps today than 40 years ago because of how my own thinking about the decolonial nature of the intersectional construct has evolved. They are worth reading for a DHCR trauma healer.

The first of these books is *This Bridge Called My Back: Writings by Radical Women of Color* (Moraga & Anzaldúa, 1981). Let me quote from the foreword by Toni Cade Bambara in which Bambara's unconscious began to be seeded with knowledge about decolonial survival strategies of the most colonized and marginalized of peoples. Bambara quotes Audre Lorde's open letter to radical, White, feminist theologian Mary Daly, who was lauded in the feminist world for her radical thinking yet relied solely upon Christian and Wiccan Eurocentric constructs as a starting point for her own revolutionary paradigms: "Assimilation within a solely Western European herstory is *not* acceptable" (Lorde, 1979/2007, p. 59, emphasis added). Bambara then goes on to describe some of the survival and resistance strategies named by the authors in the anthology: "The New Orleans African women and Yamassee and Yamacrow women went into the swamps to me with Filipino wives of 'draftees' and 'defectors' during the so-called French and Indian war . . . when Chinese, Mexican, and African women in this country saluted each other's attempts to form protective leagues" (Moraga & Anzaldúa, 1981, p. vii).

The early 1980s also saw the first of many volumes addressing intersectionality by the late bell hooks, who insisted on the noncapitalization of her adopted name, which had been that of her maternal great-grandmother. She spent her career challenging the division of women into either women or BIPOC people and, later, challenging toxic masculinity's role in destroying alliances between women who loved men and men who loved women, embracing love as a revolutionary, decolonial act.

The title of hooks's first prose work, *Ain't I a Woman: Black Women and Feminism* (1982), drew upon the famous quotation ascribed to Sojourner Truth, a formerly enslaved African abolition activist and a women's suffrage activist, who gave a speech asserting her right to be at a suffrage convention as a formerly enslaved woman, woman nonetheless, even though as an African woman she was not considered to be human, much less have a sex unless it was with regard to her availability to being raped by a slaver.

Ironically, these specific words were never spoken by Truth, who was enslaved by Dutch-speaking people in New York State. The language of this famous line represented an attempt by a White male publisher to make her sound like a speaker of English from a state in the Southern Confederacy. Thus even this famous speech claiming her womanhood among the White ladies of the suffrage movement has been colonized by the words of that White male publisher, who changed many of the details of the life that she did share in her speech so as to make it fit more neatly into stereotypes about formerly enslaved African American women, as well as the locations in which they had been enslaved (by then New York State was busily attempting to develop collective amnesia about its own history as a place where African were enslaved—and ironically, about the genocide and displacement of one of the Indigenous nations after which the location of this conference had been named, Seneca Falls).

These words are powerful and often quoted by BIPOC feminist activists as a means of underscoring the differences among women's experiences when the toxins of racism are introduced into a woman's life. The painful fact that this woman's powerful, courageous speech was stolen and colonized is a perfect example of how social pathologies—in this instance sexism, misogyny, racism, and classism—can poison even the most revolutionary of words and acts by suppressing them and putting forward the colonizer's version as truth (recall the two stories of Christopher Columbus's landing in the Western Hemisphere in Chapter 1, and more recently, laws that strip public school textbooks of the word *slavery*).

The same year the brilliantly titled anthology *All the Women Are White, All the Blacks Are Men, but Some of Us Are Brave* (Hull et al., 1982) appeared. The title says it all, even before the reader delves into the decolonial analyses of the authors; to live intentionally in the intersections requires courage because it is at those intersections that the weapons of social pathologies are squarely aimed. Well before the construct of intersectionality entered the intellectual discourse, but just after feminists who were not White Christians began to write about the ways in which their experiences diverged from those of the semiofficial women's movement, this book had an important role in decolonizing feminist thought, which in turn affected this author.

The work in my own field of feminist therapy that was instructive to me about intersectionalities was written by Val Kalei Kanuha (1990), a Native Hawai'ian lesbian social worker, educator, and activist working to stop sexual and intimate partner violence. She has also worked on decolonial efforts in Hawai'i, a land that was stolen by British and American business interests and had its Indigenous culture colonized and stigmatized, its Indigenous people nearly wiped out with introduced diseases, and its sacred places turned into tourist resorts. Kanuha comprehends intersectionality and colonialism in the marrow of her bones. She wrote as early as 1990 about what she called the "triple jeopardy" of risk of trauma exposure inherent in the intersectional identities of lesbians of color whose intimate partner relationships had become violent.

Beverly Greene (1990, 1992), African American lesbian psychologist, educator, therapist, and theorist (and a close personal friend and inspiration) followed closely on Kanuha. She was the first to discuss the specific challenges of living in the intersectional identities of African American, female, and lesbian when seeking psychotherapy. She wrote about the difficulties that women like herself encountered in finding a trauma healer who would not further traumatize them with microaggressions, disguised as psychotherapy, committed in the therapy office and perpetrated in the absence of awareness of what it meant to live at this intersectional location.

Maria P. P. Root (1992, 2000, 2004), a mixed-heritage Filipina American psychologist (also a close personal friend and inspiration) helped to found the entire field of study in the psychology of the lives and identity development of people of what was then called "mixed race." She not only tore open the boxes that assigned people to a racial category based on their phenotypic presentation, she also creatively studied what identity development was like in people whose parents did not share culture and phenotype.

Neither last nor least has been the work of one of the central thinkers of decolonial psychology, Lillian Comas-Díaz. Writing from her experience as a Latinx woman of mixed heritage, born with a disability, who grew up in Puerto Rico and, with her brilliance, infiltrated the very inner sanctums of U.S. psychology, her groundbreaking article, "LatiNegra" (1994),disrupted narratives of racism within both African-descent and Latinx communities, as expressed in the lives of women subjected to colorism. She has gone on to become one of the leading voices in the decolonial psychology movement, most recently as the senior editor of *Decolonial Psychology* (Comas-Díaz et al., 2024). It should be no surprise that her initial work in the borderlands led her here, and no surprise that my reading her work and becoming her friend, being influenced by her thinking, gave me a nuanced concept of intersectionalities well before the term came into general use.

The boxes that social scientists have chosen to define the parameters of the strands of intersectionality have been attached to both sex and melanic phenotype in many ways, thus speaking of race or sex. The prices paid by people who are born with certain gender and melanic phenotypes can be more specifically explicated in the scholarly literature because they have been studied longer. But these variations of intersectionalities are neither essential to nor necessarily inherent within most biological realities of the human body or lived experiences.

Intersectionalities challenge all kinds of phenotype supremacies, be they genital, melanic, or neurotypical—the question for the DHCR trauma healer is one of how the suffering person experiences the multiplicity of ways that they are. These identities, born from social locations and physical realities to which social meanings are then assigned have been, instead, personally or socially constructed out of lived experiences by people attempting to name themselves by their own names in the face of social pathologies which would attempt to steal their names and identities from them.

NO ONE IS BORN INTO A CATEGORY: ONE IS PLACED THERE

Simone de Beauvoir famously wrote, "One is not born, but rather becomes, a woman." (1949/1953, p. 273). So too, one is not born into a race, although one is born with melanic and related features of phenotype. One must be defined by a set of cultural norms as a particular race, which definitions vary from place to place and from era and era. One must be assigned to normalcy for having a particular kind of typical or temporarily typical presentation in the world which, in another time or place, might lead to an assignment of abnormalcy. These names are the ones given to perfectly human ways of being by social pathologies. We may believe them to be our own names before we have developed critical consciousness: "I am *x* thing, because that is what the culture around me calls me"—not a conscious thought but an internalization of the labels and the box.

These boxes and categories are not our names. Just as I know that my actual name, the one announced in synagogue when I was 30 days old, is Leah Simcha bat Shimon ben Chaim HaCohen v' Yaffa bat Yoseph and that Laura Susan was the English first-letter cognate that my parents chose because they believed that to have my real name known would put me at risk of being too visibly Jewish, born only 7 years after the Shoah, so naming our intersectionalities is a version of claiming those real names, even at the risk of putting ourselves in the gunsights, real or otherwise.

The definitional parameters of each of our intersectional identities may be informed by phenotype and/or lived experienced. They may be entirely socially constructed. It's usually some of all of these, and then there's the particular version of the intersection of Venn diagrams floating in the sea of trauma. It appears that the structural hierarchies of oppression from which the social pathologies have sprung do not want people to change their definitional parameters because the characteristics that are defined as within or outside of the protections of privilege are required by structural forms of oppression as rationales for oppressing people. Thus, the colonial narrative goes, these characteristics, be they allegedly physical or allegedly emotional or intellectual, must thus be essential to the person to whom the category is ascribed.

Whether it is rigid categories of how to be a particular gender, or the one-drop rule that enslaved the children born of the rape of enslaved women of African heritage who were themselves born of rape, or the Nazis' pronouncement that a person with one Jewish grandparent was a Jew for purposes of being murdered in the camps, the fact that for a given person a category may also feel or seem to be real, or protective, or a source of pride or comfort must be put in the context of the question of whether the definitional parameters that matter to a person were put there from the inside out, and thus reflect something indigenous to that strand of identity, or whether they are externally imposed and enforced—or some combination of both. Most importantly, from a DHCR trauma healing standpoint, is the question of what these strands of identity do for, as well as to, a suffering person.

One of the challenges for DHCR trauma healing is that we must invite ourselves and the people with whom we work to carefully, compassionately explore that question so as to remove the so-called truths created by social pathologies while keeping those truths about where danger lies that can lead to being closer to safe and, over time, to healing while knowing truth. Because these connections between bodies, phenotype, and the social constructions of identity have become so deeply entwined within a particular culture, along with the characteristics ascribed to the occupants of each category, social pathologies have functioned over time to rob people of agency in their self-definition and making it essential to acknowledge membership in categories, both those valued by the social pathology (Whiteness, maleness, heterosexuality) and those marginalized and subordinate. "You are an x" translates, within a generation or two or six, into "We are an x," with all of the toxic and devaluing characteristics stuffed into the box of x-ness by the structural oppression which created that box now part of claiming membership in the family of x. But also, "We are an x and are proud of these characteristics that only x's have, unlike our oppressors. White men can't jump!"

In order to fully heal from trauma, decolonizing the parameters and the contexts of the boxes of identities that constitute intersectionalities is a component of DHCR work, starting with the DHCR trauma healer's clear grasp of these epistemic frameworks. Critically questioning, in a respectful and collaborative manner, whether being x must mean being a target, must require acceptance of the burdens of oppression in order to be something vaguely closer to less in danger, whether one can also keep the pride in how being *x* led to creative responses to trauma, colonization, and marginalization, are among the tasks of decolonial trauma healing that rarely appear in the trauma treatment narratives.

Retelling Our Stories, Reclaiming Our Names

"Schver zol zein a Yid," it's hard to be a Jew, is a Yiddish saying I learned from my grandparents. But why, I ask, is having life be hard so central to being a member of my tribe? Why not, "You have to be strong and creative and wily and flexible to survive as a Jew," which is the version of the story I have been telling myself lately. Life was intermittently terrible and dangerous for my ancestors for about 2,000 years. It was also intermittently joyful and fun; there are some great jokes and wonderful dance tunes emerging from our far-flung exile. Survival meant being nourished by the latter and never forgetting the former.

To answer my own question, it's true that since the year 586 before the Common Era there have been increasingly long periods of time during which Jews were colonized, oppressed, and murdered by state actors or those authorized by the state. Agreed, that's hard. It's hard not to even be recognized as Indigenous people of the lands from which we were exiled and colonized.

But what if we decolonized the narrative of our collective trauma and reclaimed our Indigenous roots? What would that saying look like? Maybe, "Being a Jew means that we have had to get very skillful at surviving in all of the hard places and made us more attuned to the importance of having a just world." That's a different way to tell the same truth. It's a different version of the story which assisted me in surviving in my other marginalized intersectional identities, a methodology of changing the story which can be found in narrative therapies, which were developed through the theft of traditions of the colonized Indigenous people of Australia, who were fine with the lives they led before Great Britain decided to use their home as a dumping ground for convicts and those who lost their rebellions against British colonization in their own Scots or Irish homeland.

Changing the story of trauma at the hands of social pathologies from one of only suffering to one of survival in the face of the odds, to stories of the skills and creativity and joy with which survival was accomplished by exploring those gifts hidden in the strands of our intersectional identities, is one of the foundations on which a DHCR trauma healing practice can be built. This is a different, liberatory way in which to tell the same truths about the horrors—large, medium, and small—visited on us personally, on those like us, and on the generations before us.

Those boxes created by social pathologies not only generate and fuel marginalization and targeting, they are tools for implementing divide-and-conquer strategies, keeping oppressed people from finding common cause with one another. When social pathologies define humans into separate categories deemed to various degrees unworthy of protection, or even designated legitimate targets for maltreatment and danger, trauma becomes embedded in the heritage, cultures, and personal experiences of those whose intersectional identities are composed of these endangered categories. The trauma also comes with the message from the social pathologies: "You could have it worse, because look what happens to *y* group." The categories *x* and *y* get divided, as in the tragic story of the Hutu and Tutsi peoples of Rwanda.

As we've explored elsewhere in this volume, people have always attempted to find ways to stretch or discard the parameters of the categories of identities, with varying consequences, some of which have been marvelous and liberating, others of which have included terrible, sometimes lethal punishment by dominant groups for the crime of trying to evade categorization and, more painful still, at times ejection and alienation from their own tribe. The construct of intersectionality, conversely, helps us disrupt categories, in fact, disrupts the entire notion of categories, and says we can know all of ourselves. We can call ourselves by our own names and, in doing so, heal from trauma.

The construct of intersectionality insists that a person be known by more than what is obvious about their phenotype or visible in their behavior or dress, the place in which they live, or the accent with which they speak. Intersectionality declares that there is little that is essential about how a person ultimately defines any aspect of the body into which they are born or the body into which they grow over time, little that is essential about who they are that can be inferred from anything you can see about them.

The use of an in-depth analysis and exploration of a person's intersectionality as a component of DHCR trauma healing consequently challenges dominant social constructions of almost every variable in how human beings experience ourselves. The construct of intersectionality potentially offers people the power to define the meanings of who they are. This empowers DHCR trauma healers to make sense of distress as it is expressed through a suffering person's intersectional lenses, and also to see some of the paths to being closer to safe, and ultimately to liberation and empowerment. The construct of intersectionality disrupts identity constructs deriving from social pathologies such as mixed race (we are all of the human race) or half-breed (as if the observer, by knowing parentage, knows which DNA was expressed when sperm met egg), throws out the one-drop rule which defines any human with any known African ancestry as Black and therefore should describe most humans that way, since most of us came out of Africa. The construct of intersectionality places gender on a spectrum rather than within a binary, as it does the notion of a typically able body. In fact, it tosses the notion of a typical human into the recycle bin of history where that category belongs so that it can be shredded and repurposed into something liberating and decolonizing.

THE VERY FEW IMMUTABLES

There are very few immutable biological realities for humans. One of them is the phenotype that includes having a uterus, regardless of how these people later name themselves or present their gender orientation in the world. Humans born appearing to have a female phenotype may have neither a vulva nor a uterus if they are some type of intersex, along with those people born with what appears to be a vulva but without a uterus.

Why does this matter? Pregnancy. Humans with uteruses are the humans who can become pregnant, including through sexual violence. Women and those people who are nonbinary with a vulva or trans males with retained uteruses thus are the only humans placed at serious risk of loss of bodily autonomy by laws restricting reproductive choice. That's an immutable biological reality worsened by legal phenomena.

Any body can be raped, which is a trauma that is gendered female and as such has shame attached to it. This is because most bodies who are raped are those of natal women. But some of those are the bodies of feminine-of-center men being punished for violating the rules of toxic masculinity. Some of the bodies being raped are those of nonbinary or trans people, punishment for violating the rule that gender must be unambiguous and binary. Rape, while primarily a crime against women, is a gendered act of violent social control that says, "You are not a man or not a real man. You are not in charge of your bodily autonomy." Any child's body can be sexually abused. Any human's body can be harmed through physical trauma, intended or otherwise. The sole human immutable biological reality is that we are fragile and mortal.

So What Difference Do the Sex Phenotypes Make?

To be a DHCR trauma healer means having thought through this question carefully. A natal woman who is not intersex and whose lived experience of her gender is as woman, as nonbinary, or as transmasculine has a vagina and a uterus. These are the only humans who can menstruate, the only humans who can become pregnant and give birth. Such humans are the only ones whose reproductive bodily autonomy has always been threatened by patriarchy's goal of controlling bodies that can give birth, because of course there have always been natal women who socially present as men or as neither or both, which we now call nonbinary.

Thus, a strand of intersectionality that might not be visible, and may be incorrectly inferred from visual evidence available to a healer of souls and spirits, is that of being able or once able to become pregnant. Not all natal women with a vulva and uterus fit into that group because their bodies will not hold onto a pregnancy; calling that "infertility" medicalizes the emotional reality of that status, which may have been a source of trauma. It may have been a source of trauma that a particular natal woman or girl was among those able to become pregnant.

The Story of the Memorial Uterus

Before he claimed his identity as George,[1] a trans man, he was Sasha, a natal girl with a vulva and uterus who could become pregnant. And Sasha did become pregnant, from early heterosexual activity that was undertaken without contraceptive measures because Sasha always knew that she was George and dissociated the trauma of periods, and the uterus they came from, until the much larger trauma of pregnancy at age 15 occurred. George turned 15 in 1972, in a world where unwed mothers were sent away to give birth and their babies were taken from them, not the relinquishment of today but with a total ban on contact. The pregnancy was a trauma because it messed with George's knowledge of being a boy, because the child was taken away while Sasha/George was anesthetized for the delivery, and because Sasha/George was shamed for becoming pregnant outside of marriage.

When George began his gender affirmation process, he was surprised at how it reawakened the trauma of pregnancy and the birth and loss of a child. "I thought I would be glad to simply get rid of all that," he told his healer, Kurt, who was also a trans man but not one who had ever been pregnant or given birth. "But I find myself wondering, even at 40, whether I might want to hold onto that uterus for, I don't know, in memory of that poor kid who suffered so much." To his credit, Kurt did not interpret George's feelings about his uterus as evidence that George was not really trans, which might have been done by another, less critically conscious healer. Instead, Kurt invited George to deepen his exploration of what that uterus meant to him, and George said, "I had a dream last night that I gave birth again, only this time I kept my baby. I woke up and thought, I'm that baby, and I also need to find the baby who came out of that uterus before I can give it up, because it's the only evidence I have that Sasha was pregnant."

---

[1]Case material has been disguised to protect client confidentiality.

Finding a child taken in adoption was not an easy task in the days before the internet and home genetics testing. George was persistent, and he had social class privilege to assist him, having gone to medical school and become a well-paid orthopedic surgeon. Those medical connections were another form of privilege; they opened doors that might otherwise be closed. George knew where Sasha had given birth, and he thought he knew the child's natal sex; he recalled overhearing, in a semidrugged state, staff refer to Sasha's baby as "she." George also knew the source of the sperm: tall, brown hair, hazel eyes, musically talented, intellectually capable but dyslexic, all potentially inheritable traits.

George hired a detective and also placed ads (how very 20th century) in the local newspapers of the suburbs of St. Louis, where the birth had taken place. "Were you born in 1972 in St. Louis? Are you adopted? Are you musically talented? Smart, but struggle to read? If so, one of your birth parents would like to meet you."

Against the odds, after a year of ads and sleuthing and dead ends, a young woman named Danielle called the detective's office. "I think you're looking for me," she said. "I've known I was adopted from a very early age, and I kind of fit the description." She was taller than average for a natal woman, had brown hair, and green eyes. She had been a singer all of her life; she had been in musical theater as a kid and had gone into medicine, choosing OB/GYN as her specialty because she sensed that she could be especially helpful to pregnant teens, knowing she had been born to one.

As per the agreement between George and the detective, the latter was tasked with getting the testing done in order to confirm the likelihood that this was, in fact, George's daughter. George had picked the detective not only for her stellar references but because he knew from his lived experience in the role of a woman that it might feel less risky for his daughter to approach a woman and talk with her. When it seemed likely that Danielle was George's daughter (over time, genetic testing confirmed the case), the detective was also tasked with sharing the news: "Yes, you are probably my client's daughter. What my client wants you to know are three things. My client gave birth to you. My client never stopped loving you. And my client is in the process of transitioning to be the man he always knew himself to be. Your birth parent wants you to have the chance to consider what this all means before you make any decisions about how to proceed."

George was protecting his child, and also protecting himself; ignorance about and hatred of trans people was as potent 20 years ago as it is today, and he was unwilling to expose himself to that, not knowing who his daughter had grown up to become. It was a stroke of fortune that Danielle was a physician who dealt with women's reproductive health and who knew a little bit about trans people. She might have been raised in a family with rigid rules about femininity or negative attitudes about LGBTQ people. Instead, her parents had been relatively liberal in their views, and being a musical theater kid meant that, early on, Danielle had friends who were queer in various ways. All of these were twists of fate, all could have been otherwise.

Danielle took less than a day to call the detective back and ask to meet George, which they did in the detective's office several weeks later. It was awkward. "What do I call you?" Danielle asked George. "Uh, whatever you'd like," he replied. "This is weird," he said. "Yeah, very, very weird." And even weirder, initially, when George, an orthopedic surgeon, told Danielle, an OB/GYN, that part of his quest to find his birth child had to do with whether to have a hysterectomy as part of the gender affirmation process, and Danielle began, physician to physician, to discuss the risks and benefits to a middle-aged body of having this surgery. Then she had a sudden aha about what this all portended for George: "That was the one place you had had me, wasn't it? I get it, sort of, from my own patients who've lost a child and then were facing a hysterectomy. Now you could have both. Or either. But never again neither, George."

George had his hysterectomy. He slowly, over the years, was integrated into Danielle's family, along with two grown sons from his first marriage as Sasha, into the life of Sasha's daughter. One of his grandchildren, in primary school, drew a family picture of parents, aunts (Danielle had a sister) and uncles, and "Grandma and Grandpa and Nana and Poppy and Juju"—that last being George. "Who's that?" the teacher, well versed in the ways of modern families, asked. "My Juju, my mommy's person who had her in his uterus."

This story has unusually happy endings. There was trauma, which could heal. There was privilege, which provided power to uncover secrets, and which could have led to terrible pain had Danielle been different in some important ways. In a different scenario, George might not have been in the position of power relative to his surgeons and Kurt that allowed him to assert his desires where his uterus was concerned.

Notice the subtle elements of the intersectional identities of all parties in this narrative, not only those of George, who was traumatized by having to live as Sasha, be impregnated as Sasha, stripped of his child as Sasha, all the while knowing he was George (a name he took from a character in the play *Our Town,* one of the classics of high school theater performances), but also those of Danielle, and by inference the parents who had raised her and who were able to welcome George into their family.

Kurt, who was younger than George, was never pregnant or gave birth and had no relationship to his uterus other than the desire that it be gone as soon as was possible. His shared identity as a trans man does not mean that he shared the meaning of that intersectional space. If his own view of a "real" trans man was someone who had no desire to retain a uterus for whatever reason (although several of my acquaintance have done just that and birthed children posttransition) and had he been trained in a more traditional power-over approach to being a therapist, how might therapy with Kurt have become another layer of George's trauma from Sasha's pregnancy? Similarity of intersectional identities does not create a DHCR trauma healing experience. Critical consciousness, centering the experience of the suffering person, being compassionately curious about that person's life, their pain, their desires—those factors are the path to DHCR trauma healing work.

INTERSECTIONALITY IS A TOOL THAT DISMANTLES MASTERS' HOUSES

The construct and realities of intersectionality, used in their most revolutionary and profound ways, subvert every manner in which the various signifiers that have been used by social pathologies to distribute power and danger unequally are honored—or not, any longer. If we become able to undo the toxins exuded by the rules of structural oppression and social pathologies, trauma healing can be deeper, experienced as a transformation of a wounded person's relationships to themself and their world, when the healing experience entails a deep, thoughtful, open-minded, and openhearted exploration of how it can be made safe enough to stretch the definitional parameters of any one intersectional identity, especially identities that have been the repository of trauma.

This makes our allyships even more precious, and damage to those connections more tasty to those running the social pathologies from their perches in places of structural power. Can we tolerate our differences, our different stances, honor how people come to know and name themselves, as the older generation of critical thinkers insisted on knowing and naming ourselves? Can we look back and see ourselves in a trauma reenactment fueled almost entirely by the toxicity of social pathologies? If we can do this, be wise and compassionate, and dig deeply into a comprehension of how people come to intersectionalities that are incomprehensible to us, then we can deepen DHCR trauma healing.

A Reminder

Intersectionality as a paradigm constructs humans as complex, and not subject to external definition by anyone, even by members of their own apparent reference groups. It is a liberatory and decolonial construct about this thing we refer to as identity. Think, for a moment, about the naming of the Indigenous people of the Western Hemisphere by the European colonizers as "Indians" because these invaders made the error of believing that they had landed in India rather than having invaded a hemisphere of our planet that could not exist in their imagination. Consider the lumping all Indigenous nations into one category, which is what happens when someone has to check the box on a psychological assessment instrument for race.

An Indigenous person can check "Native American," but not Lakota or Chumash, Nooksack or Mohawk, or Tlingit, or Delaware, or Chehalis, or Duwamish, or Osage, or any of the other multitude of Indigenous nations living in North America. Each of these is a different nation, with different languages (although the Nooksack, Chehalis, S'Klallam, Muckleshoot, and Duwamish peoples, all Coast Salish nations, speak very similar languages, as did the Oneida, Seneca, and Iroquois, for example), different cultures, different meaning-making systems, all of them the original people of North America. They are none of them residents of India, for which the Western Hemisphere was mistaken by the first sets of Christian European colonizers.

The box that says "Asian," on the same assessment instrument, is the word used in American English to refer to people from East and Southeast Asia. Who is meant by this word? Does it fit a yonsei (fifth generation) Japanese American literature professor whose grandmother was of Norwegian descent and who is in a healer's office because they have recently learned more about the details of their grandfather's internment as a child during the Second World War and are experiencing intergenerational trauma?

Or maybe it's a Khmer refugee farmer referred by their nurse practitioner because no somatic provider can find a reason for the blinding headaches that have plagued them since they fled the slaughter in Cambodia to Thailand, leaving behind a family who were murdered? Or is this someone whose family came from one of the islands of the Indonesian archipelago, each of which has its own culture and language and religion, but who identifies as a pure Pacific Northwesterner because of being the third generation to be born there and yet feels increasingly alienated from the other Seattle natives, people of Norwegian descent, with whom he hikes every weekend? Will the "real Asian" please stand up? Right. The boxes on the assessment form are Christian Eurocentric categories.

If we fall back into defining a person by their melanic phenotype, as each of these people is likely to have a phenotype that fits them into the box called "Asian," we miss everything about who they know themselves to be. We miss the granularity of how trauma weaves into each of those very specific, very different intersectional identities. When we make enormous boxes based on geography and tell people, "We, the Christian European colonizers, proclaim that this is your identity," we violate their very beings, which is trauma. When we, as DHCR trauma healers, use the narrow-angle lenses that social pathologies have given us to look through rather than looking through an emotional version of the best possible space telescopes that allow us to see, at the emotional and cultural cellular level, who someone is, all of the stars in the galaxy of them, we might begin to find our way out of the briar thicket of the gender turf wars and all of the other purity conflicts that benefit no one among the marginalized and subordinated of the earth.

A DHCR trauma healer, in exploring intersectionalities with a suffering person, needs to work at this very fine and deep level of distinction, taking the yarn that creates the braid of intersectionality, teasing the threads out of the braid. An important, and often neglected, component of DHCR trauma healing is not simply liberating suffering people from unknowing their pain. It is also freeing them to know their power and their joy. To accomplish this task, which occurs recursively through the healing process and is one of the main focuses of the third phase of the three-phase model, we as healers have, I believe, an ethical obligation to honoring the true names that healing trauma-exposed people give to themselves.

In healing trauma from a DHCR liberatory perspective, it is central to our work to be able to invite all parties in the process to explorations of our intersectionalities as they relate to the experience of trauma. As we discussed in Chapter 8, addressing the topic of getting to safe enough, there is no way in which the house of being safe enough can be built without an understanding of how danger and disempowerment, stigma and marginalization, have sent toxic shards, often invisible but still leaking poison, into facets of intersectionalities. We as DHCR healers must examine the stories that the identity boxes tell us about who we are, about what we are supposed to be and not to be, and about the hidden ways in which we or our reference groups have been wounded by social pathologies.

Not an Intake Interview, Again, Please!

This is categorically not a suggestion to take an intersectionalities intake interview or create an intersectionalities genogram, although I am aware of some practitioners who use this methodology. This concept of an intersectionalities intake is something I used to suggest in teaching settings to invite students to better comprehend themselves. If you are trained in a methodology that uses genograms as a tool of self-discovery, then refashioning your methodology to ensure that intersectionality is centered will make your practice closer to decolonial. But don't make this a new intake interview!

Rather, this focus on the central importance of understanding intersection-ality is my attempt to invite you to become curious about the finest of threads, about origins of the fences that people have built around the boxes created for them by social pathologies, and then to learn how to look for the open-ings in those fences. This doubling-down on the centrality of intersectionality to DHCR trauma healing asks you to be curious about how each strand, no matter how seemingly tiny, of a suffering person's intersectionalities can hold old wounds and hidden toxins. These are the places where suffering people say to us, "I feel so stuck. Something is wrong, but what, because everything should be okay."

This discussion is an invitation to us all to know which threads of the pre-cious braids of intersectional selves were shredded by current trauma and by wounds past. All of this is in service of inviting the story of wounding and resistance and coping into the room. To move with people toward healing, we want to expand our understanding of how some components of identities became the center that held the pieces together or the strands that seemed to waft away, difficult to hold on to, leaving a person bereft, uncertain of how to be in the world, how to connect to ancestors or heritage without shame, to lived experiences without guilt. We must do this work with ourselves first, of course, and in a continuing way, so that we can recognize the ways in which the disowned or shame-filled boxes get hidden from our inspection.

A Poet Emerges From the Rubble of War

Let me illustrate with Ruth's story. This is the story of a real person, used with her knowledge and permission, written in collaboration with her and reshared here in honor of her having set me on this path of becoming a DHCR trauma healer. I first became an on-purpose trauma healer in 1983 (as opposed to having been doing it by accident from about the time I was 9) at the moment Ruth (the name she chose for herself for purposes of the article [Brown, 1986] we created about our work together when we began to meet) walked into my office, referred by the alcoholism unit at the VA hospital where I had been an intern several years earlier. It was unusual for a woman to seek care there, and not simply because so few women were veterans in 1983. That unit reeked of toxic masculinity back then. But the staff members, now my friends, knowing that I identified as a feminist therapist, thought that I could perhaps help Ruth hold on to her very tenuous sobriety.

Ruth and I spent 9 years together, through some very hard times and into some very joyful ones. In the hard times, we found that one of the gorgeous threads of her intersectionalities, which Ruth had hidden away from herself because it was vulnerable and because she had been told that it had no value because it would earn her no money, was that of being a poet.

Concurrent with our work she took a series of poetry writing classes at a community college in Seattle taught by a radical lesbian feminist, Pesha Gertler (may she rest in power), who taught poetry as a path to revolution and self-liberation. In Pesha's classes, Ruth, whose intersectional identities on entering my office were mostly those that were filled with shame, found that lost poet and then used her writing to heal herself.

Ruth was, in her own words, "a good Catholic girl." She had been a nurse during the American war in Vietnam, tending to young marines fresh off the medevac helicopters, men whose bodies were covered with burns and bullet holes. Many of them died. Many lived, scarred, broken, lost to themselves. She witnessed all of that carnage, diving under their beds when the hospital, in an allegedly safe city far from the official fields of battle, was shelled. When we met, in her early months of sobriety, she had moments when her brain took her back in time to the day when she watched a helicopter full of people she knew fall, shattered, into the sea as she sat eating lunch along the shoreline. The smells of burned flesh, especially, were with her almost constantly when she forced herself into sobriety.

From those experiences, which had shattered her beliefs about a just world and a loving divine being, and which burned into her brain as the stuff of nightmares and flashbacks, she dug out a healing image, one that came from the most painful moments of her time at the bedsides of grievously injured adolescents in marine uniforms. She told me that with burn wounds one had to be vigilant against "premature temporary closure." This meant that a nurse could not allow a wound to simply scab over, because an infection could develop in the space between the new epidermis and the gaping wound beneath. It had to be allowed to heal from within or toxins would fill the hollow space and the injured marine would die of infection. She wrote in one poem about her own experiences of attempting to unknow trauma and the prices she had paid for that, "Wounds heal from the bottom up, and the inside out. They must be kept open, inspected, if they are to heal."

No statement more DHCR about trauma healing has ever been made. Keep the wound open, don't do something that makes it look as if its all handled by putting a cover over the wound, don't ignore it and create a hollow space for the bacteria and toxins of social pathologies to occupy, no matter how painful that hollow space might be.

So we agreed that she was right. As painful as it was, almost as painful as it had been for her to witness the agony of the burned young marines she had cared for, we had to find ways to allow her wounds to come back to the light of day without putting her fragile sobriety at risk. We didn't have EMDR in the 1980s. We had our relationship, and her AA community, and going through the hell of her memories to get out to the other side of the tunnel from Viet Nam, fully planted in Seattle. She held onto my hand for dear life as she inspected her now open wounds, allowing them to heal, as she lived through flashbacks in the chair next to mine. The wounds were open. The harms done, knowable at last. The emotional pus emptied out so that the knitting back of the edges of who she was could happen.

So too with the shame-filled wounds hidden in the threads of our inter-sectional identities over which we, or the social pathologies of the culture, have attempted to place a covering that masquerades as closure; those shame-filled threads are, in our liberatory DHCR healing process, brought into the light. As carefully as Ruth the nurse would pull back the thin layer of cells trying to cover up the gaping wounds of war, trying to cause as little pain to the burned man, knowing he was nonetheless suffering unspeakable torment, so Ruth the suffering human struggled with the thinning layers of unknowing she had attempted to place over her own psychic wounds. She taught me that the liberatory and DHCR trauma healer's difficult task is to say, "I know that this will hurt like hell, and when you are ready, this is a piece of who you are that, if you can tolerate its exploration, may hold one of the keys to healing." I'm grateful to EMDR because it is something I know to offer which can make this whole thing less painful for some, not all, trauma-exposed people.

All of this "premature temporary closure," the medical terminology for covering up wounds too soon, had been done to Ruth. A psychiatrist had done the first temporary premature closure of the wounds to her psyche when she came home from Vietnam, giving her a prescription for a highly addictive benzodiazepine because she could not sleep. He sexualized the therapy, and she quit. Then she found alcohol, which quiets the same receptors in the brain and required neither a prescription nor visits to a professional where she had felt increasingly unsafe and like a failure. She kept that very thin skin over her terrible pain for 17 years.

Only her deep love for her youngest sister, Jillian (a pseudonym), who was like a daughter to her, pushed her into giving up drinking so as to be sober at Jillian's wedding. She hadn't planned to stay sober after the wedding, which is what the VA staff had intuited when they sent her my way. (As one person of my acquaintance in recovery told me, no one goes to their first 12-Step meeting thinking that they're not going to drink again. They've made a bar-gain with themselves about how long they have to do it. And then sometimes, it takes.)

No one knew what pain had been unleashed when she went to the VA and gave up the extremely effective self-medication that she had been using.

For the first few years of our time together, the fear of disappointing people, Jillian in particular, served the function of keeping her away from alcohol while together we plumbed the depths of horror that she had told no one about because each time she had tried, the listener had turned away.

Over time, she wrote her poems. Over time, she began to find connections with other humans again, with people who were not me and not necessarily in an AA meeting and who would listen to her life with the honor and care she deserved, who let her know that she could never disappoint them because they knew she was a woman of great courage. Over time she found joy again in nature, and, of course, there was poetry, and more poetry.

I can still feel the grip of her hand grabbing onto mine as her brain took her back into the horror movies of her time in Vietnam. While there were many things about her intersectional identities that I did not yet know to explore with her, we were able to open up and stretch the walls of the boxes that had imprisoned her and misinformed her about the nature of her struggle with her human responses to repeated trauma exposure and betrayal. In my presence and Pesha's, she took back the hidden gift box of her inner poet, a strand of her intersectional identities that she had dropped as impractical along her way.

I last saw her in 2016 at a memorial service for a person we had in common, another person who had worked with me on her healing, whose body had quit on her. Ruth told me then that after 33 years of sobriety, a number that she intended to stretch out to the end of her life, she was now unsure about whether she was a "real alcoholic." When I asked her about this, we exploded another one of those aspects of her intersectional identity that had been tainted by social pathologies telling lies about trauma when she said to me, "I think if I hadn't had PTSD, I would have never gotten into trouble with alcohol. I've sat in so many [AA] meetings all these years, and I've come to realize that my story is not the story of people in the rooms who didn't have trauma, although there aren't a lot of those [mutual laughter at that point]. I was medicating myself. I didn't drink before I went to Vietnam. I barely took aspirin." "Premature temporary closure?" I ventured. "Yes," she said, "I think, maybe, yes."

So Ruth's intersectional identities, which had come to include recovering alcoholic in 1983, were shifting in 2016 as she questioned what that name meant and whether it was an accurate one for her, even though she had held it up proudly for 33 years. She had had enough time being a person who remembered, but was not tormented by, her experiences to understand that her relationship to alcohol was for the most part not a thing separate unto itself, as the pathologizing culture of treatment had taught her, but perhaps a component of the intersectional identity that she began to claim in the course of our work, one she fought hard for when her application for veterans' benefits was initially denied.

Her identities as I knew them from encountering her at that memorial service for her friend, who had also been my client, 8 years before I wrote this text, identities she wore proudly, were those of a poet, a sister and daughter and friend, and someone who had come out the other end of combat-related PTSD. The combat-related part was an identity that she had been told, by the VA and by various veterans' organizations, she could not claim because she had been a nurse in a city, albeit one under continuous attack by guerrilla warriors, and not a man carrying a weapon on the poorly defined fields of war. Our team fought hard for the truth that her PTSD was combat-related to be in the paperwork.

Disaggregating the social constructs of woman, nurse, and noncombatant in her intersectional identities from her lived experiences of trauma and grief and the disruption of relationships and alienation from all that she had believed in and held dear, so that "person recovered from combat-related PTSD" could not only be a name she gave herself but also the name she fought to pull out of the structure of the VA, all were part of me learning from her to do DHCR trauma healing. Getting that combat-related designation meant better monetary compensation from the VA, a guaranteed monthly income that made it possible for her to leave a job she hated and had taken only because she was drinking and unable to function as a nurse. It allowed her the time to take the courses that in turn led her to renew her nursing license and return to work that gave her life meaning, helping people with trauma-related workers' compensation claims for the state, a role in which her intersectional identities of nurse and trauma-exposed, healing human could come together and give her a sense of meaning and purpose.

Her claiming her own name and our fighting together for it turned out to be an example of how we unknowingly decolonized those facets of her intersectionality that were being used by social pathologies of misogyny and militarism to pathologize her, and with which she had, as a well-indoctrinated member of the medical world, pathologized herself as well when we first met. Together we fought the VA to decolonize the narrative of the diagnosis given to women veterans in the middle 1980s, the infamous borderline diagnosis, and to say, "This is what combat trauma looks like in a woman, in a nurse, in a person who had heart-to-heart connections with wounded and dying men, and so absorbed their pain. And, oh yeah, someone who was under mortar attack most of the nights she was at the hospital in Da Nang, even if that was technically not a combat zone."

INTERSECTIONALITY IS FLAWED AND IMPURE IN THE BEST POSSIBLE WAYS

I'm not a fan of diamonds, which must be pure. I'm an opal kind of person myself, entranced since childhood by the way that each stone is different, each flick of fire not the same as the one next to it. I am simply not a fan of purity, whether in gems or in how humans make sense of themselves. Purity tests for humans are violence.

I watched purity tests be imposed on a dear friend who had parents from different cultures and phenotypes. The friend, who consciously identified as a member of both groups, found themself accused of being not enough of either phenotype, of not being authentically anything because they had the sense of agency, that is, temerity to insist on self-definition as both/and.

The result: this person was treated as suspect by both groups, excluded and canceled (before we had that term), despite their major contributions to psychology's understanding of intersectionality. To insist on a genuine and complex intersectional understanding of each of us—ourselves, the healers, the suffering people seeking our care, even those promulgating social pathologies who are terrified of their own shades of gray—moves us toward a truly liberatory DHCR methodology of responding to suffering in trauma-exposed people. It also means that we are refusing to use the master's tool of dividing up humans into purportedly real, immutable groups when the truest differences among us, aside from whether we can get someone pregnant or become pregnant, occur at the location of the languages we speak: some of us are in fact incomprehensible to others when we open our mouths, a problem now more easily, albeit only partially, and not always adequately, solved with a translation app

So DHCR trauma healers will, of necessity, have a both/and relationship with understanding intersectionalities. On the one hand, as DHCR trauma healers we need to develop a profound appreciation for the riches inherent in a suffering person's reference groups, not only the pains therein. This, the importance of seeking strength and joy, is the message of the original decolonial and liberatory trauma healing movements, which have pointed to Indigenous healing methodologies as perhaps more on point to the pain of Indigenous and other BIPOC people. Comas-Díaz (2010, 2012a, 2020, 2021, 2022; Comas-Díaz et al., 2019, 2024; Comas-Díaz & Torres-Rivera, 2020), one of the leading decolonial thinkers and writers in psychology, has written eloquently about this topic for decades, discussing how healing strategies from Afro-Caribbean cultures, among which are her own roots, can speak more clearly and effectively to the traumas of other members of these groups who are suffering from any kind of pain from trauma.

On the other hand, we must resist the reification of categories, particularly when that reification appears to block access to healing. "A person in this category to which I belong cannot . . .," "A person in my group is powerless in the face of . . .," "A person in my group must always . . ." are all ways in which a person has been lied to about the necessity of remaining entrapped in the externally imposed parameters of their reference group, even when it appears that the rule has emerged from within. But remember, it emerged from within a box replete with the toxins of structural forms of oppression. Reification of categories is imposed from the outside, as a means of coercion, control, and social stratification. The one-drop rule was imposed by those who enslaved and imprisoned, then raped, African women; but at times in the present this rule is used to challenge the authenticity of the Blackness of those who are light of skin or those who define themselves as some variety of Black-ish. In Chapter 11 we'll discuss in depth Maria Root's description of the multiple identity development pathways that explode the authority of categories in favor of liberating people to self-define, to call themselves by their own names.

Taxonomies Are Useful if You're a Member of the Order Hymenoptera

Among flowers, among insects, among the many diverse species on this planet, there are distinct categories, species that cannot reproduce across their lines or to do so, as with gametes from a donkey and a horse, yield mules, who are incapable of reproduction. The (many, many, too many!) sugar ants in my house do not mate with the bees in my front yard, even though both are members of the order Hymenoptera. In fact, the honeybees of the species in my raspberry forest cannot mate with other species of honeybees, much less with the yellow jackets, with whom they share markings but definitely not temperament (I talk to the former and avoid the latter like the plague, even though I am quite allergic to the stings of both). For these creatures, the categories of species membership are fixed.

For humans with our infinite variety of intersectional identities this is simply not the case; we are all *Homo sapiens*, a species that cannot reproduce with other species, but the artificial lines between so-called races of our species are just that, artificial and socially constructed, even though the truisms of hierarchies of power and dominance attempt to teach that these categories are as unbreachable as those between honeybees and mason bees. Our categories—although precious and meaningful, dangerous, empowering or liberating, or all of the above—impose taxonomies upon the species *Homo sapiens* that are flimsy and easily breached, should we be willing to try.

So do breach them. For DHCR trauma healing to proceed without stumbling over the falsehoods of social pathologies, we must simultaneously be able to dive deeply into each suffering person's intersectionalities and also be prepared to invite reconsideration, at some time in the second and third stages of the three-phase trauma healing model, of the nature of the parameters and contents of those identities.

What is riskier, and yet necessary, for a liberatory DHCR trauma healing practice is understanding humans as continuously intersectionally organized, with that organization being fluid, not fixed, no matter which reference group is in the foreground in a given moment. When we allow our model to dissect people into the variables of age, gender, or spirituality (some of the identity factors represented by the ADDRESSING acronym), we are seduced into the colonized taxonomy of dividing humans into these component parts. Female, old, living with disabilities: that's me, but not entirely me, the categories to which I belong but meaning what in terms of this particular human Venn diagram? All of the above and something else entirely.

We must also hold the space so that we can scrupulously, humbly, and collaboratively invite the suffering person to shine a light on the junctions of intersections within themselves and on the variables that have been put in the background, sometimes with intention, sometimes as part of familial or cultural strategies for being safe enough. This requires patience, skill, and attention to those moments when a suffering person opens a door, if only just a crack, for the DHCR healer's attention to hover over what is within. We must see the disowned threads, the tiny ones slipping loose from the braid, to question the shame inferred there, the names given to them that are not the right ones.

11

EXPLORING AND DECOLONIZING THE INTERSECTIONAL IDENTITIES OF SUFFERING PEOPLE

CARLA'S STORIES

"I notice you just mentioned that your mom came here from El Salvador a few years before you were born. I think this is the first time I've heard about that," I say to Carla,[1] the pale-skinned natal woman whose last name is Olson and who came into my office because she had been sexually harassed by her boss. "May I be curious for just a minute about whether that thing about your life might be, I don't know, showing up in some way in how painful this workplace experience we're talking about has been? I'm probably wrong, seems a little out of left field, and if I don't ask . . ." "Then I would never let you know," she finished. "I'm surprised I let it slip. You've got my guard down, argh."

I had just noticed, out loud, a thread that had been pushed into a corner where there were stains that looked like shame. My noticing was an invitation. I didn't pull on it very hard, just noticed that I saw it.

It led to an eye-opening discussion of how Carla had been taught to never, ever let on that she was, as she put it, "part Latina, and my mom, well, wasn't documented when she came here. I don't let anyone at work ever know that

---

[1]This case is a fictionalized composite.

https://doi.org/10.1037/0000421-012
Decolonizing Trauma Healing: Toward a Humble, Culturally Responsive Practice, by L. S. Brown

I can speak Spanish, and I sure as hell don't let them know about my background. So this whole shame thing that we've been talking about, my shame about having this White boss who keeps trying to trap me in corners and rub up against me, maybe the secret-keeping rules, maybe they're in there somewhere being activated?"

She continued, "Maybe some part of me thinks that he singled me out because he could sense that I'm not really a White girl, that Carla Olson is a kind of disguise that I put on when I'm not with my very odd family?" "Odd?" I asked. She replied, "We're like fusion cuisine, as in, lutefisk enchiladas, and aquavit-spiked horchata instead of rum in the eggnog, to give you an idea of how my mother tried to placate her oh-so-Norwegian in-laws. That's me, a lutefisk enchilada. Or I could just be making that up about it being related. I mean, what does my mother have to do with what happened at work?"

Noticing the openings to the pushed-away thread of an intersectional story that have been filled with shame by toxic social pathologies allows for a deepening and liberatory conversation about how to cleanse and rename those aspects of self. "Maybe it has nothing to do with what happened at work, maybe it could, I don't know," I say, being attentive to not setting myself up as the authority. "And, let me notice, and I could be utterly wrong, that somewhere, something taught you, taught your mother, to feel shame about who she is, and you about who you are. Or to hide it, to try to pass somehow and, eew, lutefisk anything, sorry for the microaggression."

"Yes, eew, that was not a microaggression, I think my grandparents just ate it for show and to try to show my mother what a real Norwegian eats. It's gross, we all know that." Laughter ensued. Lutefisk, for the uninitiated, is cod cured in lye, and the ability to choke some down is considered a test of Scandinavian authenticity in some parts of the world, including the Seattle neighborhood where the Norwegian independence day is celebrated every May 17. And my disrespect for this most Scandinavian of foods could have been a microaggression, and so, as a decolonial, humble, culturally responsive (DHCR) trauma healer, I caught it, named it, and offered repair so that if it had been, I would have taken a step toward being worthy of trust. We put the lutefisk back in its box. "And that sexual harassment at work, well, when it happens to you . . ."

Carla chimed in, "You're either a nut or a slut. That thing from the Anita Hill story that my lawyer had me read. And we all know that Latinas are supposed to be spicy, hot, slutty, don't we? One of the things my mother taught me is that I had to be more modest than any pure Anglo girl so that no one would ever think I was a spicy Salvadoran slut, which was the thing my father's parents called her when he brought her home, married to him, mind you, but pregnant with me. Crap. Maybe this has everything do to with how impossible it's feeling to chase away the shame. Hey, Laura, look, I didn't call it my shame, I called it the shame. I think that's a first."

Notice that Carla opening the door to one very deeply buried storyline about a hitherto invisible and well-hidden facet of her intersectional identities, whose loose thread was so thin and transparent as to be almost invisible, was a nearly explosive, liberatory step for her, an inflection point. It was a moment when she began to make the shame that had blanketed her not her shame, simply a feeling that she need not own, a feeling that perhaps had been soaked, by social pathologies, into some strands of her intersectional identities, strands that she had kept in a well-locked closet from the day she started school. This is what DHCR trauma healing looks like in practice; we pay attention to the tiny threads. We tug a little, we allow them to unspool, at their own speeds, and notice what becomes visible through the holes in the fabrics of assimilation, passing, unknowing—all the survival skills that emerge in the wake of layers of trauma.

The parameters of her intersectional identity as a woman of Salvadoran heritage had been defined by the dominant Anglo and colonial cultures by which she was surrounded growing up; Latina equals slut. They were distorted by a sexualized narrative of what it meant to be a natal woman that was reinforced by her upbringing in a variety of Christian religion that emphasized women's role as temptress and thus a legitimate target for the out-of-control sexual urges of a man. Her mother had also ingested those toxins and out of them fashioned her own well-intended parenting wisdom as to how Carla had to dress and act so as to be safe from men's inability to control themselves (but not safe enough, as evident from the workplace harassment). A DHCR trauma healer will notice how social pathologies need not do the work themselves but rather use their parasitic infestation of spaces in intersectional identities to have well-meaning, even loving, families inject those toxins into the next generation, and the next, and the next.

As the story of Carla's secret slowly emerged into our shared space, we learned that this had been a closet that her parents had built believing it would protect their family, especially their children, from bias. It was a closet whose walls were reinforced by a prohibition on Carla bringing friends home so that they would not lay eyes on her mother. Those walls were reinforced when only her father went to parent–teacher conferences, carrying the lie that Carla's mother worked in the evening (and earning lots of extra points, as a natal heterosexual man, for being such an involved parent), so that her mother's melanic phenotype and Spanish accent would never be seen or heard inside of Carla's classroom. The closet of this secret was built with all of the many steps taken by her parents to make her White, with the loving parental goals of protecting her from racist and xenophobic tropes, goals informed by the ways in which racism and xenophobia were toxins that her parents could not see in themselves but knew they wanted her protected from. The way she described her family's strategies for keeping this secret reminded me of the stories told by Jewish who were hidden and passed off as Aryan in Nazi-occupied Europe; she had to hide being Latina as if her very life depended on this charade.

The realities of her mother's melanic phenotype and place of birth were a secret that could only be known at the church the family attended, ironically, the church where her parents had met. This was a place where Carla's mother was simply one among several Latinas worshipping there, women who had been exposed to the violence of one or another fascist regime in the multiply colonized lands of Central America, women who had fled El Salvador or Guatemala in search of safety, who had lived in terror of deportation until they could somehow get documents or were able to marry an American citizen or give birth to one.

This was the parish where her father, a member of the Jesuit Volunteer Corps, which is a sort of AmeriCorps for Roman Catholic young people, was living in the rectory just after college, working to assist undocumented women like Carla's mother to get legal residency. The parish was definitely not in the part of town where he grew up and was one that his parents, whose own Catholicism had made them outliers among their predominantly Lutheran Scandinavian American community, would not attend because "Father Albert [who had officiated at her parents' marriage] sounds like a communist." "Which he probably was," Carla mused. "A liberation theology dude for sure, which was why I liked his homilies so much when I was a kid."

It was the closet of their secret that her mother built, trying to make Carla closer to safe, of her mother's own attempts to get safe enough, of her father's participation in this dynamic and the building of this closet because of how his family, and many other White citizens of Northern European descent, looked at him differently after he had fallen in love with, married, and had children with a brown-skinned woman whose English was Spanish-tinged. Because he was infected with the virus of internalized domination, with the social pathologies of racism and xenophobia that he consciously rejected with all of his heart, her father did not know how to prevent these pathologies from playing starring roles in his agreement with her mother that it was important to raise Carla and her brother, John, as White people, with blandly, definitely not Latinx names. "Although I did take Rose as my confirmation name, sneaky little me, because Rose of Lima is the patron saint of

Latin America." The DHCR trauma healer pays attention to this statement, to the ways in which a suffering person identifies their capacities to resist. "Maybe not so sneaky," I said. "Maybe just, I don't know, proud?" "Yeah, proud of a saint who worked with the poor of Lima and wasn't another virgin of something or another."

Her father knew intuitively that he had become less close to safe when he followed his heart because of how his privilege—as a heterosexual, Scandinavian American natal male, a native English-speaking citizen whose family had come to the United States by choice more than a century before he had met Carla's mother, all the privileges of his visible and foreground intersectional identities—had had some pieces pulled out of it every time he stood next to his wife. He wanted to protect his children from this experience, and he and Carla's mother did not believe that they could change the world quickly enough to make that possible.

His own trauma of rejection by his family of origin, of his loss of his belief in the United States as a fair place, of his family as not "prejudiced," to use his word, dovetailed perfectly with his wife's desires to make their daughter a "real American," because he had been taught by the social pathologies of the polite, very Nordic American city in which we all lived, that a real American did not look or sound like his beloved wife. The closer-to-safe strategies that we discussed in Marisol's story are not dissimilar to those that Carla's parents gifted her with, although Carla's father did this with the most loving intentions that a good liberal Catholic White man of his era, one a little exposed to liberation theology in his youth, could muster. And as it happened, those narratives played a part in how excruciatingly painful Carla's experiences at work had been.

I'm only going to briefly discuss the dynamics of betrayal here, which has been addressed in many earlier parts of this books as being a trauma in itself. The betrayal for Carla included the ways in which this predator at her workplace exploited his relationship with Carla's dissertation adviser to try to silence her because he knew that he could endanger the completion of her degree simply by calling up her dissertation chair and bad-mouthing her. I will mention briefly that this predator's melanic phenotype was reminiscent of the paternal grandfather whose face twisted in disgust every time he saw Carla's mother, and how that resemblance was a facet of trauma that only made itself consciously known to her later in the healing process, when Carla had been able to more thoroughly explore her intersectionalities without shame.

Carla was ambivalent about claiming her intersectional identities anywhere outside of my office. Even in her nuclear family, discussion about her

Salvadoran heritage was discouraged, "I somehow don't think it would go over very well for me to say, hey, you know, I've been talking about being Salvadoran in therapy." She felt (unnecessary) guilt about having passed for White, and she feared that she would be rejected should she try to find a place in Latinx communities. "Who in the hell is going to believe that someone who looks like me and has my last name is Latinx, seriously, really? Like, am I saying this about myself to, I don't know, find more community, or something, or, I don't know. A fraud all around, maybe?" This is an example of the purity test toxin, coming into the light.

The revelation of this piece of her intersectionalities was not a step Carla had had any interest in taking when we first met. I had to demonstrate that I might be a safe-enough person with whom to share this hint about who else she was, aside from the things she had allowed me to know: her pale skin color, her bland last name, typical for Seattle, and her all-but-dissertation status in computer science. It was her skill as a writer of difficult code that had led her into the workplace where she was subjected to repeated sexual assaults by her boss, a close friend of her dissertation adviser. It was a long time before she finally was able to call it assault. It took us a long time for her to feel safe enough to talk about the enormous burdens of the social pathologies she had internalized that were adding to the inherent toxicity of being sexually assaulted in the workplace, a phenomenon that is all about toxic masculinity and misogyny.

Her self-accusation of fraudulence, entirely a creature of the false narratives of pure categories of identities imposed by social pathologies, was a lifelong source of terrible pain, not simply something occurring at the moment when she shared the truth of her life with me. It was a label she had struggled with internally for most of the years since, as an adolescent, she had had the critical thinking skills to realize what her family dynamics were communicating to her about who she was.

What People See in a Healer Is Not What They Might Get

Of course, what is also interesting in this encounter is that yours truly, working to become a DHCR healer, has pale skin and a blandly American name: Laura Brown, one that doesn't sound Jewish at all. My total phenotype—the hair, the skin, the eyes, taken together—is the prototypical picture of an Eastern European Jew. But to anyone not familiar with the phenomenon—and Carla, a Seattle native, didn't have the data with which to read the cues since my genetic relatives are pretty scarce around these parts—I'm just another White-appearing woman with a PhD who Carla's attorney had told her knew a lot about the official trauma, sexual harassment, to which she had been subjected and thus might be a good therapist for her.

The point at which she was struggling to believe whether it would be moral for her to declare herself Latinx was the point at which I said, "Do you know that I'm a Jew? Might that disrupt your rule set here about who's a real fill-in-the-blank a bit? Or am I full of shit?" This is a type of self-disclosure that I typically don't engage in during a healing session; that information is on my website, but Carla hadn't read it, since she came via her attorney, not via a web search. It isn't usually helpful, I think, to say, "Uh, me too?" This time, though, my somatic knowing of what would undermine narratives of passing and purity was, thankfully, right.

The shock on her face said it all, and then, "Laura Brown? Jewish? I just thought you were from the East Coast," which allowed me to ask, "Would you like to know a little bit about how my family tried to get closer to safe? Because there's a reason why I seem to be so good at understanding your family's story of trying to keep you closer to safe, and it's not because I'm that great of a therapist."

Laughter, and consent. If the consent had not been offered, I would have not shared my family's stories, because DHCR trauma healers share their lives only for the benefit of, and with the consent of, those who seek healing from us. We do not offer up those stories if they are unwelcome. Carla could have just as easily told me that she had no interest in knowing any of this, maybe even been angry with me for assuming there might be any parallels—and she would have been right, if I had assessed the situation less accurately before offering what I did.

The laughter and consent were followed by a liberatory DHCR collaborative process in which each of us could expose how social pathologies had injected their toxicity into our families and both of our lives. We talked about our assimilated names, and, in my case, enjoying the shock on people's faces when I let them know that one of "those people," the Jews to whom someone was referring pejoratively, was right there in front of them our family cultures, in which our heritages were acknowledged; and the racism her mother encountered and the anti-Semitism my family was subjected to, not the same things, yet the same themes of social pathologies spanning generations. We spent most of one meeting on this. Then we returned to the more central topic of how Carla could liberate herself from these toxic narratives and, by so doing, get closer to safe and to healing, to see her authentic, complex, intersectional self as authentically whoever she knew herself to be, the authority to declare authenticity centered in her. A layer of trauma she hadn't known about started to lift, simply from exposure to light.

THE TOXIC GIFT–TRAUMA COMES FREE WITH THIS THREAD

For many marginalized and subordinated people there is trauma that is inextricably woven into some components of how the person experiences their identity, their answer to the question, "Who am I?" One of the ways in which trauma disrupts people's sense of being safe enough, or being connected to other humans in a reliable way, is that it attacks some valued aspect of identity, some foregrounded component of a person's intersectionalities. As I wrote in *Cultural Competence in Trauma Therapy,*

> Identities as defined here commonly share certain characteristics. They are delineated by values and inform values in a recursive process. Threats to identity are experienced as challenges to those values. A person's values predict their choices, the nature of their relationships, and the meanings that are made of life circumstances. Identities reflect what Comas-Díaz (2006) refers to as a world-view, an overarching strategy for understanding and lending meaning to all aspects of one's life. Identities commonly contain multiple social locations, since those identifiers visible to others tend to evolve from the more core identities held by the person, or to have informed the development of the core identities. Whether identity is experienced individualistically or collectively, which largely depends upon the cultural contexts informing identity, it is the thing that the person describes as "self." Although many writers have argued persuasively that the very construct of "self" is a Western, culturally insensitive creation, I would suggest that the sense of "I"-ness experienced by a person, whether it is the singularity described by Europeanized cultures, or the member of the family/tribe "I am because we are" version found in other contexts, is this thing I am calling identity; "self" is found in that emotional and cognitive location.
>
> Trauma has a role in shaping one's sense of self when it is a component of early life experiences and/or s embedded in the context of early development. It challenges self when it occurs later in life. Trauma is also a component of self when it is an aspect of a person's familial and/or cultural heritage of oppression, intergenerational or historical trauma. This is because trauma often lands squarely in vital components of identity from which self is constructed. Our human neurobiological responses to the various kinds of trauma can worsen the pain of trauma by undermining capacities for the kind of support and relationship that humans find healing.
>
> Internalized oppression, which constitutes the introjection of the toxins of external bias and stereotypes about one's own group emerging from social pathologies into one's beliefs about oneself or one's group (Russell, 1996) functions as a variable that creates additional vulnerabilities for some marginalized and subordinate people to be particularly affected by the next trauma. The latest trauma itself may have nothing to do specifically with the intersectional identities affected by social pathologies—it could be a car accident, which is an entirely equal opportunity thing—but it may awaken the toxins of internalized oppression because of how it shatters a person's safe-enough strategies. (Brown, 2008, p. 162)

INTERSECTIONAL IDENTITY DEVELOPMENT

Because of trauma's emotional shape-changing capacities, I have found that models of identity development that allow both for stability over time as well as recognition of transformation in context and that entirely support the construct of intersectionalities are foundational for making sense of trauma's impact on self and for operating in a liberatory and DHCR fashion when we encounter people whose sense of self seems malleable. It's also helpful to have a DHCR-informed way of considering, as healers in collaboration with the suffering person, where they are in relationship to their understanding of themselves. Rather than looking at stages of identity development, it seems to me a more DHCR way of thinking is to ask the suffering person questions like, "What age does this part of you feel like to you? Oh, and this part? And what's it like to have a part that feels like a 2-year-old and a part that feels like a teen?" This is different from asking about dissociated ego states; rather, it comes out more like, "Well, my age, the one on my driver's license, is 30. But my queer self, they're a teen, for sure."

Generally, identity instability is coded in Eurocentric psychologies as evidence of psychopathology (there's even a scale measuring this on one popular general measure of psychopathology). Decolonial trauma healing models, conversely, assume that such malleability and changeability of sense of self, as well as different ages of development in relationship to aspects of intersectionalities, are part of the typical human response to having one's certainties about the world shattered or from exposure to the chronic traumas of systemic forms of oppression.

What those models of identity development supporting a DHCR trauma healing paradigm tend to assume is that many people are likely to have apparently conflicting or contradictory intersectional identities—for example, gay and Christian—that are socially constructed by narratives of social pathologies as mutually exclusive but which are, or can be, integrated into a coherent intersectional whole by the individual. The idea of one primary identity that must exclude all others, or one invariable path toward identity development, is a wholly owned subsidiary of colonized Western psychology. When integration of intersectionalities that are socially constructed as contradictory is an unresolved component of identity development, a trauma arising from the toxicities of a social pathology is frequently, although not always, a component of the difficulties the suffering person is having in making coherent sense of all of who they are.

Trauma shatters coherence even in people who have spent the time and energy to thoroughly explore and embrace who they are in all of their intersections, who have previously had some clarity that they can live with contradictions that are only contradictory because of the dicta of some social pathology. Trauma's painful emotions, or the ways in which trauma-exposed people try to unknow their pain or the details of what has occurred, can evoke internal conflict in almost anyone, even where there had been no such difficult dialogues with self. Trauma acts to undermine the felt truths of previously held values and can block access to emotional capacities emerging from a person's pretrauma sense of self. It changes the face of the world as known, thus altering the parameters of the social context in which self is understood. If a person's intersectional identities are soaked in the toxins of social pathologies, required to be hidden, cast out, borne as a mark of shame, then trauma's typical effects worsen all of those other, paper-cut traumas that have insinuated themselves into the fabric of a suffering person's intersectional identities.

Feeling alienated from oneself and from the relational world of which one has been a part is very common in the wake of trauma. The autobiographical literature by trauma survivors is replete with stories of "feeling not like myself." As Nancy Raine writes about the anniversary of her rape, "it marked again the death of the person I had been for thirty-nine years. This woman had a history. . . . But on October 11, 1985, she died. Another person was born that day" (Raine, 1998, p. 2).

As Raine noted, her prerape intersectional identities, in which her being a natal woman was the sole point at which she felt any sense of vulnerability, identities in which she had had a life, a career, relationships, interests, and a clear sense of who she was, none of that Nancy survived the day of her rape, although her body kept on going. She barely felt herself to be a woman, much less all of the other things she had been, although all of that history and all of those facets of her intersectionalities never stopped having been true. Even as she recounted the story of her healing, she makes clear that the more-healed Nancy who wrote her book was not the same person who existed the moment before the rape.

For many trauma-exposed, suffering humans, a trauma kills or sends into hiding or exile the person they knew. A new, damaged, spoiled self, composed of old identities as transformed by trauma, informed by the toxic tropes of social pathologies comes to stand in that person's stead. The sense of "Who am I?" created by a person's pretrauma intersectional identities, if they had a life before trauma, is often so changed by an encounter with trauma that it is as if those identities, like a limb, were traumatically amputated, lost forever. For people whose life began in trauma, the sense of self as spoiled and damaged becomes a strand of intersectionality that then distorts each other strand, particularly those that might otherwise, in a person without a history of complex childhood developmental trauma, be a source of good feeling, pride, or healthy self-love.

In some ways, Carla's secret identity as a Latina is not dissimilar in its effects on her view of her successes in life to the effects of childhood complex developmental trauma. Racism and xenophobia whispered, "If they only knew who you really are," taking a bite out of the apple of her accomplishments by sowing doubt in her mind about whether she would get the same credit if people didn't think her to be White. The toxins of racism and other social pathologies are not unlike those of being horrifically abused as a child by one's caregivers, in that they permeate the person's sense of who they are and render them vulnerable in particular ways to the traumas that come next. Trauma in the marrow of one's psychological bones, whether child abuse or chronic exposure to social pathologies, makes those bones more brittle.

When trauma survivors enter a healing process they frequently come in the disguise of that new person, the traumatized one. This is a person seen as damaged goods, not only by themselves but also, sadly, by too many people in their emotional milieu. The suffering person's life is frequently replete with old friends and family who are busily trying to coax back the "real" version of this person in well-meaning, naive ways that only deepen shame about just how much trauma feels, in bodies and psyches and souls, akin to the psychological version of an earthquake measuring 9 on the Richter scale.

Their sense of themselves feels polluted by the trauma, particularly those traumas pointed directly at aspects of intersectional identity that were already marginalized in some way but about which they had previously neutral or even positive feelings. The presence of the pretrauma sense of self may be known, at the start of a healing process, only by the grief over its apparently irretrievable loss.

It is largely because of trauma's profound effect on identity and our relationships with the intersections of our personal Venn diagrams that I have found Maria P. P. Root's (2000, 2004) ecological model of identity development, which she developed in her work with persons of mixed racial heritage, especially useful when thinking about the effects of trauma on identity and the reciprocal influence of identities on the experience of trauma. Root's model incorporates the possibility of a family or cultural heritage of trauma exposure into the process of identity development and is one of few identity development models of which I'm aware that takes trauma, both individual and historical, explicitly into account as a shaper of intersectional identities. It is also one of few that explicitly assumes three important liberatory and decolonial theses. First, that identities will be intersectional. Second, that trajectories of identity development will not occur in a stage or phase or stepwise manner. And third, that a person can move from one trajectory to another, from one construction of their intersections to another, and that this is evidence only of the flexibility of a person's conceptual capacities. Let us explore the implications of this model for understanding how a decolonial and liberatory trauma healing practice operates when we make intersectionalities a foregrounded component of our healing work.

Criteria for an Intersectional Identities Development Model

Root (1998, 2004) argues that in order to develop an identity theory that takes intersectional identities into intentional account, such a paradigm is required to meet certain criteria. First, any truly intersectional model needs to account for within-group bias and oppression, the sort of expressions of internalized oppression or horizontal hostility that emerge from the purity rules of social pathologies regarding the definitional parameters of identities that were discussed earlier in this volume. In Root's original model, which refers to persons who were, like Root, then referring to themselves as "mixed race," she points to discrimination and bias against persons of mixed race within the ethnic groups making up the various sides of their heritage as an example of this kind of resistance, even within marginalized groups, to any stretching or "watering down" of the purity of the identity parameters of a group for a person to be considered a valid member of that group.

Second, such a model must construe the experience of intersectional identities, in particular, known or visible intersectionalities, as a positive phenomenon rather than a failure to make up one's mind about who one is. Root's insistence on intersectionality as a valued, normative, and typically human phenomenon differs strikingly from all other models of identity development in psychology, which treat knowable intersectionalities as pathological and the achievement of a pure unitary identity as the sine qua non of mental health. Readers can clearly see, at this juncture, Root's profound influence on my own thinking about the topic of intersectional identities, particularly as it pertains to people where trauma is already a component of some aspect of intersectionality, is targeted at one such aspect, or appears to be destructive to some component of a person's intersectionalities.

Her model next notes the importance of changes in social and political contexts and social reference groups that emerge as available to any person across their lifespan, changes that inform or transform how they code their intersectionalities. Knowing oneself to be trans in 2020 was not knowing oneself to be trans in 1990 and is not knowing oneself to be trans in 2024, where, in the larger social and political sphere, you and people like you are being vilified with greater fervor than in years past.

Finally, any model meeting Root's criteria must acknowledge the interaction of experiences in the person's social ecology, including family environment and all aspects of intersectionality in one's heritage. Root, who is also an award-winning artist with exquisite visual sensibilities, has portrayed her model graphically as a series of nested, interactive, and overlapping boxes in which these various factors are in constant interplay and in which a person's intersectionalities are in a continuous process of development rather than moving toward a fixed and apparently stable state.

DHCR trauma healing is enhanced by this and similar models of identity formation because they allow a healer to conceptualize a suffering person's identity, not only as a continuously transforming matrix of multiple knowable and as yet unknown intersectionalities but also as not requiring a fixed and stable state. Thus, with trauma, healing from trauma is not a process of heading toward a fixed end state. Rather, it is about collaboratively achieving a place where a person's distress is sufficiently lessened, their joy and capacity for being fully alive greater, their sense of being in the world having a stronger and deeper closeness to safety. Because trauma lands on and in the interstitial spaces between facets of intersectionalities, decolonial healing work with trauma survivors requires healers to rethink our paradigms for what being healed will mean.

The Identities on the Edges and in the Spaces in Between

Many people suffering distress arising from exposure to any kind of trauma exist in a liminal state with regard to their sense of who they are, one in which transition is a constant. This is not psychopathology, a point I believe requires emphasis given that precisely this way of being in the world is among the criteria for one of the most harmful of the *Diagnostic and Statistical Manual of Mental Disorders* diagnoses, that of borderline personality. What is less obvious, but equally important for the DHCR trauma healer to take into account, is the degree to which liminal identities are those emerging as a function of a posttraumatic healing process, in which identity as a trauma survivor becomes integrated in a positive fashion into other aspects of a person's intersectionalities, woven strand upon strand like a fancy braid. This is not posttraumatic growth as understood in that literature. It is making something new of oneself, in which the healing from trauma becomes connective tissue between what were previously experienced as disconnected aspects of intersectional identities.

Going back to Raine's (1998) narrative of transformation after her rape as an example of this experience of liminality, we see her moving through a multiplicity of emotional and social positions, first appearing to lose, then returning to and drawing upon her pretrauma identities in her healing process as she arrives at a place where she has never been before. What is striking about Raine's memoir, and what can be informed by Root's identity model, is the manner in which interactions between various aspects of identity and the social ecologies available to this particular trauma survivor were, to this reader, clear core components of Raine's healing process. A DHCR model is, in consequence, a transformational model of trauma healing. It is not a return to normal. It is not becoming symptom free. It is grafting this experience onto the braid of intersectionalities or detoxifying those strands of that braid in which it had become embedded.

Five Paths—and Perhaps More?

Root (1998, 2004) suggested that in attempting to have an intersectional sense of self a person has five possible strategies available. The first of these is to accept an identity as assigned by society, to check the boxes generated by structural hierarchies of oppression. This pathway involves internalizing and applying to oneself the rules created by the larger social context, including that of the definitional purity of one's categorizations. She noted that this strategy is one where, by remaining congruent with societal expectations, which is usually an attempt at creating some camouflage so as to be able to be closer to safe, a person may experience deep disempowerment and be at risk for having to continuously dissociate danger, as we discussed in several other chapters throughout this book. It's a paradox: the attempts to feel safe yield more risk. For those who have experienced trauma, having an identity constrained by the ways in which social pathologies have constructed the role of the trauma survivor may be the position occupied by many people as they enter the therapy process, an identity that feels like a prison, like something that has wiped out all previous sense of self. Raine's story of her early postrape life is an example of this pathway at work.

This is not a lesser strategy. It is not pathology. If not rocking the boat or avoiding challenging authority is seen as central to being closer to safe, it is not only not lesser, it is also wise. It may also reflect a comfort with the definitional parameters of an identity assigned to a person by the culture and its social pathologies. That assigned identity might feel like a safe haven because there is a place for it in the larger cultural lexicon, however pathologizing. When the assigned identity is one that is trauma-related, there is some risk that this particular trajectory may be problematic in some manner, as the identities that culture assigns to trauma survivors are commonly connected to the expressions of distress made by those individuals—in other words, the assigned identity is one of pathology or disorder. And sometimes, it's what works for that person, for now, for as long as needed. It is not our job as a DHCR healer to judge this trajectory. Our job is to hold the space, respect when someone calls this done, good enough, without adding "for now" to that sentence.

Theo's Stories

Theo is a survivor of sexual abuse by priests (this story is the amalgam of five similar stories and not that of any one of those men). A Franco-American natal man, whose family had come to the United States after the Franco-Prussian War, himself devoutly Roman Catholic in his youth to the point of being an altar boy, Theo had been brutally sexually assaulted by his parish priest for several years during his early adolescence. Although he had been an excellent student and a star athlete until the rapes began, he did his best to unknow what was happening until he left home for college, at which point, away from family and the rapist, he felt temporarily slightly more safe, and his distress began to become palpable and unavoidable.

This looked, to all who had known him, and in his own eyes as well, like a person whose life was falling apart. He began to increasingly accuse himself of being a failure and started to use alcohol to try to numb his distress and drown his shame, with decreasing success as time went on. He became unable to tolerate being nude in the presence of other men, and since those were the conditions in a locker room, he abandoned soccer his first semester of college, losing his scholarship and dropping out of college at the end of his first year with his academic record in tatters as well. He never resumed higher education, returning home in disgrace to begin working a series of odd jobs from which he was usually quickly fired because of his agitation around men.

He kept silent about the violations. Some of this was because of his increasingly conflictual relationship with his parents, who still had his rapist to their home for Sunday dinner. Most of his silence, though, stemmed from his deep shame. He felt betrayed by the God in which he had believed because his rapist had been the representative of the divine on earth. He was also extremely upset and confused by his having experienced erections during these same-sex violations, even though he thought of himself as attracted to women.

The definitional parameters of how to be the natal man, the component of his intersectionalities comprising the front face of his intersectional identities, had room for neither the rapes nor his erections during some of them. As the trauma strained at the definitional parameters of the box called manhood, he felt as if he were losing himself. Without faith, without family, without soccer, without his manhood, without any of those components of his intersectionalities that he had made central, he had no idea who he was aside from "a drunk and a failure."

He was lost because he only knew to cling to the disintegrating box of his manhood, desperately trying to throw off the piece of intersectionality that was the trauma of violation by another man. His attempts to prove his manhood through compulsive acts of heterosexual intercourse punched another hole in that box, as the flashbacks that showed up every time he saw his own erection effectively shut down his capacity to be sexual with anyone—not with a woman nor with himself. If he awoke to a spontaneous morning erection, he would experience terror, which was the catalyst for daytime drinking. Because the definitional parameters of the piece of his intersectionality that was "man" had been largely built out of the materials of toxic masculinity, that identity had no place for him having been raped.

He had no epistemic framework with which to imagine any ways of understanding himself other than as a man who has failed. Theo's suffering occurred at the intersection of the rapes and the prison of toxic masculinity. I met him to conduct a psychological evaluation to be included with his petition to the archdiocese for reparations. His mother, from whom he had become estranged, had reached out to him to tell him that their former parish priest's name was on the list published by the archdiocese of known sexually abusive priests whose victims could seek compensation without having to initiate legal action. In that phone call, she tearfully told Theo how ashamed she was of having welcomed this man into her home. "He hurt you, didn't he?" she asked. "Yes, Mère. Which is why I can't look you and Papa in the eye ever again."

When I met Theo his identity as a failed man was firmly fixed as the core of his intersectional identities. He described this failed version of toxic masculinity to me so eloquently that, had I not known better, I would have imagined that he had been reading Ron Levant's (1996) work on that topic. Theo told me that he was a "loser, because I never fought back. I was 14. I was as big as I am now. I was a jock. I could have beaten him up. So maybe I wanted it, because I didn't beat him up. I was weak, is what I was. A man isn't weak. A man doesn't get a hard-on when some other man has his cock up your ass." The constructions of identity assigned by toxic masculinities to men who are raped, and consequently perceived as failures within the definitional parameters of that social pathology, had infiltrated Theo's core sense of who he was.

Theo's healing would require more than a decade of work with an intersectional feminist trauma therapist to whom I referred him after the evaluation, during which time he met and married a Latina natal woman, herself a survivor of childhood sexual abuse. Their relationship was rarely sexual, something that allowed each of them many experiences of getting closer to safe while in the close physical presence of another person who never shamed them for the intrusive pain of their respective experiences of violation. One of their few completed experiences of lovemaking led to parenthood, which was the ultimate healing experience for Theo.

He contacted me shortly after his daughter's birth to tell me that Sarah's appearance in his life had suddenly changed him. "I quit drinking, Dr. Brown. I quit canceling sessions with Teresa, I did EMDR. I'm a father, Dr. Brown, and I can protect this little girl. That's my job, that's why I didn't kill myself, so that Sarah could be here." He now sends me emails from time to time with pictures of his daughter next to her certificates for being on the honor role, of her in her volleyball uniform, at her martial arts classes—"because my kid is going to know how to be safer than I was." Theo feels pride in Sarah, and pride in his being a good dad. "Sarah's father" has become his primary identity. And that leads us to Root's second trajectory, because that is precisely where Theo, in his healing experiences, has landed.

Root's (1998, 2004) second trajectory of intersectional identity development is one of identification with one visible aspect of identity, in which other aspects of identity are made peripheral or even denied. "Sarah's father" is an excellent example of this, because this trajectory is an active choice. It may involve placing the least vulnerable or, as in Theo's case, the most highly valued intersectional identity in the foreground. This identity variable becomes a shield of sorts, allowing a positive distance from the places where the wound scars dwell. It is a closer-to-safe identity development trajectory.

Although on the surface this might seem to be precisely what Theo did before the birth of his daughter, during which time he accepted assignment to a singular and damaged identity, one whose toxic definitional parameters he did not know how to escape, what differentiates this strategy, according to Root, is that it is one in which a person makes a choice rather than accepting an assignment. Theo chose the identity of Sarah's father.

In making this kind of choice, a person might have examined the definitional parameters of the box they are fitting themselves into. Theo had not; he had simply discovered this new identity the first time he held his daughter and found it to be one that liberated him from his old toxic identities, even while drawing upon what had been good in them—he was doing "man" correctly, at last, as "good father." Some people question definitional parameters of an identity that had previously been rendered toxic, and through that questioning process become able to free themselves from toxic rules deriving from some form of structural hierarchies of oppression. Some people find ways, through some sort of liberatory process, which may or may not involve engagement with some sort of formal trauma healing, to expand the parameters of an identity that had felt lost to trauma, embracing a liberation from the narrow places imposed by social pathologies. For a trauma-exposed human, choosing to foreground the least vulnerable strand of their intersectionalities, done with full consciousness of that choice, might entail putting the experience of trauma in the background. This trajectory might be seen as a sort of contemplation stage of change; the person knows that they have been exposed to trauma and harmed by it. Just for today, they are deciding to find ways not to unknow or numb themselves but rather to put energy and focus onto the chosen facet of intersectionality and experiment with that being the path to healing.

The task for a DHCR trauma healer working with a person who has chosen this trajectory, and who is now unable to avoid the distress that they had hoped to put behind them, involves first honoring the work done to create this new positive identity and affirming and validating all that the suffering person has done in their experiment with this healing strategy. Because this person is once again in distress, they may be struggling not to fall back into the narrative of failure or shame that is lurking in the traumatized components of intersectionalities that they had hoped would have healed simply through the embrace of the new, chosen identity.

Jordan's Stories

Being pushed by the reemergence of distress into the action stage of change is often catalyzed by the appearance of intrusive recollections of trauma. Jordan's story exemplified this identity development trajectory. What follows is her individual story, which she gave me permission to write about. A Euro-American natal woman, a lesbian from a blue-collar family that had held up the toxic social pathologies of misogyny, racism, and toxic masculinity as truths, she had experienced severe and repeated trauma and neglect from very early in life. Finding a refuge in her studies, at which she excelled despite the daily struggles she faced to dissociate nighttime events so as to appear to be normal at school, she described how she made a conscious decision to leave her past behind; in her 20s she moved as far from her childhood home as was possible while still remaining in the Lower 48. In the Pacific Northwest, she reinvented herself as a therapist and activist. She came out as a lesbian and formed what was to be a lifelong partnership of many decades with another feminist activist. She created her new identity and, until a few months prior to coming to work with me, had made "working-class dyke feminist therapist" her intersectional identities of choice.

She came to see me because she wanted to be and could not become pregnant. What she held onto as her foreground identities were her roles as activist and healer, and those were the sole aspects of who she was that she was willing to let me see, in addition to the pesky problem of not being able to get pregnant, a problem that turned out to be a permanent state of affairs because she had polycystic ovary syndrome (PCOS), which renders many women unable to conceive.

Being a trauma survivor had been relegated to a distant corner of her self. But while sharing her life story with me, she mentioned in passing that she had been sexually abused when young, then stated, as firmly as I've ever heard anyone say it, "I've dealt with that." Her energy was very clear. This was a line that I was not invited to cross, and so, in my 1985 self, not yet liberatory but endeavoring to be egalitarian, I did not cross it until it shattered and spilled out onto my carpet a few weeks later.

What she did not tell me at our initial meeting was that the fertility treatments on which she was embarking, the constant poking and prodding and genital invasions—to which one of her abusers, a physician, had also subjected her—was making intrusive distress from the trauma of her childhood break through, pushing past her chosen identity as a strong and powerful woman. This painful and increasingly unavoidable distress, in the form of horrific nightmares and multiple episodes of terror and intrusive images occurring during the day, exploded the walls of the intersectional identities she had constructed and chosen as her shield.

That identity, as she had built it with, unknowingly, the messages of misogyny and patriarchy regarding who was powerful and valued and who was worthless, had had no place for her to have been vulnerable and violated. Similar to Theo, but in the version that was replete with misogynist messages about who a "strong woman" should be, the definitional parameters of her chosen identities were ones that she had assumed would be protective against the toxicities with which she had been raised. Her attempts to unknow the pain of her first 18 years, the details of which she never forgot, by raising the shield of her new chosen identity had stopped working because, as it turned out, becoming a mother was to be the capstone to that shield. Instead, attempting to become pregnant had opened the door to her demons.

Stigma is ascribed by structural hierarchies of oppression, by patriarchy and misogyny, to those who are raped, not to the rapists. Stigma and shame are assigned by those same social pathologies to those who have been abused, not to the abusers. Because of the immense shame heaped on children like the child Jordan had been, her tenacious grip on the new identity she had built for herself, the powerful woman who lifted up others, could not coexist with the pain defining the lived experiences of her first 18 years when it burst like a flood of sewage through the dam of that new chosen identity.

Until her encounters with medical care broke through what had been a fairly effective strategy of creating a new identity, which itself existed on another planet from the one in which she had spent her first 18 years, she had been able to live for a time as if the planet on which she had spent those

18 years simply did not exist any longer. On that planet, where she had been a girl told that she was pregnant by a doctor/rapist, who then invaded her 12-year-old uterus to "abort" her, where she was then raped again and again by that man and others, her unknowing methodology of literally dis-associating herself from herself had been an enormously effective one. "I knew it was happening, but I just floated above it and watched. I felt sorry for that poor girl."

Dissociation from the emotions of her violations, along with the safer spaces of school, had propelled her from a painful and problematic childhood and adolescence into an adult life in which her talents and competencies defined her to her social and emotional networks. It had given her the illusion that she was safe, that she had escaped relatively unscathed. Then the fertility treatments put her on a transporter beam back to that planet of pain and violation, the one that she thought she had escaped from.

This pain, through which she held onto me and her wife, and eventually the son to whom her wife gave birth, like a drowning woman in a tsunami, was something she had had to unknow in order to feel closer to safe. She had had to believe herself to be on the planet of safe enough to go through a graduate program, shielded enough to be a witness the pain of others, safe enough to allow her wife close enough to her to allow her heart and body to open to that woman.

Then she lost this version of being closer to safe because it was a shield built on sand. We had to collaborate to build a sturdier shelter in which she could weather the long-delayed windstorm of self-hatred that had been growing in ferocity behind the walls of her new identity. This meant revisiting that girl she had been and wrapping the shield of compassion and power from her new chosen identity around that suffering child.

Jordan and I worked together for 3 decades, until the week before she died. She had a type of cancer that went undiagnosed until she was deep into the fourth stage of metastasis. She had had the symptoms for 4 or 5 years, but because one of her intersectional identities was that she was fat, like many women with PCOS, the possibility of renal cell carcinoma was rendered invisible by the toxin of fat phobia that infects every aspect of the medical world. That toxin killed her.

Her physicians only saw a fat woman and so ascribed every single symptom of this cancer to something related to that particular socially stigmatized intersectional identity. The medical dismissal of her repeated attempts to get answers to the somatic realities of fatigue, inability to tolerate carbohydrates, and persistent weight gain despite hours of exercise every day were all treated with advice to lose weight, a narrative that continued it was too late for her life to be saved. The cancer was only diagnosed by accident when a lab value for calcium came back elevated. The most common cause of this kind of lab result is a parathyroid problem, but instead the CT scans that followed revealed already widely metastasized cancer.

She suffered through chemo and radiation, knowing that they were only a holding pattern giving her a little more time until her inevitable death. She was finally able to be angry at the medical establishment, which both protected her abusers, even when she reported their crimes, and then also neglected her concerns because all they could see was her size. Similar to many people with complex trauma who soothe their trauma-disrupted neurobiology with food, similar to many fat people, the lethal disease that killed her was invisible to medical doctors who could only see her body mass index. To a person, no physician credited what she told them about how many hours a day she exercised or how carefully she watched her caloric intake. She was fat when she died too.

I saw her for the last time 8 years before I finished this chapter, 2 days before her death, as she lay in a hospice bed, forever unconscious, her head bald from the last useless round of chemo. The only solace for my grief, and that of her wife and son and their extended family of choice, was that in the almost precisely 30 years between the first time she stepped into my office and the day of her death she had been able to reconcile her deeply conflicting intersectional identities into a whole, loving, and passionate human being who embraced all of who she was and all of who she had been. She had embarked on Root's third trajectory of intersectional identity development.

Jordan had become able to be all of who she was—a lesbian feminist blue-collar activist, mother, wife, survivor of horrific childhood complex trauma, swimmer, writer, proud in an absurd way of having survived long enough to die of cancer, not at her own hand, not because she was suicidal from her childhood trauma. In the 2 years between diagnosis and death she had come to insist on joy, on connection, on being fully alive even as she knew that she was dying. She had become able, just in time for her cancer diagnosis, to refuse to see her childhood horrors and her adult strengths, the pains of her life and the joys of it, too, as contradictory. She had fully entered Root's third trajectory for intersectional identity development, one in which the person's self-definitions, and the fluidity of categories, come to predominate, and the toxic either/or rules of social pathologies are cast aside.

Root's (2000, 2004) work portrays this third trajectory for intersectional identity development as an active, creative, agentic strategy in which some component of a person's intersectionalities become the source and core from which others emerge, remaining fluid and responsive to who this person knows themselves to be. This trajectory is inner-directed and, in consequence, will rarely be a case of "who you think you see is some of who you get," as this is a space of liberation from categories imposed by social pathologies.

This is a trajectory in which the exposure to trauma may not take the foreground in identity, but one where the trauma-exposed person will have found pathways to interrogate the meaning of that experience. They will have, most likely, experienced some kind of healing, formal or not, that has detoxified the trauma exposure from assignments blame and stigma. This person may have "proud survivor" in the foreground, as did Jordan, or not. Having healed from trauma will likely never be completely invisible, and the person themself will decide where in the picture of self that detail fits. The fluidity of this trajectory of the construction of intersectionalities has liberated such a trauma-exposed person from the scripts imposed by structural hierarchies of oppression as to how to be all of who they are, including a person once affected by trauma and not held in its grip any longer.

We now explore Root's (1998, 2004) fourth strategy for intersectional identity development, which can best be characterized as "throw out the cookbook and grow your own identity." This strategy actively challenges the ways in which humans have been previously assigned identities due to phenotype or circumstances of birth and engages resistance to social pathologies at a deep level. In this intersectionalities trajectory the person is not simply "who you see is not what you get," but "I define myself; not you, not the strands of my intersectionalities, not a social pathology, not my trauma. I am who I know myself to be, remaining connected to my communities in the ways that I decide."

Eugenio's Stories

Eugenio[2] was an artist whose collages of found objects were deeply symbolic stories about his life under the Chilean military junta, a fascist regime embodying every single form of social pathology, one placed in power by the social pathology of U.S. imperialism, which funded the overthrow of the democratically elected government of socialist Salvador Allende. Eugenio's parents, members of the Socialist Party, had come to Chile from Germany to escape the Nazis, and the family had been active in leftist causes. Many of his friends from art school were among the desaparacidos, the disappeared ones murdered by the junta. He had fled to the United States after sudden release from prison, where he had been tortured physically and mentally. After a period of allowing his body to heal as best as possible, he returned to his vocation as an artist. He became acclaimed for his work, respected as a teacher and an elder in his community.

When interviewed about his collages as part of a retrospective honoring his many decades of work, he said that what he had realized while in prison was that nothing was more important to his sense of himself than his artistic

---

[2]Case material has been disguised to protect client confidentiality.

vision. It was the thing he had held in his mind above all else during the years of torment. "Yes, I was tortured. I do not want to be thought of as the torture survivor artist, or even as a socialist artist, although I am one. I do not want my experience to be seen as exceptional. Many people have been tortured, and you do not fete them. You are feting the artist. Yes, this trauma lives inside of me, every moment of every day, how could it not? It has taught me things I never knew I needed to understand about how to be an artist. It has taught me, most importantly that for me, the artist is first, always, and must be first, always, even on those days when my brain tries to take me back to my cell." He challenged anyone who suggested that he was in denial about the horrors of his experiences to "look at my work—there you will see the truth about horror."

He told his physician, someone who had had to take a decade to earn Eugenio's trust, given that some of the torturers were doctors, that he indeed suffered from nightmares about his experiences. "Every day for all of these years I have grieved the deaths of my friends and comrades, the loss of my homeland, of being able to speak my native language when I go to buy groceries. My parents had raised me to know that the world was not a safe place for me, but oh, Dina, my friends. . . ." He asked her for medication to help him sleep, because "everything else I can bear, but sleeplessness sends the artist away, and that is not something I can accept." He was no stranger to therapy, given that his mother had been a psychoanalyst. But psychotherapy was not the methodology that he trusted to be healing for him. He refused to allow anyone to pathologize him. Eugenio knew that the illness had been the horror of the junta. In creating his own identity as the artist, an identity that was the amalgam of everything he was, and yet was none of those things either, he was his own liberatory healer.

Toward a Symbolic Identity

Root's (1998, 2004) final strategy for living in intersectional identities is what she describes as the creation of a symbolic identity. Symbolic identities do not exist in any form recognized by any extant forms of intersectional identities. The person on this trajectory is someone who has managed to resist all of the rules and toxins of social pathologies, even if they have been trauma-exposed. They have a name for who they are that has never existed before.

This strategy might at first glance look like the closer-to-safe methodologies of assimilation or passing by persons whose various strands of intersectionality might be otherwise invisible. But to create a new category for oneself, in which intersectionalities are not simply intersecting but instead allowed to generate this never-before-seen thing, the metaphor for which might be swirls through many different paint colors all in one container, is to cast aside all definitions. Symbolic identities are frequently fluid, rejecting binaries and socially constructed categories that have been laid on top of phenotype or even lived experience.

It appears to me that psychologist Nick Walker exemplifies this. She is a trans woman, proudly autistic, or as she calls it, "neuroqueer" (N. Walker, 2021). Neuroqueer is the symbolic identity that she has created to name herself as she knows herself to be, because no other extant identities were the ones she saw in the mirror. She has not attempted to change her presentation to conform with expectations of how a person with a female sex phenotype would appear. Her name has remained the same. She does not appear to have attempted to erase evidence of having been a male sex phenotype before she uncovered and claimed her transgender orientation.

She created the construct of neuroqueerness to describe who she, and other people in her affinity group, are. She lives at the radical edge of the autism self-acceptance world, challenging other autistic people to be more radical in their insistence on receiving respect.

I don't know Walker personally. I know that within the worlds of her various intersectional identities many people, including others trans people and other autistic people, do not accept her symbolic identity because of her refusal to play by the usual definitional paradigms. She has been quite publicly unwilling to "play nicely" with those who do not share her standpoints to make them more comfortable. I don't know whether she has a trauma history. She has not shared one in her written work so far. Yet I also know that autistic people experience all kinds of trauma, from stimulus and social overload within their own brains, from the stigma and microaggressions aimed at them for simply being authentically autistic in the world, from having had to mask. Trauma is not part of Walker's story as she tells it to the world. Exploding all categories is her story. She has built a new identity, a new word, and invited into it those who find that it reflects them, too.

Root's trajectories of intersectional identity development point clearly to the truth that there is no one way for a person to experience intersectionality. There is also no one way in which trauma folds into or informs those processes. Her model is profoundly decolonial, because there are no stages or phases, no less or more mature place in which to land, no better or worse way of creating a sense of who one is out of the possibly enormous strands of intersectionality. Thus she disrupts the narratives of mainstream identity development paradigms which claim that there is a right way to experience intersectionality or a right way for trauma to be a component of intersectionality.

Eugenio is not in denial. Walker is not pretending to be trans simply because she does not present typically female as prescribed by the culture in which she lives, nor is she pretending autism because she has a PhD in psychology and can make eye contact and sustains loving and intimate relationships with other humans.

CONCLUSION AND MOVING FORWARD

When we deeply understand a person's intersectionalities and the role that trauma has played in forming or deforming them, making them foreground or hidden, then we can ask the liberatory questions in the DHCR trauma healing process. We can, collaboratively with the trauma-exposed person, explore toxic internalized messages while we are also working together to find a way for their body's human responses to danger and relational disconnection to come to a state of regulation, comfort, and ease. In this exploration we will have also learned more about what safety means for this suffering human, and how safe enough can be achieved without the loss of aliveness, joy, power, agency, and meaning making.

So now let us turn to the question of how we decolonize the healing process itself. Because none of what has come before in this book will matter if the healing process itself does not meet criteria for being decolonial and liberatory. What I will ask you, my readers, to do next, is to suspend your allegiances to everything you know about what psychotherapy is meant to be. I invite you to set aside all of the pedestals on which liberation, feminist, queer, and critical psychotherapy theorists have been placed. Create some space for the bumpy ride that I've been on for the past decade. This time we, the decolonial healers, the liberation and feminist and critical and queer psychologists, are asking the questions of what meets criteria—in this case, for making a healing methodology one that can live in the DHCR universe.

12

CRITERIA FOR A DECOLONIAL, HUMBLE, CULTURALLY RESPONSIVE PRACTICE OF TRAUMA HEALING

Making the Grade

If we consider carefully the possibility that an individual's failed psychotherapy may center around a systemic corruption of a relationship that should be basically trustworthy, then our current practice of psychotherapy becomes suspect, or open to questions.

—A. G. Rogers, *A Shining Affliction* (1995, p. 318)

So having thoroughly critiqued and interrogated the problems of trauma therapy as usual, having offered some examples of what decolonial, humble, culturally responsive (DHCR) trauma healing might look like in practice, having delved deeply into the foundational constructs of safety and intersectionality, we arrive at last at the question for which the rest has been prelude: How do we know if what we're doing is DHCR work? What follows are immodest but not particularly humble proposals about how we, as DHCR healers, can set criteria, albeit ever evolving, for whether a particular trauma healing practice passes through that filter of which I wrote in Chapter 1. Can this thing be DHCR? Can the toxins in the roots of whatever it is be sufficiently neutralized or discarded in the service of making a trauma treatment into a DHCR trauma healing practice?

https://doi.org/10.1037/0000421-013
Decolonizing Trauma Healing: Toward a Humble, Culturally Responsive Practice,
by L. S. Brown

ABOUT NOT DROWNING IN THE SEA OF PSYCHOTHERAPY ALPHABET SOUP

In this third decade of the 21st century, trauma healers can draw upon an enormous and constantly expanding menu of interventions, many of which are proclaimed by their lead teacher to be the thing that will finally truly heal trauma-exposed people from their suffering. There is quite the alphabet soup of these things, a bigger bowl every year. Some of them present their primary value to traumatized people as being scientific or evidence-based because they are the spawn of various randomized controlled trials (RCTs) that excluded almost everyone suffering from exposure to trauma. Others in the soup point to their focus on the body—somatic approaches—as giving them superiority to other treatments, which is one of the emerging trends in the trauma healing field, especially among people seeking a path toward acknowledging the ways trauma represents itself in our neurobiology. Attention to the body is good; the way in which many of these approaches have appropriated various healing modalities and strategies from Indigenous healing methods of colonized cultures without giving credit where due is problematic for a DHCR healer.

Other of these therapies derive from more psychodynamic or humanistic paradigms. Again, absolutely nothing wrong per se with any of this. The challenge for DHCR work is whether or not the core of the thing being done can survive passing through the filters created by DHCR lenses.

There are so many of these trauma treatments around right now that it's dizzying for this retired trauma healer to keep track of them all. I get at least two flyers in the mail every day advertising training or certification in something or another, not to speak of the near tsunami of online announcements via email or social media of classes and workshop related to trauma. It's as if trauma has gone from being the orphan of the mental health world to its golden child, and everyone wants to adopt that child after neglecting it for so long. Most of the things advertised do seem to help some people some of the time. None of them are the new miracle, which they often claim to be. And none of them describe consideration of anything related to intersectional identities, colonization or decolonial practice, or liberatory perspectives. So a DHCR trauma healer has to search with an electron microscope at times for what might meet DHCR trauma healing work somewhere.

Any one of this multitude of interventions can contribute only a tiny fraction of the elements of the healing relationship between a suffering trauma-exposed person and a DHCR trauma healer. The best data, based on decades of research on what makes psychotherapy work—and this is research done within the colonized paradigm but by skeptical participants from their perches in academia who are just a bit subversive—show that any given intervention only ever accounts for between 8 and 10 percent of a successful outcome of the whole shebang (Norcross & Wampold, 2019a). So learn all the techniques you wish, and you'll get 10 percent.

The just listening, bearing witness, and holding the space—the ways of being a healer that I've written of much earlier in this volume in the discussion of the missed opportunities in the world of trauma healing, the things that W. H. R. Rivers did and his patient Siegfried Sassoon described helping him so much (Jamison, 2023), the ways of being that are central to DHCR trauma healing—account for much more of the rest of what heals people's souls.

Attention to intersectional identities as an element of what makes for good trauma healing has not been a focus of formal study yet, to my knowledge, because my buddies who have been quietly subverting the RCT model of what makes for good therapy will cheerfully acknowledge that they haven't looked very hard in that direction. (Disclosure: John C. Norcross and Bruce Wampold are my friends, and I consider them possibly unwitting coconspirators in the decolonizing project, the saboteurs inside the walls.)

Despite research findings indicating that the relationship is the crucial element having been easily accessible for more than 2 decades, most trauma healers will never have heard of these findings because they are rarely taught in the halls of academia. Because they sense that something was lacking in their graduate training, most trauma healers will have had or will pursue training in one of the official trauma healing methodologies in an effort to deepen their capacities and the range of what they have to offer the people who seek their care. Plus, they usually come out of their degree programs feeling, and rightly so, utterly unprepared to work with someone who has been trauma-exposed, and certainly not in any sort of culturally responsive way.

Take, for example, me, a therapist who went to graduate school in the 1970s when trauma wasn't even mentioned; I pursued this path toward trauma-related skill development in a manner consistent with my professional cohort. I'm trained in eye movement desensitization reprocessing (EMDR) at level 2, then learned to do brainspotting. I know several mindfulness-based approaches, particularly acceptance and commitment therapy (ACT), and am very influenced by functional analytic psychotherapy (FAP), even though it is not formally a trauma healing modality. Relational psychoanalysis and emotion-focused therapy (EFT) are also hovering in my clinical and intellectual background, EFT particularly because it's a cousin of gestalt therapy, which was the therapeutic modality that most appealed to my younger self; I pursued additional training from two faculty members who were newly converted to gestalt therapy in my graduate program and then through a yearlong course that I attended evenings during my internship at the VA hospital. Like almost all psychologists of my cohort, I can do cognitive behavioral therapy (CBT) and exposure therapy, as those are what I was taught in a program that had one early adopter of pure behaviorism and one follower of Albert Ellis among the faculty. I draw upon some elements of dialectical behavior therapy (DBT) skills, which, no matter what it says in the books, is really a way of working with very traumatized people whose neurobiology is activated in the absence of the person ever having been soothed sufficiently. Quite the collection of stuff, eh? And all of this wraps into being a liberatory intersectional feminist therapist.

As I say to healers who consult with or are trained by me, the usual result of getting older in our field is that one becomes more integrative and less orthodox, and I am certainly no exception to that norm. Nor, in my opinion, should any DHCR trauma healer be worshipping at the shrine of any one intervention, no matter how authoritative the source who taught it to you, no matter how effective it seems to be with most of the people who are seeking your care for their trauma-induced suffering, more of the time than not. One size never did fit all, and if by this point you haven't gotten the message that the suffering that people experience from the varieties of trauma exposure is hugely individual, variable, and informed by all of their intersectional identities, then I haven't been adequately redundant, despite fearing that I have been too much so.

Ergo, a DHCR trauma healer will be doing something, some flavor off the menu of what's available in your era of learning, to offer trauma healing. The challenge is to offer it so that whatever you're doing meets the criteria, as it were, for being DHCR (and I know, my own addition to the alphabet soup). This is the central concern of what follows in the last chapters of this book. What are those criteria, and how might some of the items on the menu of alphabet soup meet those criteria?

I'm going to apologize in advance for the fact that my menu is not some scholarly version of the book-sized kind found at IHOP or Denny's or your local diner. It is limited by my own, still growing knowledge base about what might be in a healer's repertoire and by the limitations of my training, the stage of professional development I'm in now, and the feedback I've received over the years from the real experts—the people suffering from exposure to trauma. There are probably approaches for trauma about which I know nothing, or have never heard about, that meet criteria beautifully. Write to me about those, please; my email address is on my website, which you can find easily with any search engine. If I'm around in another decade to do a revised version of this book, and I agree that they meet criteria, I'll comment on them. That is, if I'm still thinking this way. I cannot give you a script or a list. I can offer you some ways to think about what you've learned to do, what you think you might want to learn, and then let you loose with those criteria in mind.

I am also not going to do an analysis and critique of each of the various trauma healing methodologies known in the Global North. That's an entirely other book. I do want to bow deeply to the importance of integrating some knowledge, not simply of somatic practices, but of the specific neurobiology of trauma and attachment and how that emerging knowledge might be integrated into DHCR trauma healing (Porges, 2011; Porges & Dana, 2018). An important component of the DHCR model rests on our increasing understanding of these human systems, since, as I have been noting throughout this volume, they define the responses that we have to all kinds of trauma as completely human, built into human neurobiology.

The reality of the neurobiology of trauma and attachment, the reality that these experiences live in shared human neurons and parts of our brains and bodies, even though they are experienced and expressed through the lenses of intersectionality and the sociopolitical context of the trauma-exposed person, are a necessary foundation for the depathologizing project at the core of DHCR trauma healing. While the distress will present in different ways from person to person, depending on how parts of their brain that are not specific to trauma response are organized, that is, their basic neurotypy, as well as how they express distress through the frameworks of their intersectional identities, I do not believe it possible for a healer to feel secure in promoting the depathologizing principles of DHCR practice without knowing something about the neurobiological underpinnings of human distress. So please, do get educated in that material in whatever manner you best learn. To go from the weakness model applied to traumatized soldiers in World War I to war neurosis in World War II to posttraumatic stress disorder (PTSD) in the third edition of the *Diagnostic and Statistical Manual of Mental Disorders* to understanding that this is not a disorder, these are human responses to the traumas of social pathologies requires having a foundation for that last statement that is more than just a political opinion. It's nice to have the brain scan data support my politics.

DHCR CRITERIA: AN IMMODEST PROPOSAL

In developing this quite immodest set of four criteria for whether an official trauma healing intervention can be considered a DHCR trauma healing modality, I have drawn heavily on the thinking of feminist, mujerista, womanist, queer, critical, and, of course, other decolonial and liberatory healers. Nothing I am proposing in this section has not been proposed by someone else, in some form already. I am, rather, integrating from what has spoken to me the most clearly, hoping to preserve the essence of whatever it is that is informing me. I will be wrong in some ways and miss some important criteria.

Enough equivocation (or perhaps, not enough humility?). Notice that this tentativeness, as well as the chutzpah to enunciate these criteria, have all emerged from parts of my own intersectionalities: the White part that believes that what it thinks is right, the natal woman who was taught uncertainty, the Jew who learned to always say, "But on the other hand, this other scholar interpreted these words as meaning this other thing entirely," the trauma healer who has learned that no one size fits anyone quite well but that each person, if given the tools, will knit a warm healing garment that does fit them well. And the part of my intersectional identities who is, I believe, the last piece of who I am: the longtime trauma healer remembering what the experts—the suffering people who honored me with their presence for more than 4 decades—taught me.

Elements of a DHCR Trauma Healing Experience

I have a lovely acronym to help you remember the elements of any DHCR trauma healing experience: PIEN. These are not the criteria; these are the elements that must show up at some point in the work after a methodology has met the criteria. Such a practice must attend to the political (P), by which I mean the structural hierarchies of oppression from which social pathologies spring; the intersectional (I), the ways in which trauma is woven into the suffering person's intersectional identities; the existential (E), the ways in which trauma in this person's life raises existential and spiritual challenges and dilemmas; and the neurobiological (N), the ways in which the various aspect of the neurobiology of trauma exposure, attachment, and social engagement are being expressed in the distress, the unknowing experiences, and/or the difficult behaviors that the person brings into your office. Table 12.1 might help the more visually inclined remember this acronym. The arrows indicate the multidirectionality of each of these variables, one affecting the next, which affects it back, and so on.

FIRST CRITERION: DHCR TRAUMA HEALING MUST SUPPORT A DECOLONIAL FRAMEWORK

While this seems self-evident, it is not. Some of the newest, most apparently leading-edge trauma therapies for which ads arrive in my mailbox speak a lot in the language of diagnosis and pathology, particularly, ironically, the more body-based approaches. These interventions seem to have clear notions of what

TABLE 12.1. The PIEN Elements of a DHCR Trauma Healing Experience

The arrows indicate the multidirectionality of each of these variables and how they affect each other continuously.

Political (P) 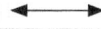	Existential (E)
• What is this person's history of being colonizer/colonized/both? • What is happening in the current socio-political context, and how does that relate to the intersectional identities of both healer and sufferer? • What are the power dynamics in the healing relationship, and how can they be shaped to be more liberatory and collaborative? • A necessary foundation for any and all decolonial work, no matter how it is conducted.	• What are the existential and spiritual meanings of this trauma? • What effects does this trauma have on the person's ability to make meaning or participate in spiritual practices? • A necessary component for the "mourning and remembrance" component of Harvey and Herman's three-phase model (1996). • Development of critical consciousness happens here and also back in P.
Intersectional (I)	Neurobiological (N)
• What are this person's intersectional identities, and how do they conjugate them? • In what ways has trauma infused some or all strands of intersectionality, or not, prior to the "official" trauma? • In what ways did trauma appear absent? • What does the suffering person represent to the healer because of what is known of their intersectionalities? • What does the healer represent to the suffering person because of what is known of their intersectionalities? • What do each of their intersectionalities do to frame the view of the healing experience?	• What is this person's neurotype? • What neurobiological trauma response systems might be involved in how this person's suffering is manifesting, and how might that inform all parties about what the nature of the trauma might have been (fear, attachment, betrayal, continuous, escapable or not, and so on)?

Note. DHCR = decolonial, humble, culturally responsive.

constitutes health and its absence. These so-called new things have not, for the most part, broken from the very old notion that trauma-exposed people are having symptoms and need a diagnosis, rather than having a human response occurring within their intersectional identities. Nor do they take sociopolitical realities into account.

Giving up the use of diagnosis and pathologizing humans instead of oppressive social systems is a necessity if a healing practice is to be considered

DHCR. This is the "P" part of the PIEN criteria, and it's the entry criterion for DHCR work. If you can't do a particular methodology without diagnosis nor without treating the distress and the unknowing strategies as pathology, you're going to have to consider how to rethink the epistemic framework. You've got to have the political awareness of colonization and its effects to do DHCR work. That's one thing about which I'm absolutely certain.

Taking Our Old Paradigms to the Mikveh

This doesn't mean that, if you practice within one of these frameworks, you cannot do decolonial work. Rather, as it was incumbent on me, and on all of us who came before, it is necessary to interrogate our approaches to trauma healing to discover what is colonial within them. This can feel strange, particularly when whatever paradigm has informed our work has felt, to some degree, revolutionary, upsetting some dominant paradigm or another. Somatic work is supposed to be upsetting talk therapy, but not when it's being conducted as if the body in question isn't living in a traumagenic social and political reality replete with social pathologies.

In the Jewish tradition in which I was raised, and which informs a lot of my worldview despite my long-ago departure from most of its prayers and rituals, there exists an apparently benign yet potent cleansing ritual. It's that of the mikveh. One goes to the mikveh, the ritual bath, which must have some "mayim chayim," living water, water from the sky or a natural body of water, making up what is in that tub, not only water that flows easily from the tap. For a ritual that began in a place where rain rarely falls, the meaning of having something alive and wet as central to what makes that water healing and cleansing should make us sit up and pay attention to the question of why that rule was put in place, even if the roots of this ritual of cleansing have been lost to habit. I think the mikveh is meant to enliven.

Observant Jewish women go to a mikveh after each menstruation. My observant Jewish, radical feminist, heterosexually married graduate school companion, lacking access to a mikveh, dipped herself in a lake, even in the freezing rain of winter in southern Illinois. Observant Jewish men go to the mikveh before each Sabbath, when they greet the "Sabbath Bride." Those becoming Jews by choice are dipped in the waters of the mikveh—three full-body immersions for anyone visiting, not washing away sins or previous beliefs but soaking themselves in what is Jewish. Some Jewish survivors of sexual abuse and assault have found that going to the mikveh, often for the first and only time in their lives, has been a surprisingly potent component of the reconstitution of their embodied selves and a reconnection with the place in their intersectional identities where this violation occurred at the hands of some other

Jew, a family member, whose sexual assaults drove the toxins of the social pathology of misogyny deep into this strand of intersectionality, sometimes creating decades of alienation.

The baptismal rituals of Christianity are, after all, nothing more than a version of the mikveh in which Rabbi Yehoshua (aka Jesus) and his followers cleansed themselves (Pelikan, 1997). John called the Baptist was making a mikveh in the Jordan River, an operational definition of mayim chayim. Baptism is the appropriated, colonized version of a mikveh, an appropriated version forced on the Jews of Andalusia and the Algarve who wanted to remain and not leave their homelands after the Catholic Reconquista, "conversos" who later found themselves burned at the stakes of the Inquisitions of Spain and Portugal because their Jewishness hadn't been sufficiently cleansed out of them. An appropriation, no longer a cleansing and return to wholeness but a renunciation of evil, of "Satan and all his works."

DHCR trauma healing requires us to take our ways of doing our work to a sort of mikveh. We aren't trying to burn down relational psychoanalysis or EMDR or internal family systems (IFS) or sensorimotor processing. Rather, we are cleansing and softening our trauma healing methods in the mikveh of the living waters of a decolonial framework. This means going through our terminologies and constructs in order to cleanse them of nonliberatory, or even antiliberatory, ways of understanding the human response to trauma exposure.

We need to have the courage to seek out and name the places in the healing arts we have personally been practicing that have been corrupted and colonized. This is the epistemic analogy to how the person entering a mikveh first clips each nail, washes and combs their hair for any substances lingering in it, and consequently allows the body to be fully exposed before being washed in the healing and cleansing waters. I've already said that we need to let go of the words *psychotherapy* and *therapist* and *client* and *patient*, that we need to stop using a diagnosis to name the pain that people experience in their utterly human responses to being exposed to all of the kinds of trauma. These steps clip the nails.

Combing through the hair though can be harder because hair is denser. Things hide in it, as anyone who's been surprised by a spider creeping around in their locks after a stint in the garden or who has picked lice out their children's hair can testify. This finecombing is where looking at our practice through the PIEN framework can be helpful to us.

What might this finecombing look like? Let's take, for example, because I know enough about it, EMDR. Let's say that the trauma from which this person is suffering, and for which they seek care, is that they were the victim of a hate crime based on their melanic phenotype. Something I would do as a decolonial step, before offering EMDR, would be to engage with this person, as described at many places earlier in this volume, around questions of our intersectionalities. So in this case, combing out the "I" in PIEN. What do we represent to one another? What, if any, other components of intersectionalities were harmed by this hate crime? Was it a crime of betrayal, of someone's failure or unwillingness to protect? What do I, the healer, represent to them? Which leads to the finecombing step, all of this before I even mention EMDR, of inquiring into the presence or absence of active social pathologies in this person's life, the "P" criterion. How much hate speech are they exposed to in daily life? How much insidious traumatization through the news or social media? Here, we begin some discussions about being closer to safe, which is existential, the "E," and also a component of setting up the EMDR protocol in a way that is respectful of this suffering person's realities. We talk, somewhere in here, about how their suffering is manifesting, which gives me information that I in turn share about the neurobiology of their trauma response; the "I," and back to the "P" again, looking at how power is equalized in DHCR trauma healing by not making information the sole possession of the healer.

Okay, I've combed out quite a few spiders here. I have not said, "EMDR is something that some people who've had your experience have found helpful. I'd be glad to tell you about it, or give you a book about it, or help you understand it in some other way," which is a power-balancing statement, but insufficient. What I have done instead, before ever saying this line, is to comb out assumptions about intersectionalities and power and social pathologies. Then I get to introduce EMDR. I've already learned that this person has had experiences of safety in their family home, and so I tentatively offer them the safe place exercise. Had I learned that they had never experienced safety, I would go to what other clients have taught me and request an image of a beautiful space, "real or imagined, it doesn't matter."

Only then do I get to try out the EMDR protocol, paying very careful attention to what is happening. While EMDR practitioners are trained to do a certain set of things in a certain order, DHCR trauma healing practice, by centering the experiences of the suffering person (the "P," the politics of trauma healing work), will follow the lead of the suffering person through EMDR even more than is standard—and EMDR does a pretty good job already of putting the client in the lead more of the time than some other approaches I've learned to use.

Then we're back to "I," intersectionalities and being safe enough, closer to safe: What do we need to make time for such that this person can leave the healing space and return to the world of the quotidian, in which the hate crime occurred, knowing how to be safe enough, closer to safe? Drawing on what we learned before we even began EMDR, as we combed it out, we might utilize an EMDR protocol for creating an internal sense of safety, an image of a nurturing or protecting person or symbol to which this suffering person might turn, on which they might draw when confronted with the unsafe realities of that world beyond the healing space.

This is simply one example. Notice that a lot of the combing out happens before, during, and after whatever the official healing thing is. Notice that combing means looking for each of the PIEN variables because if one is neglected, it's likely in there tangling things up and pulling them away from a decolonizing direction.

Cleansing Trauma Healing From the Fearful Acts of the Parent/Founder

To support a DHCR framework, our healing methodologies must be taken to the intellectual mikveh that is the development of a critical consciousness in ourselves, about ourselves, about our theories and methodologies. Critical consciousness is not only for suffering people we work with. We need, as healers, to start humble, as we've been discussing in this entire volume. The more experienced we are, and thus the more likely to be proposing a "new" model of how to do our work, the more humility we are likely to need, especially those of us who, like me, prided ourselves on integrating liberatory principles into our work as if somehow we were more progressed than our peers. Oy, arrogance. Which leads us to the second criterion.

SECOND CRITERION: DHCR TRAUMA HEALING IDENTIFIES DEVELOPMENT OF CRITICAL CONSCIOUSNESS IN ALL PARTIES AS EVIDENCE THAT HEALING IS OCCURRING

Throughout this book we have explored this construct, central to a DHCR model and shared with liberation theology and psychology (Comas-Díaz & Torres-Rivera, 2020), feminist theory (G. Lerner, 1994), and general decolonial psychology (Comas-Díaz et al., 2024). The suffering person, in the healing process, learns "I am not the problem, and I have the power to be a part of the solution." This phenomenon is both political and existential—the existential meaning of grasping that social pathologies are the problem and the source of suffering.

In a DHCR healer such a consciousness must always be present, in a two-track manner. We both eschew any narrative of the suffering person as the problem and do this for ourselves as well when the healing process goes through its expectable turns of the spiral. We are not failing when a person's suffering does not abate in the face of chronic exposure to danger, when we are in a long struggle to get close enough to safe in the presence of that chronic danger. We are doing decolonial healing work where we are not skipping the steps of telling the truth, not creating conditions in which a suffering person must pretend to us that they are fine when all indicators are that they are not. We, the DHCR healers, need our own critical consciousness wrapped around ourselves at these times when someone says, "PTSD can be treated in 12 sessions," and the voices of the social pathologies creep into our heads and tell us what imposters we are.

This kind of consciousness has informed everything I've written earlier in this volume, expressed in my locating the problem of trauma in social pathologies, not in suffering people. The PIEN framework is central to the manifestation of critical consciousness. Holding an understanding of social pathologies, of one's own intersectionalities, of the existential dilemma of being safe enough, and, importantly, the ways in which one's distress and one's unknowing are simply the human neurobiological response to trauma, betrayal, and threats to attachment and connection constitute the foundations on which critical consciousness can take root in the trauma-exposed person and also be integrated into a preexisting trauma healing modality.

As healing proceeds, critical consciousness grows and works to detoxify the suffering person from the poisons of social pathologies. As my colleague and friend Christine Courtois (2020) said eloquently in the title of a book she wrote for people suffering from trauma exposure, "It's not you, it's what happened to you." I would add to her wise words, "And what happened to you happened because of a social pathology of some kind even if it's hard to see the direct connection just now. An individual may have done something to you; they were empowered to do it, taught that it was acceptable to do this to you, by a social pathology that they believed protected them." When a suffering person integrates that epistemic framework of critical consciousness into their own way of knowing themselves in the world and takes on the "P" (political) in the PIEN framework, healing cannot help but move forward.

Liberation psychology speaks of conscientization, feminist therapy of consciousness-raising, decolonial psychology of moving away from coloniality. "Woke" is a way of narrating this process through an Afrocentric lens. In many marginalized groups there are culture- or context-specific Indigenous terms for this experience of becoming awake, to the truth, to the pain of oneself and one's communities, and to the possibilities for healing and change. It is possible that, for a suffering person in whose strands of identity there is a construct that speaks to critical consciousness, part of the "culturally responsive" in the DHCR model invites the healer to be curious about what words or ways of being would communicate critical consciousness from the suffering person back to themselves: the "I" (intersectionality) in the PIEN formula.

What a person calls this awakening can be important, and what they call it is something to which a DHCR trauma healer needs to give careful attention, because in the subtexts of that term are paths for liberation, the taking back of power, healing. In a DHCR healing model it cannot be skipped at any phase of the trauma healing process. For instance, in several cultures with which I am familiar, including my own, "remember" is the word that says, "wake up." Rastafarians and Jews alike sing of "remembering Zion" as a symbol for freeing ourselves from the social pathologies that oppress us.

For most models of trauma healing to meet this criterion of creating critical consciousness they will have to drop their reliance on diagnostic labels and pathologizing language about people's distress. Even most of the best work on polyvagal theory's application to healing, or on the neurobiology of attachment and its manifestations in people's distress in their interpersonal worlds, still speaks of people having human responses to disruptions in those neurobiological systems as having something wrong with them somehow and offers treatments for the distress that take no account of the political and social realities that have activated the neurobiology of distress.

We have to learn to cast this language of political and social neutrality, as well as the thinking that has informed it, aside if we are do to DHCR work. It's difficult to get over the habit of referring to someone's borderline or narcissistic tendencies, to describing a person as having obsessive compulsive disorder (OCD), or to have a notion that there exists a human typical from which certain human brains have strayed into atypical. It's necessary to change how we speak, which changes how we think, which changes how we speak, which changes our maps of the suffering world.

This criterion thus underscores the importance, for a DHCR trauma healer, no matter their modality, to be grounded in knowledge of the "N" of the PIEN model, the neurobiology of trauma and attachment from which all of the distress and the strategies for unknowing naturally emerge. If I can continuously remind myself that the suffering sitting with me is not a pathology of that neurobiology but rather a typical human expression of it, then I am less likely to fall back into the pathologizing epistemologies of my training. "This distress is as natural in response to trauma as is breathing" is a useful slogan. When I hold this epistemic framework, I am then in a better position to remain tethered to my own hard-won critical consciousness and to bring it to the healing process as much as possible. Therein lies the irony of the apolitical nature of much of what is being written and taught in the neurobiology of trauma space.

This task of using critical consciousness at every step of our practice is not a simple goal to accomplish. When I am frustrated with what is happening in my work with someone, or even when I am frustrated by the behaviors of various other human beings who stumble onto me, I am likely to fall backward into pathologizing thoughts and language. I was raised in all of the social pathologies present in the United States from midcentury, when I was born, through the present moment 70 years later. Sometimes this is me engaging in code-switching, so that the person with whom I am speaking can engage their default mode and its cognitive shortcuts, or, actually, so that I can engage those cognitive shortcuts for them and not have to give the entire decolonized version of what I am saying. This is all evidence of how little critical consciousness is part of "therapy speak," and how thoroughly pathologizing epistemologies of social pathologies have colonized us.

A question before us is how to continuously evoke critical consciousness if that is not the place where a suffering person wants to go. Since DHCR work is client-led, it's not like we can do what some people have suspected me of doing, that is, give people a lecture about how what they're dealing with is really all about fill-in-the-blank social pathology—in my case, given that I am infamously a feminist therapist, patriarchy. But this is not a dilemma if we remind ourselves that we don't have to offer the PIEN model in the order of its letters.

We start where the suffering person is, which is most likely in the "EN" (existential and neurobiological) portion of this mnemonic. This is a liberatory, egalitarian, collaborative DHCR healing process that we are offering, and humility is central to DHCR healing practice. The suffering person is not interested in, may even actively reject, critical consciousness at this moment in our work together. We follow them; we engage in a both/and with this suffering person, holding onto our epistemic framework and not pathologizing, marginalizing, or demeaning theirs, without going into an intellectual power-dominance stance: "Here, let me educate you, and then you will understand that you are not the problem." Don't laugh; sometimes, when we are trying to learn how to infuse our work with critical consciousness, some of us, like yours truly, have been caught doing this at early stages of career development.

An example of this challenge of DHCR work is Mimi,[1] who came to see me because she was depressed and her primary care doctor had suggested I might be a good fit. We are both Jewish, both middle class, both originally from the Midwest of the United States, both professional women. It was extraordinarily simple for me to see how her depression was her body and mind's way of screaming, "enough, enough, enough," to the years of misogynist realities she had endured, at home and at work. But when I offered some vaguely feminist suggestions about how that might be part of her depression, she shut me down, and fast. "I know you're a feminist therapist, Laura, and that's fine for you. You don't have to live with a man. Or work with men. You're in charge of

---

[1]Case material has been disguised to protect client confidentiality.

your life. I need to get better, and I do not want to blow my life up to get there. So can you work with me? Because if not, there are probably plenty of other Jewish fortyish therapists in town. And I do need a Jewish therapist because I think that my loud mouth is part of what gets me into trouble. At least at work."

Since I was, if not DHCR, at least at that point a somewhat experienced feminist therapist who held fast to the notion that the client was the expert on her own life, not me, I said, "Okay, I'm in. Your goals are the only important ones here, Mimi. Let's focus on your goals." I apparently shocked her because she began to cry and said, "No one has ever been interested in my goals, ever. Not one damn time in my life. Not my parents, not my husband, sure as hell not my boss."

I knew that this was the beginning of critical consciousness, and I wisely did not get too greedy. I passed the tissues and stayed in the mode of empathy and holding space. I invited her to know what she knew and feel what she felt, which are ways of being powerful, and not silenced, silencing being a political thing called patriarchy. I didn't say that, not then. I thought it, and knew it, and stuck with my commitment to making her not the problem in our work.

It was an interesting first 6 months. Mimi would come into the office and rid herself of what I thought of as the latest round of toxic sexist garbage from her husband or her boss. I continued to hold space and offer empathy. I learned very quickly not to offer anything resembling a commentary: "Laura, that's more of that feminist stuff that I didn't come here for." "Mimi, you're right. I'm sorry. Let's get back to what's going on for you."

Then there was the day when she walked into the office and said, "Okay, time for the feminist stuff. I'm good at pattern detection, and there are some patterns here I've been seeing that I really didn't want to talk about because I really didn't want to see them. Do you promise not to say you could have told me so?" "Well, duh, no, I'm not going to do that. I'm not always a great therapist, but I'm not here to scold or judge you."

Then she launched into the patterns that she'd been telling me about, stopping at intervals to ask, "That's sexism, right? I'm not making it up, am I?" "Uh, yeah, that sure does look like a duck, Mimi." We had that kind of back-and-forth for several weeks, and then she came in, her energy low. "Now that I know, what in the hell am I going to do?" Critical consciousness is hard to have because it leads to the desire for change and, as was true for Mimi, the knowledge that the changes had to start with her.

Stages of Change Reconceptualized—From Self-Blame to Critical Consciousness

This is a wonderful time to remind ourselves of the stages of change paradigm, a potentially depathologizing epistemic system. A person in this model is not resisting, or avoiding, or deflecting. They are at a particular point in their engagement in the process of healing. While I take umbrage with the notion that a person needs to move from the stage of "I am not the problem" to "Yes, I have a problem and should do something about it," DHCR practice can appropriate and transform it. Let's simply rename it "Stages of Considering Critical Consciousness."

As Carl Rogers (1961) noted more than half a century ago, the work of healing needs to be tailored to meet where people are:

> It is the client who knows what hurts, what directions to go, what problems are crucial, what experiences are deeply buried. It began to occur to me that unless I had a need to demonstrate my own cleverness and learning, I would do better to rely upon the client for the direction of movement in the process. (p. 99)

DHCR words, eloquently written.

So let's consider his paradigm applied to critical consciousness, remembering that people move around a spiral with these stages of change, rather than in straight lines. We begin with something not usually in the model, a construct developed by interns I worked with when I supervised a training clinic that was a proto-DHCR setting. They called this the "anticontemplation" stage of change. What this looked like was some version of "I don't know why I have to be here! I hate therapy! Therapy never works! I hate you! I hate that I need to be here!"

In a DHCR practice framework, this kind of opening salvo should inform several things. First, this person has likely been harmed by therapy and the mental health industrial complex and probably pathologized for their refusals to comply. Many of the folks who came in the door at our clinic in this stage of change arrived with the label "borderline" attached, had been "fired" by previous therapists. They felt helpless and were in stunningly high levels of distress. Second, we at the clinic had to start from precisely where this suffering person was, with simple validation—not empathy, as that was often suspect, seen as bait that a therapist would offer, followed by the switch of rejection when the suffering person failed to respond to whatever was on offer.

Our clinic saw people who were very poor, many of them had been through the meat grinder that is community mental health, a system whose entire name is one large lie, as it is not about the communities in which it is situated, and certainly does not do anything to improve so-called mental health. The people working in it are often heroic, exhausted, and simply unable to handle having 80 people on their active caseloads. One of the most difficult steps toward critical consciousness for the people who walked in our door in this stage of change was for our clinicians to know this and never ever to explain away the problems of the system that suffering people felt betrayed and stigmatized by.

Instead, the anticontemplation stage DHCR response embodying movement toward critical consciousness is something along the lines of: "It truly sucks that when you hurt this badly, you end up in a place like this because you're poor. You have less than zero reason to trust me or anything I say or do. What I wish you would tell me is what makes therapy not work for you, please, so that maybe we don't do whatever that is—that is, if anything ever has worked." This is validation, from a PIEN standpoint. P = the social pathology of classism, which consigns the poorest people in distress to systems that do not help them. I = Intersectional identity of being a person living in chronic poverty. E = the suffering person's existential dilemma, the degree to which they feel trapped, feeling as if there is no choice because they are in so much pain. N = the healer offering ventral-vagal connection, noticing the neurobiology of this highly activated person. Lather, rinse, repeat, in the colloquial term that one of my favorite media commentators, Rachel Maddow, uses; the directive to do this over and over again until the trauma is cleansed, because doing this once, or three times, or for 6 months, may not be what informs this person that this healer, and this healing setting, might be safe enough to have the topic change from "I hate therapy" to "I still hate therapy, but you're different, so let me tell you where I hurt."

Now back to the original model, and to the precontemplation stage, which is the place of "I don't have a problem. Other people have a problem with how I am." This is really a reversal of a DHCR perspective, because we don't think you have a problem; we do think you're marginalized and subordinated and suffering because social pathologies devalue you.

In a DHCR model, this might sound like: "I keep getting into difficulties with people at work because they say I have White privilege. I just immigrated here from Denmark 5 years ago. I didn't participate in any of this stuff; in fact, it's hard for me to be living in the United States and know that it was built on genocide and slavery. But I wish that those folks at work would see it my way. I'm an immigrant, and they treat me like I'm some White American."

How do we invite this person to critical consciousness when they are quite clear that the problem is other people's problem with their lack of critical consciousness? This stage can be particularly challenging for a DHCR healer because we can see, quite clearly, how this blond-haired, blue-eyed, pale-skinned Danish person whose English is ever so slightly accented in a way that people find charming has a lot of White privilege.

This is not White fragility such as DiAngelo (2018) has described it. This is not willful ignorance. It might look and feel that way, and the DHCR healer has to pay attention to intersectional identities and listen to this person emphasizing a particular aspect of theirs—immigrant. Confronting this person about being in denial or saying, "Look, you have White skin so you benefit from White privilege whether your ancestors built it or not" is neither DHCR nor likely to be effective. What we're hearing is an absence of critical consciousness, and our challenge is to find a way in.

A question a DHCR healer might ask this person is, "How might you look inside of yourself, at the person you are, the immigrant from Denmark, to better understand what makes it hard for you to be perceived in this way, to understand how other people perceive you as having White privilege?" In other words, we begin with the P and the E, the political meanings of being an immigrant, the existential dilemmas of this invisible marginalized identity. "What do you imagine they are seeing, or not seeing, in you?" Or, rather than asking this person to check their privilege, asking them, "How can you deepen your understanding and empathy for the people who perceive you in this way by understanding what about this makes you feel invisible?" And there may be a little neurobiology thrown in; is this issue activating the sympathetic nervous system (SNS)?

Because to take that step, to invite this person in the precontemplation stage of critical consciousness development to stand in the experiences of those they are feeling unjustly judged by, means that we are inviting them to empathy and to see themselves through the eyes of others, eyes that see what the world sees first and offers privilege to, rather than eyes that cannot yet see the kid from Ishøj, a working-class town in the exurbs of Copenhagen, built in the 1970s where only a few farms and a small village once stood, a place synonymous with the Danish version of being a hick.

It's the job of the DHCR healer to invite this person to help both of you see that kid, by asking, "Can you look inside of yourself to see who they cannot see?" This opens the door for the healer to discover that kid from Ishøj, who was smart and passed exams and went to university and took on the veneers of sophistication that enabled this person's assimilation into the educated classes from which this person did not come. It allows the blossoming in the healer of empathy for that kid, which then opens the door for inviting empathy in for that kid in those who cannot yet see that kid, and can see only those aspects of intersectionalities in which that kid is wrapped.

With empathy, the seeds of critical consciousness may be sown. In the PIEN framework, P, the social pathology of White supremacy, comes in through the topic of privilege. By acknowledging the very central component of this person's intersectional identities, which is their being a recent immigrant with a history of being a child living in poverty in their home country and being the poor kid among the well-to-do at university, I acknowledge their experiences of marginalization and alienation which are invisible to most others. It's easy to miss immigration trauma in the psyches of people whose forward intersectional identities appear to be replete with privilege, easy to not know what intersectional identities they have carried from home. And if we miss the I in this person's PIEN, we'll create a rupture in trust.

Why? Because, as all of the nearly accent-free immigrant colleagues of mine have talked about with me over the years, no matter how much one is not perceived as an immigrant, no matter how charming one's accent or pale one's skin, no matter how fluent one is in what may be their third or fourth, not second language, there is always an experience of otherness. "I have this nanosecond pause in my brain when I'm speaking English where I have to translate it out of Spanish," said one woman from Latin America whose phenotype is European and who was very upper class at home. A friend who came from Sweden for graduate school has talked about how homesick he gets in the winter for the ways in which the yuletide is celebrated.

By validating the I, the intersectional, the foreground intersectional identity where pain resides for this person, we also do something for the N, the neurobiological experiences of feeling misunderstood and unseen, by seeing and offering ventral vagal connection. And then back to the E, the existential question of how can we see in ourselves what others see, and what is still invisible to us?

The contemplation stage of the development of critical consciousness is often marked by the presence of guilt, shame, self-hatred, or some combination of all of the above, with these painful feelings attached to some or several facets of the person's intersectional identities where privilege accrues or where a person's present circumstances disconnect them from a culture or social class of origin.

This suffering person, in addition to being trauma-exposed, which is why they are in the room with you, is on the verge of critical consciousness and so far, in many instances, is turning the critique primarily on themselves if their primary intersectional identities are those of groups privileged and not marginalized in the culture in which they currently live. Those are the guilt and shame presentations. Self-hatred or seeing oneself as a failure, an imposter, or a fraud are more common in the contemplation stage of critical consciousness development. Here, the person is saying, "There is a problem, and the problem is me."

This may or may not present as an expression of a person's intersectionalities. It is equally, if not more likely, to show up as some kind of painful trauma-evoked suffering. Like Ruth, whose story I shared in Chapter 6, many people in the contemplation stage of critical consciousness are hurting because they have internalized toxins of social pathologies and believe that if only they were different in some way—stronger, a different set of identities— they would be fine and not suffering from being exposed to trauma. There is often guilt and shame over the methods they have used to attempt to unknown their pain or even unknow the trauma itself. Several things are absent for people at this stage of critical consciousness development.

First, there is usually no inkling that the problem lies in social patholo-gies, since it requires the development of critical consciousness to be able to identify those dynamics. Second, there is often a sense of utter powerless-ness, expressed as hopelessness, helplessness, and sometimes the desire to kill themselves. The notion that healing is possible seems like a page from a fantasy novel. There may be, depending on the person, some sense that some of their pain emerges from having been targeted in one or several facets of intersectionalities but not the belief that having distress in response is simply human. As my colleague Micheal Kane, an African American trauma therapist for the past 40 years, describes it in his blog Loving Me More, the obstacles for members of his community to even imagine that it would be okay to seek emotional healing are so woven into the narrative of having to be a strong Black man or woman that simply walking into his office is perceived as evi-dence of having failed the community.

Self-blame and shame in the wake of trauma are so pervasive, no matter what the trauma has been or what the person's intersectional identities might be, it can sometimes be hard to see these as evidence of being in a contempla-tion phase. The standard stages-of-change model would likely identify such a person as being in the action stage, given that they are seeking therapy. Because we are talking about critical consciousness development, however, a DHCR healer needs to see what the person's suffering tells us about the presence or absence of that consciousness.

This process of critical consciousness development is core and founda-tional to the healing process. Developing critical consciousness in a person who knows they are in pain and sees themselves as the problem weaves almost seamlessly into the first of the three phases of trauma healing, the getting to the phase of something resembling safer. Why? Because in order to challenge the illusions and myths of safety and transform that narrative into the storyline about getting closer to safe (Herman, 1992), we invite a suffering person to discover that they are not the problem, that their distress is human, that their difficulties with allowing themselves to notice how not safe they are are fully human, and human in ways that are informed by their intersectional identities.

So the three-phase model of trauma healing proposed by Harvey and Herman (Harvey, 1996; Herman, 1992)—creating safety, processing the trauma, and making existential sense of life—and the stages of critical consciousness devel-opment dovetail here. They become the main course of the work of healing. This is where a DHCR healer can offer the suffering person the menu of healing practices that are available, always doing so in the context of raising consciousness, of placing the pathology in structural forms of oppression, of identifying distress as human, not pathological. If what your offering as a healer keeps these things woven into the work that you are doing, then your practice will meet criteria for a DHCR practice.

Are there action and maintenance stages in the development of critical consciousness that are part of the DHCR healing relationship? My answer is yes and no and maybe. The contemplation stage looks very much like the first two stages of the three-phase model of trauma healing, and all of that is very much like the action stage of the original stages of change. The recursive nature of trauma healing, which can be seen in some of the clinical examples given throughout this book, demonstrates how these two stages of development of critical consciousness blur into one another.

Jae's Story

For example, a suffering person, who we will call Jae, seeks care because they have realized that their strong desire to be emotionally vulnerable with other people has eluded them. They have just turned 40. They feel enormous shame; they tell the healer that they have been a failure at relationships and wonder if this thing that seems simple for so many other people is somehow out of their reach.

First touch with this person, who is in the place of "I have a problem and I believe I am it," goes like this: "It has to take a lot of courage to even walk into my office given how badly you feel about yourself. I'm curious if you are willing to tell me about who you are aside from this painful topic? Because we will get to that, and I have a hunch, which could be wrong, that we will learn more about the nature of this painful thing if we learn more about you." Notice, first touch does not immediately take the invitation to go into a narrative of pathology and also, as we will talk about more below, does not immediately enforce the healer as an authority, but offers a hunch, a hypothesis, rather than a certainty.

What does this DHCR healer learn about this suffering person named Jae? The healer learns that what appears to be phenotypically visible—that this person has White skin and appears female in body—is accurate. Their only known ancestry is European and, as the important first invisible strand of intersectionality, identifies as nonbinary, not female, "although I would love to have a kid, to be pregnant, to be in a relationship that will last long enough. I'm terrified that I'm out of time."

We learn that Jae is very proud of the work that they do as a physical therapist assisting people who have had traumatic brain injuries and that doing their work well is one of their few joys in life. We also learn that Jae works overtime most days, takes weekend and holiday shifts, and is thus rarely not at work, even when they are attempting to be in a relationship, and that Jae grew up in a well-to-do family. "And that was a big part of the problem," they tell the healer, "because no one believes that what was going on in my family could possibly be going on in the family of two college professors."

What was going on was that this suffering person and their siblings were being exchanged in a family sex trafficking ring, something shockingly common among the people who came to me for care over 4 decades. "My own parents never actually touched me. They handed me off to other families in exchange for the other kids. I know, it sounds like a really bad made-for-TV movie. But it was my life. And I didn't protect my brother and sister, and I was the eldest. I didn't fight back, or at least not after one of the other fathers beat me so badly that I ended up with a pretty bad concussion, which is why I work with other traumatic brain injury (TBI) survivors, because I know what it's like to come back from that and mine wasn't that bad. I didn't try hard enough to get a teacher or the cops or someone, anyone, to save us."

We learn that Jae did everything in their power to unknow this horrific abuse, this complete absence of safety anywhere in their young life, increasing the intensity of those attempts to resist knowing terror by restricting food, running for hours at a time, cutting on themselves, and putting the memories of what had happened "away in a box in my mind" until they had their physical therapy license. "And I guess because I became a professional with a duty to report child abuse, some part of me woke up and reported my experiences to me. That's the best way I can describe it. And then the flashbacks and the nightmares, wow, a barrage. I'm pretty sure this is true. My siblings think I'm nuts. And I'm pretty sure this is why I'm so screwed up."

So in the first touch, which went on for several months, Jae allowed the healer to know some important pieces of their trauma. Being trafficked as a child by one's own parents has multiple layers of plain old ordinary trauma: sexual violations enabled by the parents, physical abuse, terror, attachment trauma, betrayals, all wrapped up into one stinking package of hell.

There is the apparent moral injury trauma as the child Jae grew old enough to believe that they could do, should do, something. This is the moral injury of the adolescent sexual abuse survivor who has the completely developmentally typical belief that they can and should do something about the bad behaviors of the adults who still control them and who also control the narrative about the adolescent with the rest of society. In this instance, when adolescent Jae went to law enforcement, their parents were able to completely sabotage them, telling the police that their daughter had some serious mental health problems and had been reading too much true crime fiction: "You know how teenage girls are, so dramatic."

This last speaks to the aspects of intersectional identities and social pathologies that gave power to the perpetrators. They were White, upper-middle-class college professors, respected and respectable. They knew what to say and how to say it. These are the social pathologies of ageism—don't believe a 13-year-old—and of classism, in which the perpetrators' privilege gave them credibility, screened them from suspicion, and even allowed them to include a medical doctor in the family trafficking ring who dealt with any injuries inflicted on the children in this group, including the terrible beating given this suffering person. The social pathology of misogyny, which creates narratives of girls and women making false accusations, and the social pathology of racism—their Whiteness protected these perpetrators—were also factors here. The so-called false memory movement's narrative used all of these social pathologies, adding the extra zinger that the girls (i.e., grown women) from these nice middle-class White families with highly educated parents were being induced to make false accusations by therapists who were feminists.

Part of the first touch was the healer saying, somewhere around the third session in their second week together, "Okay, Jae. Here's the thing. I can offer you some things pretty quickly that might reduce how much distress you're having, and I can tell you about those so that you can make some choices. And there's something I'm going to say now, and keep saying, because I have a hunch you won't believe it. You are not to blame. You are not screwed up. You are in terrible pain, in the ways that human beings are designed to be in terrible pain when these kinds of terrible things are done to them. You are not the problem."

The healer said this at the beginning of that meeting because she knew that Jae would need some time to take in what the healer had just said. What Jae did was begin to shake, tremble, sob gutturally, fall out of the chair and onto the floor. The healer asked, "Can you hear me, Jae?" When a tiny nod of the head ensued, the healer said, "I'm not going to ask you if you want me to come physically closer because that's probably above your pay grade right now. May I sing to you?" Small nod of head.

Polyvagal theory (Dana, 2018; Porges, 2011; Porges & Dana, 2018) has posited that the sound of a woman's singing voice assists humans in moving from states of either activation or freeze, both of which seemed to be happening in Jae at that moment, and into ventral vagal connection. The healer was aware by then that Jae had suffered terrible abuse through touch and violation of their space and believed that to offer any kind of physical closeness so early in the relationship would lead to a fawning response, one in which Jae said yes when what they meant was no way, no how. Singing was a way that the healer could access ventral vagal without touch. So she sang a melody without words, from Bach's unaccompanied cello suites. No words, because the healer did not know what words might feel dangerous, and introducing another language might feel like a gaslighting attempt. Singing a melody that the healer posited might feel connecting was her best guess.

This is the action stage co-occurring with the contemplation stage; Jae believed themselves to be at fault, the healer offered the first challenge to that, the P, the critical consciousness, which is the human politic, and then engaged in ventral vagal connection, which is a healing practice, the N of the PIEN framework. Notice how the two stages of development of critical consciousness cannot be separated, as with each step of development of critical consciousness in a trauma-exposed person there is likely to be a letting go of whatever unknowing strategy had been in use, which leads to new overt distress, which is an invitation for the healer to offer something that is the best possible match for where the suffering person is in every way, tailoring the healing to meet the suffering person.

As the healer sang the melody, Jae began to quiet. The healer continued singing until Jae sat up, got back in their chair, and said, "Well, that was, I don't know. Large. Can you say what you said before again, please? I promise not to freak out, okay?"

"I wouldn't call what you did freaking out, I would never put down your feelings like that," said the healer. "You had a human response, and you can have it again if that's what shows up. And again . . ." the words on the first step to critical consciousness: "You are not to blame. You are not screwed up. You are in terrible pain, in the ways that human beings are designed to be in terrible pain when these kinds of terrible things are done to them. You are not the problem."

Jae seemed to freeze in their chair this time and asked, in a tiny voice, "Can you please bring that blanket over from the couch and give it to me. Do NOT put it over me, just give it to me." Reciprocity of power was emerging, which we'll discuss in the section on the next criterion; the healer had intuited a boundary and respected its possible presence, Jae had felt that somehow and spoke a boundary: Do not touch.

I hope this story illustrates that the final stages of change in the development of critical consciousness are intertwined and recursive. Sometimes people enter trauma healing already somewhere in the borderlands between self-blame and critical consciousness. Sometimes people come in sounding as if they have critical consciousness, but it becomes apparent over time that it was only a few layers deep, never touching core feelings of shame and self-blame. Sometimes getting to the action stage of critical consciousness, in which one is certain that one is not the problem, requires getting to the place where the pain and suffering and difficult behaviors are sufficiently in the rearview mirror that the person can focus their attention on this deepening way of understanding the difficulties of their life. Sometimes it's not apparent that the person has gotten there even when they tell you they're ready to go. Sometimes we plant seeds whose fruits we only know about much later, or never.

I'm not sure there's a formal maintenance stage of development of critical consciousness because I don't usually get to know what happens in people's lives when they say goodbye to me. Sometimes I get a card or an email that lets me know that this person has internalized, and is now passing on to others, the critical consciousness that emerged in our work together. Most of the time a healer does not have the opportunity to know this piece, and that is the nature of trauma healing: we engage with someone until they are ready to say goodbye. It is the grief inherent in our work.

THIRD CRITERION: THE RELATIONSHIP BETWEEN HEALER AND SUFFERING PERSON IS LIBERATORY

When I was developing feminist therapy theory I used to write about "egalitarian" relationships, which were one step better than how things were outside the world of intersectional feminist therapy. Today, though, I think that egalitarian falls short of the DHCR mark because although the idea spoke to the notion that the healer/therapist needed to do whatever was possible to lessen the power imbalance in the healing/therapy process, there would always be some imbalance because of the power invested in the role of the therapist.

This is a tricky dynamic to disambiguate. A DHCR healer does have responsibilities to themselves, their communities, the healing relationship, the suffering person, and the suffering person's communities. Because trauma-exposed people frequently enter healing relationships in places of great pain and confusion, it is not hard for someone in the healer role to exploit the temporary needs of the suffering person to be able to lean hard on the healer, to make the healer very central in their life. Volumes have been written about trauma transference and countertransference; my wise colleague Constance Dalenberg, in her brilliant (and sadly out of print) book, *Countertransference and the Treatment of Trauma* (2000), points out the findings of her research, which were that one very good way to predict that a therapist/healer is going to do something to endanger themselves, the healing process, and/or the suffering person is for trauma to walk into the room of someone utterly unprepared to encounter trauma.

One way to protect against anything overtly bad happening is to create a framework that mirrors the strict neutrality of classical psychoanalysis. Mind you, research on psychoanalysts (Chesler, 1972; Gabbard, 1989; Pope et al., 1994) has determined that most of them break this frame; the therapists who sexually abused their patients (mostly women, mostly trauma survivors) have included a large number of people, mostly men, trained in classical psychoanalysis. As bait on the hook for a suffering person desperate to be affirmed as worthy of love, they would often use the ruse: "We are breaking the rules together because you are so very special."

Some people who ascribed to the notion of egalitarian relationships sadly used that framework as an excuse to exploit the suffering people with whom they were working. Intersectional feminist therapists were so alarmed by these developments among our colleagues that we wrote a special feminist therapy ethics code, which spelled out that "egalitarian" did not mean "equal," nor did it ever allow for sexualizing the healing relationship.

All of this suggests that to have a DHCR healing encounter, we have to parse the meanings of the construct of a liberatory relationship. We have to go beyond the simplistic power analysis of therapist being powerful, client being less powerful, and thus we should make it all more equal. That wasn't a terrible starting point, because an analysis of the power dynamics between healers and trauma-exposed suffering people is absolutely necessary for there to be a liberatory relationship.

I suggest that we begin by telling the truth about the power dynamics in the relationship in a more complete way. There is power as dominance; there is power as nurturance, as connection, a sharing of resources to promote growth. There are the dynamics of the roles and of the intersectional identities of the people occupying those roles. There are the effects on the healing relationship of what is occurring in the present social context. There are the ways in which each person's power shifts and changes across time during the healing relationship. All of these power dynamics are fluid, not static.

Telling the truth about the suffering person's powers to make choices is a first step toward becoming liberatory. If a healer says, "The way I work is *x*, and I do only that. If that doesn't sound like a good fit for you, let me know, and I'll give you names of people who also do other things. I can understand if you need to go away and take some time to decide without me around," that statement is not a nonliberatory statement. It's telling the truth so that the suffering person can make a decision and has the power. It's also liberatory because the healer says, "I will not leave you out in the cold," and because the healer recognizes the covert power of their presence on the suffering person's abilities to discern what the right choice is for them.

Conversely, saying "Only *x* can heal trauma" is a deeply nonliberatory statement because it asserts power as dominance over the truth of healing and steals choice at a very vulnerable time in a person's life. If you're a suffering person and a so-called expert says, "You must do this in order to stop suffering," it's very hard to say, "No, I'll see someone else." It is easier for a suffering person to say no thanks when the healer is honest about the specifics of what they offer without declaring their way to be the one true way to get out of pain, and when they remain present with the person until that trauma-exposed individual has found the right place to be.

A next step is to be more radical, as healers, in the honest embrace of our own vulnerabilities. This is the humble in the DHCR trauma healing model. This does not mean that a healer does not have the right to privacy about their life, because we do. Instead, it means holding an alive awareness of those vulnerabilities as we engage with a suffering person, rather than protecting ourselves from that awareness with the notion that we are oh, so different from the suffering person sitting with us.

Laurie Anne Pearlman and Karen Saakvitne (1995) wrote eloquently about the reality that when a healer does openhearted work with suffering, trauma-exposed people, the healer is affected and also suffers, experiencing what they called vicarious traumatization (VT). VT's effect is to pierce any veils of difference and invulnerability that a healer might have used to try to shield themselves from the truths about the world.

VT, when allowed by a healer to be felt within themselves, can create less imbalance of power. Experiencing VT and allowing ourselves to feel it in our bodies and psyches and hearts as we work means knowing in all of those deep places that we, healers, are not immune, that we too struggle with reminders that safety is illusory. VT allows us to resonate deeply with the suffering that is in the room with us, to allow ourselves, if only for a brief time, to experience a shared embodiment of that pain. The concept of projective identification in psychoanalytic thought, wherein the suffering person cannot tolerate their pain and somehow psychically hands it over for the healer to experience, is precisely this thing, except that in the DHCR framework it is not evidence that a suffering person has borderline dynamics. It is, instead, an experience of emotional solidarity between healer and sufferer. In solidarity, there is liberatory potential.

Where this is leading is to the notion that a liberatory healing relationship is one in which the healer holds the strands of power dynamics lightly, but ever-present in awareness, interrogating their own work for the subtle ways in which they might assert dominance power that seems like no big deal, yet which adds up over time. We do not liberate the relationship from the colonial rules that have restricted the potentials of trauma healing by rebelling against them or throwing them off, leaving only a vacuum in their place into which anything or nothing might accidentally emerge. At each step of the way the DHCR trauma healer considers where the power lies, how not to steal it by accident, and when we do steal it by accident—because we are human ourselves in that same recursive process of critical consciousness development—we name that we have engaged in dominating behavior and offer repairs.

Let's go back to Jae's story for a moment. What if the healer, instead of singing a melody, had said, "This is a song that a lot of other people have found soothing," and sung that. True confession time: that singer is me, and I have done that, until one brave person said, "I don't find that song helpful at all. Could you sing this other song instead, please?" Deciding what song to sing and choosing one without words was already taking some power because I picked an actual melody I knew rather than simply singing improvised notes. Had I still been doing the "other people" narrative with a person who was barely able to speak, much less protest, I would have been asserting dominance, the power to know what would be soothing, the song I had sung until the brave person told me no, not that one.

It's pretty subtle stuff, this attention to the strands of power dynamics. It's getting up close to the fabric of the other person, so close we can see the threads from which their intersectionalities, trauma, ways of unknowing, and ways of being safe enough are constructed, which ones sturdier, which ones gossamer. Jae then felt empowered to tell me to give them the blanket and what not to do with it (although they later said to me, "I have no idea where I got the notion that I could tell you what to do and not expect to be smacked," which we were then able to unpack).

FOURTH CRITERION: SUPPORTS BEING RADICALLY COLLABORATIVE

I've written a lot before this, in my previous work on feminist therapy (Brown, 2017, 2018) about the importance of the feminist therapist, who has morphed over time into the DHCR healer being collaborative with the suffering person. I've even given some examples in various places in this book of what it might look like, done by this particular integrative, decolonial, liberatory intersectional feminist trauma healer back before I added intentional decolonial awareness to what I was doing in my office. But here I haven't quite operationalized what precisely I might mean by this term.

Radically collaborating with a suffering person in a manner that sweeps away the false authority of the healer's role means something quite different than merely offering a choice, when choice is as much of an illusion in the suffering person's life as is safety. I touched on this above in talking about power dynamics in the healing space. Radical collaboration requires that the healer has deeply grasped the way in which the power of their role can turn into dominance and subtly undermine the suffering person's ability to collaborate and to advocate for what they want. In radical collaboration we do not begin the discussion of how to proceed by offering multiple choices and then immediately starting in with whichever of their proposed strategies the suffering person picks in that moment. We give space and time.

Radical collaboration instantiates the preferential option for the suffering person by putting their voice first. The healer engages, in various encounters of first touch, in a process of codiscernment with the suffering person. What has been helpful and not helpful in their life? If they struggle to know, what do they imagine might be helpful? What do they hope that the healer might offer them? What do they fear the healer might do? All else must be made subordinate to the imperative that the healer patiently awaits the knowing of the suffering person as that person enters the collaboration.

Putting the voice of the suffering person first is different from being person-centered. The person-centered therapist has decided a priori to do a person-centered approach to therapy. While this model makes much room for the voice of the client and is a theory that is a precursor to the DHCR trauma healing model, it's still being offered in a top-down way, whose starting point is the healer's preferred intervention. It's not liberatory if the healer decides to empower the client, because when the healer is the one who makes this decision without collaboration, they've decided from the position of the invisible power imbalance, from the position of a benevolent dictator saying, "This will be good for you." A firm commitment to radical collaboration, to the preferential option for the voice of the suffering person, is required for DHCR practice to occur.

But what, you may ask, do you do with the person whose suffering has led them to the words that come with the other-than-contemplation stage of the development of critical consciousness, or even people on the starting edge of the contemplation stage. It's so seductive, when a healer hears variations on the theme of "I don't know, you're the expert, that's why I'm paying you" in response to the space created for their voice, or "I don't know what would help, nothing helps" to offer something not quite radically collaborative.

What's a DHCR healer to do? Get curious. Ask, "Can you remember ever feeling differently? When you did, what were you doing? What else was happening in your world?" Sometimes that answer is that a particular substance helped, "but I can't do that anymore because it messed up my life." The suffering person has offered a clue about the chemicals in, let's say, cannabis interacting with their brain in a way that was helpful. The liberatory healer explores that in greater depth: "How did cannabis help?" "It made me less anxious." "It made you feel less anxious, okay. What did less anxious feel like? How come cannabis stopped helping? Has anything else you've done in your life gotten close to its helpful effects? Do you think there would have been ways to keep the helpful effects without your life not working in the ways you tell me it made your life not work?"

This is commonly referred to in the motivational interviewing (MI) and other similar approaches as the use of Socratic questioning. In MI, the questions are set up so that the person gets to the "right" answer, which is that they get motivated to stop using a substance. In the radical collaboration of DHCR trauma practice these questions have a different goal, which is to invite the wisdom, knowing, and thus power of the suffering person to emerge. To reuse the menu metaphor, the suffering person's responses will point to which menu items might be offered when it's the healer's turn to join the collaborative encounter.

On the other end of the spectrum a person may come to a healer with a well defined notion of what should happen, thanks in part to the ubiquitous availability today of online information about trauma healing in its various forms or due to their own prior experiences. Radical collaboration does not entail a healer's automatic compliance with the suffering person's request for thing x, even if that is precisely the modality with which the healer is most comfortable. We don't simply comply, because that takes the healer out of the collaboration and also makes opaque the rationale for the request for thing x.

Instead, radical collaboration asks the question, "Tell me what about thing x has appealed to you? Oh, that it seems as if you don't have to talk much about feelings. Tell me, is it important to you that we not talk much about feelings? Can you help me to understand what that's about for you?" The suffering person may have decided that they wish to experience as little emotional vulnerability as possible on their road to having less pain, and for this person, emotions are the equivalent of way too vulnerable.

This is information that can support a genuinely liberatory DHCR trauma healing relationship. Here's an intersectional identity, "Do not want to be vulnerable or feel painful emotion," one of the intersectional selves that emerges from trauma exposures, from social pathologies, from other intersectional identities, from existential dread, in other words, from many facets of PIEN. This is where a healer can join the conversation, perhaps sharing the information that it's likely going to be very difficult to do pretty much any trauma healing practice without some emotions showing up.

"When your feelings emerge, how do you want us [importantly, not me, the therapist, but us, the relationship] to respond to that? Would you like to know some things I have available in addition to thing *x* that some people have found helpful in living with emotions effectively? Not now? Okay." A dialogue ensues, the dance of collaboration in which the subtleties of power are seen, heard, felt, and responded to with care and intention by the healer, and without dominance. The healing practice moves onward having set a norm that the suffering person's voice is in the lead, that the suffering person defines what words are helpful, which might do more harm. Rather than the old Gestalt therapy intervention where the therapist says, "Let me feed you a line," DHCR practice has the healer asking the suffering person, "Tell me the words that will work for you, please."

The degree to which this is a departure from psychotherapy as it has been practiced, even by those of us who claimed the various liberatory modalities, may make full-on engagement in radical collaboration challenging. After all, the most liberatory of trauma healers have spent years in school, becoming licensed or certified, declared the expert, given permission to be dominant while also kind. For many of us who had not yet sufficiently interrogated the deep and subtle corruption in our discipline, it was the best we could do to offer multiple choice.

This is where that H in DHCR informs us. Humility. To practice humility in this radical manner may seem at first as if we are pretending not to have our expertise and skill. This is absolutely not the case. We are being humble precisely where disguised or disowned power in the healer is most deadly to the suffering person's ability to develop a sense of personal authority early in the encounter, at the point where we genuinely know very little about how this suffering person is going to give up power in order to stay in relationship with us.

The skill to create the space for the voice of the suffering person, the expertise to inquire in a manner and with language that is attuned to the intersectional identities of the person in the room, the emotional capacities inherent in listening well enough to have a pretty good hypothesis, albeit not a rigidly or firmly held one, about what the next step will be in eliciting the voice of the suffering person—these are all high levels of skill and expertise, requiring practice, discipline, and peer support in order to implement consistently. To not know, to rest in the humility of not knowing, allows for these relationships to be healing no matter what we do.

Death and Other Extreme Conundrums

For each liberatory therapist, certain stories of suffering may be more seductive to the therapist's desire to leap into the "here, let me help you, I know what to do" component of therapy-as-usual. Suicidality is definitely one of those narratives that is extraordinarily difficult to respond to in other than an authoritative, if not authoritarian and controlling, manner. A suffering person sitting in our office telling us that they want to kill themselves is usually a frightening thing for a healer to hear, and these are often words that magically transform DHCR healers into frantic therapists, trying to do something that will keep the other person alive, and ourselves out of trouble with the licensing authorities. Yet if we want to set our liberatory commitment from the very first encounter, we need to apply radical collaboration even, and perhaps especially, with this topic.

A suffering person who comes in our door with plans to kill themself may seem only to be able to collaborate radically at the level of saying that they would like to live but don't know how. Nonetheless, radical collaboration at this life-and-death juncture is possible. "What has kept you alive until now? When you wanted to kill yourself before this, how did you save your own life?" Notice the wording—"How did you, the suffering person, find the resources with which to save your own life? How did you have that power?" the DHCR healer asks, without telling this suffering person, who feels powerless, that they are powerful. Because in these life-or-death moments, the suffering person feels utterly lacking in power, having only the power to die. So overtly saying to that person, "This is a way you are powerful," may be felt as an insult, an invalidation of the phenomenology of the suffering person, the healer acting as if the suffering person's internal reality is invisible to them. The DHCR healer has to know that there is power there, and also not invalidate the lived experience of the person who wants to be dead.

We do have a responsibility as healers to develop some kind of safety plan. The answers to the above and similar questions are going to lead to the most effective version of the safest plan possible for forestalling suicide, one that will fit this suffering person like a glove rather than the one-size-fits-all safety plan that the therapist has learned in suicide prevention courses. We collaborate. We soothe our fear. As my colleague Tyson Bailey says, we learn to invite Death to tea and have a conversation with us. We become transparent about our fear, and the reasons for it: "I am afraid that if you kill yourself, you will let the people who harmed you win. I am afraid that you will let the social pathology win. I am afraid that my heart will break."

What about the person who is dangerous to others? Here is where the liberatory commitment to the welfare of the larger community broadens the lens of radical collaboration. Let's leave to the side for just a moment whatever legal mandates may exist in your jurisdiction to put shackles on that person, please.

I am reminded by this question of my work with a person who lives with dissociation and had an ego state that would drink to well past the legal limit. Another ego state that would emerge when there was enough alcohol present to invite that one out of its cave. That second ego state, "Whee, free at last," would usually get in the car and drive, quite drunk, after dark.

Each of these ego states was developmentally rather young and not very good at comprehending consequences, consistent with their developmental level. So I attempted an effort at collaboration from my 2010 version of self, in which I learned a great deal about how poorly this goes if one doesn't put the suffering person's voice first. What I did was go into a controlling maternal mode of faux collaboration in which I spoke of the grave consequences of driving drunk and expressed my worry for the safety and well-being of the person. That was not received well, to put it mildly. The ego states involved told me that they saw me as threatening them with prison time and trying to tell them what they could or could not do. Wrong about threat, right about trying to control them.

I owned up to the fact that I was trying to control them, which I knew to be a stark departure from my usual approach to working with them and which made me feel a lot less safe at a moment when they needed me to feel safe enough to them. And then I asked a more correct than not question, which was an unknowing radical collaboration. What did they think was happening that got me frightened enough that I was trying to control them for the first time ever? Back and forth we went: "You don't approve of us drinking!" "Well, you're right, I don't love it that you drink as much as you do. And . . . if you stayed home and didn't drive, I wouldn't be going into worried-controlling mode." "You're trying to control us!" "You're right. I'm scared and worried. What is important to you about being able to drive after you drink?" "No one can tell us what to do!" "Okay, correct. Will you answer my question, though, please? What makes driving after you drink so important? I don't understand." "Uh . . . no one can tell us what to do. We've never run into anyone yet, so why are you worrying?"

This discussion between me and two young places in this person opened up a profound and previously unidentified and unaddressed wound from the severe neglect that this person had experienced in their childhood. The parent who was at home would stand by and watch while siblings hurt them, sometimes even abused them, doing nothing to intervene. They had internalized the belief that no one would ever care whether or not they were harmed, and they experienced my expression of worry about the consequences of driving drunk not as protective, since in their emotional lexicon there was no such thing as protection, but as controlling. This was very large. Rage and then grief emerged.

This insight, which showed up only because I belatedly backed off and ceded the floor to this person's voice(s), became a focus for years of work. My demonstration that I could call foul on myself and be completely transparent about my motives also allowed this person to restore me to the status of a probably safe person, and eventually collaborate with me on their safety while drinking, because safety while drinking became something that mattered to their entire dissociative system.

They did not immediately stop driving while drunk. They did, however, start to come into their sessions telling me about having read or heard news stories about accidents caused by drunk drivers or the sentencing of a drunk driver, asking, "Is this what you're worried would happen to me?" "Yup, that, uh-huh." They told me that they had begun to Google the topic to make sure that it wasn't just my word that they had to rely on, something for which I responded with clear evidence of happiness, "Yay, you didn't simply believe it because I said it!"

Eventually these younger parts came to understand consequences better and stopped driving drunk. They realized that they had the power to keep other people safe, to keep themselves safe, to protect themselves and other people from harm. This was a kind of critical consciousness for this person, the dawning awareness that they were not the problem, and they could become the problem and had been treated as the problem for so long in their dangerous family that they took for granted that they would, of course, be the problem once again and that now they had a choice to not be the problem for someone else. Or the problem, period.

But what about an imminent risk of harm or threat from the person whose suffering leads them to violence against others? Many of us are bound by legal mandates to protect potential victims. As DHCR trauma healers we have a moral commitment to the welfare of the suffering person and also to their community. What this means coming from us may look quite different from how this mandate is operationalized by folks in the mainstream.

This might—not necessarily, but might—be the sole situation in which we cannot absolutely radically collaborate, when the moral injury done to a person already is so great that they are considering doing further moral injury to themselves by doing harm to others. Ironically, the person throwing themselves into the risk of moral injury through doing harm to others may seem to be the ultimate in the practice of a social pathology. Yet they are likely to be the person already most harmed by the social pathologies whispering lies in their ears.

The prison terms being meted out to those who perpetrated the insurrection against the US Capitol are stark evidence of this kind of price paid by the most vulnerable who have believed lies of social pathologies that they are empowered to harm others. I am personally aware of one person among them, a young person whose family sought to get that person care in 2020, in a vain attempt to woo them away from one of the groups preaching social pathologies and leading the attack on the Capitol. Through networks of connection, their frantic attempts to get their family member to help reached me. Their attempts were for naught because the social pathology taught that it was in the right and that the loving family were "sheep," fooled into believing in the rule of law. That person is now in prison for many years. That's an enormous price; had this person been in therapy and saying what was being said to the family, a DHCR trauma healer, if there was no agreement to collaborate on keeping safe enough, would have approached law enforcement, and this person might have been home on January 6, 2021.

So, too, the terrible moral injuries suffered by members of the military required to engage in violence against others, and the manner in which those moral injuries traumatizes these people beyond the trauma of combat and is destructive to their capacity to rejoin society, is painful evidence of the dangerousness of social pathologies to all parties. Some of those so injured return home filled with SNS activation that they are unable to soothe and which spills out as violence against those close to them or to their communities, especially when interactive with social pathologies of toxic masculinities, racism, homophobia, or xenophobia, enacted most frequently on the bodies of those closest to them.

Being collaborative differently with an individual at risk of behaving violently toward others does not mean that we immediately move away from DHCR trauma healing principles. We have to soothe our own SNS that is activated when we hear certain words, because we will not make wise choices from an activated position. Carefully and as collaboratively as possible assessing the threat risk to the suffering person and the rest of the community, we then, if it is possible, invite this person, whose suffering is very great, first to coregulate with us so as to reduce the hyperactivation of their SNS.

Then, and only then, we might begin to invite collaboration as how to stay safe from arrest, incarceration, long-term loss of freedom and choice due to incarceration, or even death. That's how to talk about it—"Keep you safe from all of this, none of which you deserve no matter how terrible you feel about what you did in Iraq." No person wishes themselves imprisoned, unless the lies of hopelessness and the pain of moral injury in which they have already cast themselves outside of society are shouting in their ear. No person wishes themselves stripped of their human and civil rights unless the wounds of their trauma have taught them that they ought to be punished and that hurting more people is a way to get punishment for the harm they did with impunity when in uniform. Doing violence against others is more likely than not to lead to those undesirable outcomes. Thus there is an implicit shared goal present in most cases, that of keeping the suffering person free and alive, and freed from additional moral injuries incurred if they harm another being.

What if you do have to engage in stringent and controlling measures because this particular suffering person simply does not have the capacity to collaborate on keeping themselves (and by inference, all others) safe and free? Ironically, this may be one instance where framing this suffering person's neurotype to the world as "mentally ill" rather than criminal may be the least not-liberatory thing to do. Psychiatric incarceration is only slightly preferable to incarceration in the criminal legal system. That slight difference between being turned into a felon and losing most of one's rights and being labeled as mentally ill and only losing the right to legally buy a weapon for a while in some states can make large differences in a person's life over the long term.

Intersectional identities and social context need to be taken into account in how any outside authority is brought into the mix to create safety. Calling law enforcement to deal with a Black, Indigenous, or person of color (BIPOC) person who is lost inside of their mind and unable to be safe enough for others is dangerous to that person in almost every instance. Keep in mind the episode in Florida where an African American therapist ran out into the street to protect his confused and disoriented White client and was shot by a police officer who assumed that the therapist was being violent instead of protective. Recall the time when a disoriented BIPOC man in Arizona was shot by law enforcement who feared him because he was of color and confused.

Let me call out the name of Tommy Le, whose family's police misconduct case I worked on, the details of which are very much in the public record through numerous media reports. This physically small, 20-year-old Vietnamese American man, disoriented one night, was shot multiple times in the back while fleeing sheriff's deputies in a Seattle suburb, carrying only a pen. Law enforcement immediately put out the lie, to the media and thus to his family, that he had been threatening the deputy who shot him with a knife, and thus the deputy was justified in shooting him, multiple times, in the back. But there was no knife. No threat. Simply a disoriented young man of color with a pen.

The most well-meaning law enforcement personnel are rarely trained to use nonviolent methods in their dealings with people whose grasp on shared realities is tenuous. Many of those holding legal guns have been affected by social pathologies about mentally ill people being dangerous, not to mention the social pathology of racism, which will make those guns go off so much more quickly when the person is BIPOC, embodying what Henry Louis Gates referred to as the "badness of Blackness," the assumption that Black bodies are dangerous ones.

It will be important to consider the intersectional identities of this suffering person, as well as those of any intended targets of violence, in developing a strategy for keeping all parties as safe as possible. Calling law enforcement to ask that they inform a BIPOC person that they are at risk of being a target of violence may be putting the intended target in harm's way from law enforcement as much as they might be at risk from the person in your office. Calling the target yourself to say they are at risk and need to take steps to get safe may be a more DHCR manner in which to proceed.

In a difficult situation such as this, the liberatory therapist's radical collaboration may primarily consist of thinking through, in collaboration with as many supportive DHCR colleagues as possible, how not to point the systemic violence of social pathologies against the suffering person who is contemplating violence. We do have a responsibility to create safety and freedom for that person and for the community. A DHCR model is not solely concerned with the individual. If the community is unsafe, then the individual cannot be liberated.

Sometimes we have the hard decision of collaborating with this person's present and future needs to be safe and free, making those components of the emergent needs to protect people from violence, either from the person in your office or from undertrained or misguided law enforcement actions. Collaborating with the community to create safety for this person and their intended targets is yet another component of commitment to some form of radical collaboration even in the most trying of circumstances.

This likely means doing a fair amount of advance planning, when possible, finding who the alternate emotional crisis responders are or where, within marginalized communities, there are safe havens for people who cannot keep themselves safe from themselves for a while. These structures are rare. But as the number of suicide by law enforcement grows, the moral injuries done to those with their hand on the trigger are, as of this writing, beginning to create collaborations between law enforcement and the communities they have harmed, in some places, however tentatively.

MOVING FORWARD

So here we have a foundation for DHCR trauma healing practice. In the last chapter of this book, we'll go into more detail about specific DHCR healing practices and how to integrate DHCR principles into your work as a trauma healer.

13 AREN'T THERE ALREADY SOME DHCR TRAUMA HEALING METHODOLOGIES?

And What Can We Learn From Them?

There are indeed already decolonial, humble, culturally responsive (DHCR) trauma healing methodologies. Few of them have been specifically articulated as such to date, aside from some very group-specific Indigenous healing practices that are meant to be offered within the context of a particular colonized and traumatized Indigenous community (see, for example, Comas-Díaz et al. [2024] and her description of Indigenous healing methodologies in the Western Hemisphere). They have not been subjected to randomized controlled trials, nor have they been systematically studied within the Christian Eurocentric epistemic of colonial models of healing. And yet they are powerful, effective trauma healing methodologies. They have been developed in the Global South, and they teach lessons about how to conduct DHCR trauma healing. I even had a go, earlier in my development of these ideas, at writing about feminist therapy's contributions to trauma healing, in which some proto-DHCR constructs are articulated (Brown, 2017).

https://doi.org/10.1037/0000421-014
Decolonizing Trauma Healing: Toward a Humble, Culturally Responsive Practice,
by L. S. Brown

TESTIMONIO

Testimonio is one of the few trauma-specific healing strategies that, while developed by liberation psychologists specifically to work with survivors of state-sponsored terror and torture in Latin America, appears to embody a DHCR trauma healing methodology with decolonial principles built into it, rather than having those principles integrated later (Aron, 1992). It exemplifies the PIEN framework. It is political (P), explicitly so, in addressing the malfeasance of a rogue nation-state. It is explicitly intersectional (I), as it must invite suffering people to address ways in which traumas inflicted by a state actor, such as additional trauma inflicted while being extrajudicially detained at Guantanamo or being kept for years in solitary confinement after a wrongful conviction are destructive to much of what the suffering person formerly experienced as self, while the DHCR trauma healer is usually not someone who shares any of this particular lived experience of trauma. It is existential (E), as it directly addresses questions of why me, why not me, and moral injury arising from the very fact of having lived through what killed others to whom the suffering person was connected through family and community. Finally, it is neurobiological (N), as the presence of the healer as a nonneutral witness to the testimony creates conditions for coregulation that can reduce the often chronic overactivation of both sympathetic nervous system (SNS) and dorsal vagal trauma response system.

Liberation healers, many of them psychoanalytically trained psychiatrists and psychologists prior to the Pinochet regime in Chile that overthrew the democratically elected government of Salvador Allende, developed the construct of testimonio, or taking testimony, based on observations made by trauma healers from the Jewish world that people who had survived the Shoah were helped to grieve and work through some aspects of their trauma through being invited to give testimony, either in formal legal or informal psychotherapeutic contexts.

Cienfuegos and Monelli (1983), who published under the pseudonyms of Lira and Weinstein in order to protect their identities from the repressive Chilean regime in which they lived when they first wrote and who first published about testimonio, were aware of the powerful effects of witnessing the terrible experiences of people traumatized by organized hate. They began to experiment with offering this in Chile following the U.S. CIA-sponsored coup leading to the ouster and death of Allende in 1973, a coup followed by the establishment of a brutal military dictatorship headed by Augusto Pinochet, a man later found guilty of war crimes against his own population.

The Pinochet regime rounded up people en masse, imprisoning them in a soccer stadium with no shade, water, or food. The regime tortured individual people. It arrested people and killed them, as later learned, by throwing them into the ocean from planes, creating the phrase "los desaparecidos," the disappeared. The regime targeted large groups of people in the first days of the coup: intellectuals, artists, socialists, students, psychologists, people whose worldview before the coup was frequently one of being safe enough.

No one was safe. One of Chile's most famous singers of the time, Victor Jara, was among thousands held captive in a sports stadium before the military tortured and murdered him, throwing his body into a street in Santiago as a warning to all that none were safe. Pregnant prisoners were held until they gave birth, their children given to army officers and other regime supporters, then they were among those dumped alive into the ocean. Much of the population living in Chile's urban centers was exposed to mass trauma, chronic traumatic terror perpetrated by the state, meaning that victims had nowhere to turn to seek justice. Testimonio was developed in this context.

An irony of Cienfuegos and Monelli's (1983) earliest work to create testimonio, which was being developed while the Pinochet regime was still in power, is that the authors published under pseudonyms due to their own risk of becoming one of the disappeared. Testimonio is described as a "treatment of choice" for this group of people whose trauma was due to persistent, inescapable, state-sponsored terror, a phenomenon that replicates, on the larger social level, the experiences of children living trapped in families with dangerous caregivers, those who develop complex trauma responses and coping strategies. What makes testimonio unique in the trauma healing world is that it explicitly integrated psychological and sociopolitical elements, an analysis of how abuses of state power were components of larger social systems of corruption and social pathologies. Testimonio aimed to reduce suffering, with a focus on empowerment and the exploration of how to return social justice to the life of the traumatized person.

Since it was first developed and disseminated, testimonio has been offered to people outside of Chile who have also experienced state-sponsored terror, such as individuals seeking political asylum or refugees from conflict zones. Because the focus of this deeply DHCR trauma healing practice is with people who have been targeted by a dangerous regime and barely escaped with their lives, while most healers practicing it have not also lived through the same trauma but may be workers in asylum or refugee settings, its practice involves a willingness by the healer to develop a heightened consciousness of the fragility of social orders and the dangers that might suddenly appear in the middle of the quotidian life of any human being. Trauma healers practicing testimonio outside of Chile are now less likely to have shared culture or experience with this suffering person.

The core value of this DHCR trauma healing methodology is that of witness and belief regarding the role of authorities as sources of danger, not protection, of betrayal, not loyalty, in the life of trauma-exposed humans. This requires a nuanced attention to dynamics of power in the healing relationship, with careful attention to anything that might look, feel, or sound like coercive control to the trauma-exposed person suffering the effects of the abuse of power by state actors. Notice the parallels: states, parents, families, and institutions are meant to protect their members. Transforming from protective to dangerous, from allied to abusive, all are themes in these traumas. Thus testimonio offers a model of DHCR trauma healing that may be brought into a variety of trauma healing situations.

Testimonio's practitioners position themselves as a nonneutral ally, affirming that what was done to the suffering person was wrong and entirely undeserved, and most importantly, as a witness, someone who takes the testimony of the suffering person. This stance of nonneutrality in the face of trauma was articulated very early in the world of trauma healing by wise thinkers like Herman (1992) and Ochberg (1988), and then was swept away by the advent and colonization of the trauma world by Eurocentric epistemics that insisted on neutrality. Testimonio, a DHCR trauma healing methodology, reinforces these early insights about the necessity that a trauma healer take a clear stance that what occurred was wrong, that it was not the fault of the traumatized person in any way, and that the healer will witness the story without judgment of anything that the suffering person did or did not do, said or did not say, in order to survive to give their testimony.

Commentators on testimonio practice have all emphasized the importance of having such healers be unflinchingly grounded in facing the objective realities of a terrorist state such as that experienced by the survivors with whom they work. Similarly, when applying this DHCR methodology with people whose experiences were not state terror but rather family terror, trafficking, institutional betrayal, or other forms of trauma, the healer must be similarly firmly planted in the no-excuses zone. Self-blame is common in all of these suffering trauma-exposed people, because if one blames oneself, one might find the inflection point in the story where one might have said or done something differently, which would, in turn, have changed the outcome.

In testimonio practice, the healer listens to the self-blame and notes and remembers it, not to interrupt and challenge the narrative but to engage later, if invited, with the suffering person about how self-blame was an attempt at empowerment. This is a radically different way to respond to self-blame than what is typically prescribed in trauma treatment as usual, which is to challenge it. Instead, the healer identifies it as an attempt at finding power in the midst of the worst forms of powerlessness, a reminder that the potential for reclaiming power might be present when it has felt utterly lost.

Testimonio functions not simply to give the survivor a voice and a setting in which the experience of terror is witnessed and in which a healer is present to hold the space, neurobiologically coregulate past terror, and soothe somatic shutdown so that the traumatized person may experience reconnection with another human once again. Testimonio also operates to validate the survivor's phenomenological experience that this trauma represents an objective moral wrong for which no excuses can be made.

Again, notice that this DHCR trauma healing methodology is one that is not simply for those traumatized by state terrorism or violent acts of colonization. Validating the phenomenological experiences of moral wrong and, sometimes, of being forced to inflict moral injury on oneself is not unique to those traumatized by state terror. It is part of the trauma experienced by many suffering humans exposed to inescapable abuses of power or contexts in which their suffering is silenced and denied on behalf of upholding the reputation and power of institutions.

An explicit goal of testimonio is that it is decolonial for its participants. It is not intended simply to be soothing. It creates a held space that allows the toxins of the rogue state, the abusers of power, the betrayers, the disappearers, the silencers, to be leached out of the soul and psyche of the traumatized human through the power of being listened to, being engaged ventral vagally, seen and heard, felt and connected with in a nonintruding, nonprescriptive manner. A testimonio may be offered in a formal healing setting or may occur sponta-neously in the context of community or close connection. What is important is witnessing and joining in the principle that what was done to this person was a moral wrong, inexcusable, a crime.

Being witnessed in this nonneutral manner returns a sense of power and moral agency to the person who has been traumatized and whom the state power has attempted to strip of their humanity. It reignites the desire for change and justice where being a target of state terror and abuses of power had often left people in a state of despair, plagued by feelings of helplessness, hopeless-ness, and guilt that they had stayed alive while friends and comrades died or suffered terribly. Testimonio addresses the moral injury inflicted on this group of traumatized people because it confirms that even though the traumas done to them and others were perpetrated under the color of law or in families or other institutions in the name of upholding allegedly legitimate authority conferred by a social pathology on the perpetrator of the trauma, that such actions are no less morally wrong and reprehensible. Testimonio affirm that what was done was perhaps even more immoral and reprehensible, as these traumas represent a profound betrayal of a function of a nation-state or of a family or protective institution, which is to create just lives for its citizens, its family members, its faithful adherents. In testimonio a suffering traumatized person tells the truth that a nation-state or a family or a protective institution should not engage in capricious, vengeful punishment of those who said the "wrong" things, not indulge in capricious abuse of the bodies and spirits of those who were inescapably vulnerable to a caretaker not bring down hellfire on those who opened their souls to a person or institution who represented divine authority. Notice how testimonio, a DHCR healing methodology, speaks to all suffering trauma-exposed people who have experienced betrayals, failures of protection, abuses at the hands of those who were trusted to be the keepers of safety, of order, of openness of spiritual space.

The therapeutic technique was derived not only from Cienfuegos and Monelli's (1983) awareness of the healing power of the testimonies given by Shoah survivors but also, more directly, from observations of the public testimonials of those affected by state terror and repression. Examples of public testimonials include the Madres of the Plaza de Mayo of Argentina, who gathered weekly during the reign of the military junta with photos of their disappeared children and grandchildren to publicly demand an accounting from the government.

In recent years, social media has been used as a form of testimonio. For example, Facebook pages set up to demand justice for unarmed victims of police shootings or women who have been raped by prominent individuals constitute a 21st-century electronic modality of public testimonio. The #MeToo movement created a space for collective testimonials, ones that more resembled the consciousness-raising groups of 1960s second-wave White feminism in that those witnessing were also those traumatized, not neutral witnesses, rather an expanding collective of witnesses saying, "Me, too," to stories of sexual violation and exploitation.

In testimonio when used as a form of trauma healing in the space of a DHCR healing, the trauma-exposed suffering person is invited to develop a rich and detailed life narrative in which the injustices to which one has been subject and their effects on that individual are given a prominent place, not one that abolishes the remainder of the person's life story, and also a place that, for purposes of the healing work, foregrounds the ways in which the person has been the target of abuses of power that harmed them and their communities. One healing value of this exercise is seen in creating a forum for the survivor of state terror to reaffirm values and principles that have been compromised by the trauma to which the survivor and the survivor's communities have been subjected by an institution posing as a representation of law and moral authority. In testimonio, survivors take back moral authority and assert the primacy of their own ethics and values.

This focus in testimonio on the recapture of moral authority is a foundational component of this particular DHCR trauma healing methodology because one of the systemic effects of state terror on communities or continuous trauma in dangerous families or institutions is the sabotage, by the abusers of power whoever they might be, of community values of compassion, care, and respect, of personal values of decency, love, and connection.

When a state, the ultimate legal authority, or a religious authority, often in collusion with the oppressive state, or parental figures who traffic rather than nurture a child in their care, sometimes in collusion with a religious authority, when any of these power figures authorized by social pathologies and systemic forms of oppression sanction rape, kidnapping, murder, and extrajudicial execution of dissenting voices, then the moral scaffolding of a community, a family, a religious community is destroyed, and members of the community or family may turn on one another, helpless as they are to take action to genuinely liberate themselves from the authorities raining terror from their positions of power in the social hierarchy.

Striking examples of this phenomenon can be seen in many colonized Indigenous communities, where extremely high rates of within-group violence occur in the context of colonization by a U.S. government that practiced or sanctioned many forms of state terror on Indigenous populations. Intergenerational trauma from betrayal of entire Indigenous nations that signed agreements in good faith with the U.S. government only to experience betrayal, violence, and degradation expresses itself in ways described earlier in this book. Entire communities whose neurobiology is responding to continuous traumatic terror then engage in various strategies to calm those somatic experiences, which look from the outside like high rates of overuse of substances and high rates of intimate partner and sexualized violence. That this is reenactment of the violence done to the communities of Indigenous people is generally invisible; sexualized violence on the bodies of Indigenous women, and their murder after such violence, remains a constant in the lives of Indigenous communities. To engage in DHCR trauma healing work in these places requires unflinching witnessing by the healer of the continuing truth of how these communities are being harmed, including harms inflicted by larger Eurocentric cultures of which the healer is a part.

This latter is as much the case for healers of color who are not Indigenous, nor is the equation a clear one. Formerly enslaved men became the buffalo soldiers who were tasked with murdering Indigenous people and forcing them off their lands. Indigenous people bought and sold the bodies of Africans. Asian American and Pacific Islander persons were brought into the mix as competitors for scarce resources. White supremacy pitted each group against the other, undermining potential alliances that are today still broken, even as attempts are being made to heal those wounds. Thus a healer of color cannot assume that they can enter the Indigenous space and not learn of their own or their community's complicity, any less than would a healer of European descent. Training to practice testimonio requires the kind of deep dive into one's intersectional identities and, in particular, the aspects in which one subjugated group has been pitted against another so as to deflect resources from liberatory activities, as discussed in the first four chapters of this book, particularly Chapters 3 and 4.

The therapist in testimonio work takes a stance of moral nonneutrality, affirming from the start that what is being told is evidence of criminality perpetrated by those meant to enforce the law or protect the vulnerable. Becker et al. (1990) describe this as the "bond of commitment" in which the healer agrees to stand in solidarity with the suffering trauma-exposed person, affirming the injustice of what has been done and providing a completely safe container for the testimonio to take place. Agreeing to fearlessly witness and absorb, with an open heart, that which the trauma-exposed person has suffered is another component of testimonio; the stance of healers in testimonio is that they give up the privilege of not knowing of atrocities. Becker et al. (1990) explicitly frame the ways in which the person expresses their pain as the intended consequences of the state terror to which the survivor has been subjected, a DHCR paradigm for a "symptom."

In this space, healer and speaker acknowledge the truth: that an explicit goal of the infliction of the trauma in these instances was to prevent the survivor from ever threatening the social, familial, or institutional status quo. The trauma-exposed suffering person is left in a state of complete dorsal vagal freeze coupled with chronic SNS terror activation, both of these engendered by threat of revictimization should the suffering person find within themselves the capacity to resist in some way. Silencing is also accomplished via the energetic debilitation of the entire body and spirit and the draining of personal and community resources, wrought by the trauma itself. Thus, in testimonio, survivors are given the feedback, when asked for, that their distress is not a sign of pathology in any way. Even though most such suffering people would qualify for the diagnosis of posttraumatic stress disorder (PTSD), and if seeking asylum or recompense through a legal system may require being given such a diagnosis in order to reach safety or receive reparations, a DHCR healer would of course not define any of this distress or anything done to manage the distress as disorder. Testimonio is the original framework for placing the pathology at the location of the perpetrator and the systemic forms of oppression that enabled, encouraged, and protected the abuses of power that caused harm.

Another component of testimonio is the importance of it being led entirely by the suffering trauma-exposed person. Their stories are told at the speed and with the details necessary for that person to frame the trauma and its continuing aftermaths in the contexts of ordinary life. Narratives of trauma elicited from survivors in order to satisfy the needs of others—be they therapists, immigration officers, or curious and sympathetic supporters—are unlikely to have a healing effect because they are performances, demanded by others for their edification, and suffering traumatized people often sense this voyeuristic undertone when the listener pulls for details of a trauma story that the suffering person does not wish to share but feels coerced to offer in order to get closer to safety.

Offering the opportunity to engage in testimonio is differentiated from assuming that having suffering trauma-exposed people recount their experiences on demand will be helpful. For a healing practice to truly embody the values of testimonio, the suffering person must know that the healing process will be an act of solidarity. The DHCR trauma healer witnessing testimonio has consequently the moral obligation to witness in an active, engaged manner with the survivor, following their lead.

Writing as Healing

Many aspects of testimonio are mirrored in other, non-DHCR practices, such as that promulgated by Pennebaker (1997), who has published an evidence base for the use of writing down the trauma narrative as a therapeutic intervention. Similarly, prolonged exposure (PE) therapies, when done with an awareness on the part of the healer with regard to the social and political contexts informing the trauma and the intersectional identities of the traumatized person, can utilize the development and narration by the suffering person of the story of their trauma, in their own words and at their own pace, in a supportive context as a means of reducing the fear and anxiety classically conditioned to the trauma experience and providing counterconditioning.

But to make these into DHCR healing practices the healer would need to return to questions regarding whether what they are offering meets the criteria outlined in Chapter 12. Is critical consciousness being developed, for example? Simply because some components of trauma treatment as usual appear to mirror some aspects of testimonio does not make them DHCR trauma healing, and healers trained in these official methods must take care not to be seduced into believing that they are doing DHCR work in the absence of foregrounding DHCR principles.

What sets testimonio apart, and thus makes it a truly DHCR trauma healing practice in every way, is its focus on not simply recounting of the traumatic event, as would occur in PE or writing, but essentially and importantly, on the social justice violations that were a component of the trauma and the recovery of meaning, agency, and values by the suffering trauma-exposed person.

These moral and political elements are central and not optional for a practice to be called testimonio. Testimonio is trauma healing that is decolonial at its very core.

LATINX HEALING STRATEGIES

Lillian Comas-Díaz (2022; Comas-Díaz & Jacobsen, 2024), a leading thinker in the fields of liberation and decolonial psychology, has proposed models for healing work that arise specifically from Latinx experiences. These models are of value to all DHCR healing practice because they derive explicitly from the experiences of colonized persons, no matter which specific Latinx group (and they are many and diverse) is being drawn upon.

Comas-Díaz discusses using the liberation psychology strategy of calling back the spirit, a specific form of identity reformulation in which a person's previously devalued and often traumatized, marginalized intersectional identities are brought forward, centered, and healed of the toxins of oppression. She noted that this practice involves the affirmation of a marginalized person's cultural roots and the practices deriving from those roots that a person may have rejected, felt shame about, or hidden in pursuit of the false safety strategy for assimilation, which was discussed at many different points earlier in this volume.

Comas-Díaz also suggests the use of a perspective-taking strategy called *sabiduría*. This healing methodology is similar to that found in many long-colonized and pervasively traumatized cultures. It reframes life's vicissitudes as opportunities for spiritual development and healing that would not have occurred in the absence of the wound. She proposes that Latinx persons have a "cosmic locus of control," (2006, p. 441) in which neither self nor other is perceived as ultimately in charge. Rather, power is seen as coming from divine sources. Notice how similar this is to the role of the Black church in some communities of descendants of formerly enslave persons of African descent, communities that have been chronically subjugated and traumatized; this is a form of critical consciousness in healing in which the power of the suffering person is amplified by that person's relationship to a divine.

This is not a passive stance of the situation being in the hands of the divine, which is how Eurocentric colonizer models for understanding relationships with a divine have biased the thinking of many healers trained in Western, logical positivist, and antireligious perspectives. Rather, it is a paradigm of a partnership between the suffering, traumatized person and a powerful, beneficent energy so as to persist with engagement in the struggle to heal, even while systemic and structural forms of traumatizing oppression continue to manifest daily in the life of the suffering person. When a DHCR healer can enter into this framework with a suffering person of any intersectional identities who has a sense of a relationship with this kind of transpersonal partnership in healing, then the CR—the culturally responsive—component of the work may be deepened by following the lead that Comas-Díaz offers.

Comas-Díaz also discusses at length how to work collaboratively and integratively with Indigenous healers. In Latinx cultures these persons might be identified as santero/as or curandero/as and may be other practitioners of syncretistic spiritualities found within Latinx cultures, noting the powerful influence of spiritual themes in Indigenous understandings of emotional well-being that were present in the Indigenous cultures colonized by Spanish and Portuguese invaders from the 15th century onward. Her model, which draws from her focus on people for whom being Latinx is a central component of intersectional identities, is consistent with the notion of deauthorizing the Eurocentric standards by which healers are presently admitted to the practice of healing traumatized wounded souls.

All of these are constructs that Comas-Díaz presents as necessary for emotional healing in general, holding as a constant the presence of pervasive trauma in the lives and heritages of the Latinx people of whom she writes. But specifically as to trauma, Comas-Díaz (2006) noted that

> although dissociation is clinically viewed as a dysfunctional reaction to trauma, *La Raza* worldview considers dissociation an adaptive response. Indeed, individuals' responses to racial and ethnic trauma through dissociation may not signify avoidance, poor self-esteem, or learned helplessness. On the contrary, they may indicate cultural resilience in interacting within a hostile environment. (p. 442)

In other words, Comas-Díaz's description of dissociation dovetails precisely with discussions at many points earlier in this volume as to the necessity of unknowing danger in order to move through the world and not be paralyzed by fear.

It is worth noting how much of the work already done to develop DHCR trauma healing modalities has come from the Latinx communities: liberation psychology, Latinx healing, testimonio, decolonial psychology. Other work presenting already developed or developing DHCR trauma healing practices has emerged elsewhere in the Global South.

ENGAGED BUDDHIST TRAUMA HEALING PRACTICE

An example of another DHCR healing practice which has been developed over the past 2 decades and more by an American psychologist (Norsworthy & Khuankaew, 2004, 2006, 2008, 2020), whose intersectional identities include

White skin, growing up in financially marginal circumstances, being lesbian, and being an academic (Norsworthy), and a Thai social justice activist, whose intersectional identities include being lesbian, a public intellectual, and a psychotherapist (Khuankaew & Norsworthy, 2005), is engaged Buddhist healing work.

Although only the names of these two authors are attached to this practice, it was in fact developed in continuous collaboration with traumatized people. These authors would sit in listening sessions with people who were not necessarily seeking assistance for healing, persons with very extensive trauma exposure, including experiences of sexual assault, ethnic cleansing, refugee experiences, and other forms of pervasive and persistent trauma. What the authors and the people with whom they collaborated in building their theory had in common was their practice of Buddhism. What Norsworthy brought to this process as a model of how to do DHCR work was that although her own practice of Buddhism was long-standing and deeply rooted, she was aware that, unlike her coauthor and the participants, it had not informed the totality of the cultures in which she lived. Thus, she stood in the position of beginner's mind rather than as the expert from the Global North come to harvest the insights of the Global South so that she might take them away, as colonizers took away the human and natural resources of the Global South for many centuries, giving them an official-sounding new name and claiming to have "discovered" something.

In an article written on the occasion of her receipt of the APA Global Humanitarian Award, Norsworthy was transparent about how she started her work in Thailand and, later, Burma, replicating the roles of Western/Global North person as expert with hegemonic knowledge and Thai person as helper who would translate but had little to offer of value (Norsworthy, 2017). This transparency models what is necessary in DHCR trauma healing practice: a DHCR trauma healer must be attentive to and aware of ways in which these kinds of other than conscious assumptions about who is the expert enter into everything done by people trained in Eurocentric trauma healing modalities.

AND IT'S NOT ONLY FROM THE GLOBAL SOUTH

While they have struggled with desires to become part of the mainstream canon, intersectional feminist, mujerista, and womanist healing practices have been the proto-DHCR models on which this author's DHCR trauma healing epistemics have been founded. All of these practices are grounded in critical consciousness, emphasizing the truth that the personal is political (Brown, 2018; Bryant-Davis & Comas-Díaz, 2016).

These healing practices arose from explicitly political sources; the work of intersectional feminist, mujerista, and womanist activists who included people working in the world of the healing of wounded souls and spirits. All of the healers from these traditions focused on the pathologies of systemic and structural forms of oppression, and womanist and mujerista healers were the crucibles in which feminist therapy reemerged as an intentionally intersectional practice.

Because many healers from these traditions worked with suffering trauma-exposed people, particularly those whose traumas were inflicted in gendered and intimate spaces, careless assumptions have been made that healers from these traditions work solely with women or with survivors of sexual or intimate partner violence. What is more accurate is that healers from these DHCR traditions utilize their deep understanding of the nature of abuses of power as mirrors of the colonized, Eurocentric cultures in which they and the suffering people with whom they work exist. Consequently, as this author (Brown, 2018; Comas-Díaz & Brown, 2016) has commented, these DHCR healing practices are, like testimonio, grounded in the healing of trauma through liberatory means, in which the lived experiences and voices of those who are suffering are centered.

CONTEXTUAL TRAUMA THERAPY: NOT INTENDING TO BE, BUT APPROACHING DECOLONIAL

In the literature on working with traumatized persons that is not positioned as coming from a decolonial or liberatory perspective, it has been refreshing to find the work of Steven N. Gold (full disclosure—a good friend). This work is growing into something that could easily be the first decolonial-sounding trauma healing paradigm emerging from not quite the mainstream of the trauma healing world but close enough, given its author's prominence as a past president of two trauma healing organizations and the first editor of the journal *Trauma Psychology: Theory, Research, Practice, Policy*. Hiding underneath these very mainstream credentials, however, is a revolutionary and, if read carefully, decolonizing paradigm for trauma healing with persons who have grown up with experiences of attachment trauma, betrayal trauma, and emotional deprivation during childhood and are now seeking trauma healing as adults. Gold is calling this paradigm contextual trauma therapy (CTT).

Gold wrote,

> CTT recognizes that among survivors of prolonged child maltreatment, each individual comes to therapy with a unique constellation of factors [or as I would say, with a unique set of intersectionalities]. Each has been influenced by a distinct personal history; family background, trauma history, pattern of diverse gender, racial, sexual orientation, national origin, and religious identifications and experiences; psychological difficulties, developmental deficits; and adaptive strengths. (2020, p. 5)

Gold structures CTT around the intersectionalities of the traumatized person; as he puts it, "a defining feature of CTT is arriving at an awareness of these aspects of the client's experiential background and how they shape the client's functioning and sense of self—rather than structuring treatment primarily around diagnostic categories and corresponding predetermined interventions" (ibid.).

Gold goes on to emphasize the importance of the therapist following the lead of the traumatized person and collaborating with that person on the direction that the trauma work will take. Notably, he is willing to call out the therapist-centric practices of applying "interventions" to people without understanding all of their intersectionalities, which in his case includes a strong focus on early experiences of emotional deprivation. His discussions of how parents in marginalized groups may be unavailable for a child because they are dealing with financial, housing, and food insecurity is remarkable for its weaving together of the experiences of that child, which are traumatizing, and complete empathy for the no-win situation of parents affected by structural and systemic forms of oppression.

Thus, while Gold does not set out to be decolonial, it is my sense that CTT is deeply decolonial in how it thinks about suffering people, healers, and the process of trauma work. It may also provide a door through which more cautious trauma healers might move toward more overtly political and decolonial trauma healing practices. Because Gold spent 3 decades listening carefully to people who experienced the many varieties of "illegitimate" trauma—emotional deprivation, neglect, frank abuse, betrayal, attachment trauma—and thus focused his work on people who are now described as having complex trauma, he allowed himself and his work to be shaped and changed by those suffering people.

CONCLUSION

This is not an exhaustive list of extant DHCR trauma healing practices. I have offered descriptions of these as examples because they are the ones with which I am most familiar, and they serve as clues to the curious who are in search of a DHCR healing practice in which they may ground themselves. Notice, and remember, that each of these extant practices grew spontaneously from a context of layers of historical, political, and colonizing social pathologies, and each formed spontaneously into a healing practice without having to meet the criteria for assessing whether something derived from the world of trauma therapy as usual might be able to be transformed into DHCR work. These are examples of what happens when healing is decolonial from the very beginning, if not early in the development, of a healing practice.

Writing from the perspective of one who was present almost at the creation of what is now called intersectional feminist therapy and who participated actively in its development over the past 50 years to the point where I am misidentified as a founder of feminist therapy (which I was not; I was just the catchiest writer among us), I can attest to how difficult it is to grow a DHCR practice and not be drawn into the epistemics of colonized and colonizing methodologies. I have been present at the struggles, within communities and within myself, as to how to continue walking the path that has led me, at last, to the DHCR vision. When I read what I wrote 10, 20, 30, and 40 years ago as I first entered the space of feminist therapy scholarship, I have to have compassion for that younger self rather than cringe at how indoctrinated into colonized epistemics I then was.

So too, as you search for ways to engage in DHCR trauma healing, have compassion for those who came before. Consider that some of the most brilliant minds in the world of trauma healing were passed by because they were liberatory and genuinely revolutionary at a time when few were willing to hear them. Be willing to be set on the margins; in fact, celebrate a little if that's where you seem to be situated by your commitments to DHCR trauma healing work. You are not alone; you will simply need to take some time to find your people. I am one of them—not a leader, simply one among them.

Look in the mirror. Start with yourself. As I continue to attempt to do, practice humility and compassion as you seek to uncover the ways in which you have been drawn into participation, collusion, been used by colonial epistemics, by the false promises offered to us all in the trauma healing world. Then do that again, and again. When you go to a conference and sit there thinking, "I am weird," make sure you have your DHCR buddy in place to call or text or email about your feelings of alienation. This can happen to anyone; the first time I gave a talk about decolonial practice, I was the keynote speaker at a prestigious conference. I was met with silence, with people leaving the room. The leader of the organization, who had invited me, had read my speech in advance and refused either to introduce me or ask someone else to do so. I had to work hard with myself and my hurt feelings to remember that in the 1930s world of leftists there was a thing later referred to as being "prematurely anti-Fascist"—in other words, knowing that the social pathology of fascism was dangerous and worth fighting against before the leaders of various leftist groups found it convenient to take that stance. Being decolonial is inconvenient, as I learned that day. So it might be inconvenient for you. When it is, come back, read these lines, and know that you're not alone (and at least you're not up in front of 200 people glaring at you like you've just landed from another planet, invading their nice, cozy, "let's talk about six interventions with borderlines" convention—and I'm not joking; there were about that many presentations along those lines at this conference).

I am grateful to the prophets who came before me, to Audre Lorde and Adrienne Rich, to Ignacio Martín-Baró, to those who travel with me—Lillian Comas-Díaz, Beverly Greene, Kathryn Norsworthy, Thema Bryant—who continue to call me to pursue justice in my work as a teacher, a writer, in the ways in which I can be a DHCR trauma healer today, everyone who has ever sat with me, all of my students. I am grateful to every suffering person who took the risk to open their hearts to me. I seek forgiveness from the ones whom I could not see or hear clearly enough, and I forgive myself for having been able to do, to see, to hear, only what was possible through the lenses that I wore at that time.

This practice of humble gratitude, of self-forgiveness, does not excuse us from the continuing practice of critical consciousness, from the ongoing work of discovering how we may be allies to those who our lives make marginal. Self-forgiveness is not an excuse. It is wiping the lenses clear of shame so that we can delve more deeply, see more clearly, the ways in which we have been colonized, the path toward an expanded critical consciousness.

Healing from trauma, despite its ubiquity, despite its power, despite the ways in which it is woven into systemic and structural oppression, despite the presence of social pathologies—healing from trauma is possible. DHCR trauma healing offers, I hope, a path toward that healing.

References

American Psychiatric Association. (1987). *Diagnostic and statistical manual of mental disorders* (3rd ed., revised).

American Psychological Association. (2017a). *Clinical practice guideline for the treatment of posttraumatic stress disorder (PTSD) in adults.* American Psychological Association.

American Psychological Association. (2017b). Multicultural guidelines: An ecological approach to context, identity, and intersectionality, 2017. https://www.apa.org/about/policy/multicultural-guidelines.pdf

American Psychological Association. (2019). *APA guidelines for psychological practice for people with low-income and economic marginalization.* https://www.apa.org/about/policy/guidelines-low-income.pdf

Anderson, A., Chiczuk, S., Nelson, K., Ruther, R., & Wall-Scheffler, C. (2023). The Myth of Man the Hunter: Women's contribution to the hunt across ethnographic contexts. *PLOS ONE, 18*(6), e0287101. https://doi.org/10.1371/journal.pone.0287101

Anzaldúa, G. (1987). *Borderlands: La frontera: The new mestiza.* Aunt Lute Books.

Appiah, K. A. (2022, June 7). Can I withhold medical care from a bigot? *New York Times Magazine.* https://www.nytimes.com/2022/06/07/magazine/withhold-medical-care-racist-ethics.html

Aron, A. (1992). Testimonio: A bridge between psychotherapy and sociotherapy. In O. Espin, E. Rothblum, & E. Cole (Eds.), *Refugee women and their mental health: Shattered societies, shattered lives* (pp. 173–189). Haworth Press.

Bailey, T. D. (2023, August 3). *Exposure begins with "hello."* Presidential Address, Division of Trauma Psychology. Presented at the Convention of the American Psychological Association, Washington, DC, United States.

Barry, E. (2023, April 25). She redefined trauma. Then trauma redefined her. *The New York Times.* https://www.nytimes.com/2023/04/24/health/judith-herman-trauma.html

Becker, D., Lira, E., Castillo, M., Gomez, E., & Kovalskys, J. (1990). Therapy with victims of political repression in Chile: The challenge of social reparation.

Journal of Social Issues, 46(3), 133–149. https://doi.org/10.1111/j.1540-4560. 1990.tb01939.x

Bhatia, S. (2021, August 12–14). Decolonization and coloniality in psychology: Neoliberal subjectivity and narratives of Indian youth [Paper presentation]. In L. Comas-Díaz (Chair), *Decolonial psychotherapy: Healing in context* [Symposium]. Convention of the American Psychological Association, online.

Boston Women's Health Book Collective. (2011). *Our bodies, our selves* (10th ed.). Suffolk University Press.

Brand, B. L., Schielke, H. J., Schiavone, F., & Lanius, R. (2022). *Finding solid ground: Overcoming obstacles in trauma and treatment.* Oxford University Press. https://doi.org/10.1093/med-psych/9780190636081.001.0001 https://topddstudy.com/researchteam.php

Braun, B. G. (1988). The BASK model of dissociation. *Dissociation: Progress in the Dissociative Disorders, 1*(1), 4–23.

Briere, J., & Scott, C. (2014). *Principles of trauma therapy: A guide to symptoms, evaluation, and treatment (DSM-5 update)* (2nd ed.). Sage Publications.

Brodkin, K. (1998). *How Jews became white folks and what that says about race in America.* Rutgers University Press.

Brown, L. S. (1986). From alienation to connection: Feminist therapy with post-traumatic stress disorder. *Women & Therapy, 5*(1), 13–26. https://doi.org/10.1300/J015V05N01_05

Brown, L. S. (1994). *Subversive dialogues: Theory in feminist therapy.* Basic Books.

Brown, L. S. (1997). The private practice of subversion: Psychology as *tikkun olam*. *American Psychologist, 52*(4), 449–462. https://doi.org/10.1037/0003-066X.52.4.449

Brown, L. S. (2007). Empathy, genuineness—And the dynamics of power: A feminist responds to Rogers. *Psychotherapy, 44*(3), 257–259. https://doi.org/10.1037/0033-3204.44.3.257

Brown, L. S. (2008). *Cultural competence in trauma therapy: Beyond the flashback.* American Psychological Association. https://doi.org/10.1037/11752-000

Brown, L. S. (2009). *Feminist therapy.* American Psychological Association.

Brown, L. S. (2017). Contributions of feminist and critical psychologies to trauma psychology. In S. N. Gold (Ed.), *APA handbook of trauma psychology: Foundations in knowledge* (pp. 501–526). American Psychological Association. https://doi.org/10.1037/0000019-025

Brown, L. S. (2018). *Feminist therapy* (2nd ed.). American Psychological Association.

Brown, L. S. (2021, August 12–14). Decolonial liberatory intersectional feminist therapy. In L. Comas-Díaz (Chair), *Decolonial psychotherapy: Healing in context* [Symposium]. Convention of the American Psychological Association, online.

Brown, L. S. (2023). Who's afraid of Anne Frank? Or why White Supremacists should fear this book. *Journal of Critical Race and Ethnic Studies, 1*, 128–133.

Brown, L. S., & Courtois, C. A. (2019). Trauma treatment: The need for ongoing innovation. *Practice Innovations, 4*(3), 133–138. https://doi.org/10.1037/pri0000097

Brownmiller, S. (1975). *Against our will: Men, women, and rape*. Simon and Schuster.

Bryant, T. (2023). Psychologists must embrace decolonial psychology. *Monitor on Psychology, 54*, 8.

Bryant-Davis, T. (2005). *Thriving in the wake of trauma: A multicultural guide*. Rowman and Littlefield.

Bryant-Davis, T., & Comas-Díaz, L. (Eds.). (2016). *Womanist and mujerista psychologies: Voices of fire, acts of courage*. American Psychological Association. https://doi.org/10.1037/14937-000

Burton, M., & Guzzo, R. (2020). Liberation psychology: Origins and development. In L. Comas-Díaz & E. Torres-Rivera (Eds.), *Liberation psychology: Theory, method, practice, and social justice* (pp. 17–40). American Psychological Association. https://doi.org/10.1037/0000198-002

Caplan, P. (1995). *They say you're crazy: How the world's most powerful psychiatrists decide who's normal*. DaCapo Lifelong Books.

Cassingham, B. J., & O'Neill, S. M. (1993). *And then I met this woman: Previously married women's journeys into lesbian relationships*. Mother Courage Press.

Chesler, P. (1972). *Women and madness*. Doubleday.

Chesler, P., Rothblum, E. D., & Cole, E. (Eds.). (1995). *Feminist foremothers in women's studies, psychology, and mental health*. Harrington Park Press.

Cienfuegos, A. J., & Monelli, C. (1983). The testimony of political repression as a therapeutic instrument. *American Journal of Orthopsychiatry, 53*(1), 43–51. https://doi.org/10.1111/j.1939-0025.1983.tb03348.x

Clance, P. R., & Imes, S. A. (1978). The imposter phenomenon in high achieving women: Dynamics and therapeutic intervention. *Psychotherapy, 15*(3), 241–247. https://doi.org/10.1037/h0086006

Clifton, L. (1987). *How to carry water: Selected poems*. BOA Editions Ltd.

Coale, H. W. (1998). *The vulnerable therapist: Practicing in an age of anxiety*. Haworth Press.

Comas-Díaz, L. (1994). LatiNegra: Mental health issues of African Latinas. *Journal of Feminist Family Therapy, 5*(3–4), 35–74. https://doi.org/10.1300/J086v05n03_03

Comas-Díaz, L. (2006). Latino healing: The integration of ethnic psychology into psychotherapy. *Psychotherapy, 43*(4), 436–453. https://doi.org/10.1037/0033-3204.43.4.436

Comas-Díaz, L. (2010). On being a Latina healer: Voice, consciousness, and identity. *Psychotherapy, 47*(20), 162–168. https://doi.org/10.1037/a0019758

Comas-Díaz, L. (2012a). *Multicultural care: A clinician's guide to cultural competence*. American Psychological Association. https://doi.org/10.1037/13491-000

Comas-Díaz, L. (2012b). Psychotherapy as a healing practice, scientific endeavor, and social justice action. *Psychotherapy, 49*(4), 473–474. https://doi.org/10.1037/a0027820

Comas-Díaz, L. (2020). Liberation psychotherapy. In L. Comas-Díaz & E. Torres-Rivera (Eds.), *Liberation psychology: Theory, method, practice, and social justice* (pp. 169–186). American Psychological Association. https://doi.org/10.1037/0000198-010

Comas-Díaz, L. (2021). AfroLatinx: Decolonization, healing, and liberation. *Journal of Latinx Psychology, 9*(1), 65–75. https://doi.org/10.1037/lat0000164

Comas-Díaz, L. (2022). Decolonization: A personal manifesto. *Women & Therapy, 45*(4), 304–319. https://doi.org/10.1080/02703149.2022.2125617

Comas-Díaz, L., Adames, H. Y., & Chavez-Dueñas, N. Y. (Eds.). (2024). *Decolonial psychology: Toward anticolonial theories, research, training, and practice.* American Psychological Association. https://doi.org/10.1037/0000376-000

Comas-Díaz, L., & Brown, L. S. (2016). Multicultural theories. In J. C. Norcross, G. R. VandenBos, & D. K. Freedheim (Eds.), *APA handbook of clinical psychology: Theory and research* (pp. 241–272). American Psychological Association. https://doi.org/10.1037/14773-009

Comas-Díaz, L., Hall, G. N., & Neville, H. A. (2019). Racial trauma: Theory, research, and healing. *American Psychologist, 74*(1), 1–5. https://doi.org/10.1037/amp0000442

Comas-Díaz, L., & Jacobsen, F. M. (2001). Ethnocultural allodynia. *Journal of Psychotherapy Practice and Research, 10*(4), 246–252.

Comas-Díaz, L., & Jacobsen, F. M. (2024). Decolonial psychotherapy: Joining the circle, healing the wound. In L. Comas-Díaz, H. Y. Adames, & N. Y. Chavez-Dueñas (Eds.), *Decolonial psychology: Toward anticolonial theories, research, training, and practice* (pp. 295–320). American Psychological Association. https://doi.org/10.1037/0000376-013

Comas-Díaz, L., & Torres-Rivera, E. (Eds.). (2020). *Liberation psychology: Theory, method, practice, and social justice.* American Psychological Association. https://doi.org/10.1037/0000198-000

Combahee River Collective. (1977). The Combahee River Collective statement.

Combahee River Collective. (1983). The Combahee River Collective statement. In B. Smith (Ed.), *Home girls: A Black feminist anthology* (pp. 272–282). Kitchen Table: Women of Color Press.

Courtois, C. (2020). *It's not you, it's what happened to you.* Telemachus Press.

Courtois, C. A., & Brown, L. S. (2019). Guideline orthodoxy and resulting limitations of the American Psychological Association's *Clinical Practice Guideline for the Treatment of PTSD in Adults. Psychotherapy, 56*(3), 329–339. https://doi.org/10.1037/pst0000239

Crenshaw, K. W. (1989). Demarginalizing the intersection of race and sex: A Black feminist critique of antidiscrimination doctrine, feminist theory and antiracist politics. *University of Chicago Legal Forum, 1989*(1), 8.

Dana, D. (2018). *The polyvagal theory in therapy.* W. W. Norton.

Danieli, Y. (1980). Countertransference in the treatment and study of Nazi Holocaust survivors and their children. *Victimology: An International Journal, 5*(2–4), 355–367.

Danieli, Y. (1988). On not confronting the Holocaust: Psychological reactions to victim/survivors and their children. In *Remembering for the future, Theme II: The impact of the Holocaust on the contemporary world* (pp. 1257–1271). Oxford: Pergamon Press.

Danieli, Y. (Ed.). (1998). *International handbook of multigenerational legacies of trauma*. Springer. https://doi.org/10.1007/978-1-4757-5567-1

de Beauvoir, S. (1953). *The second sex* (H. M. Parshley, Trans.). Jonathan Cape. (Original work published 1949)

Denmark, F. L. (1995). Feminist and activist. In P. Chesler, E. D. Rothblum, & E. Cole (Eds.), *Feminist foremothers in women's studies, psychology, and mental health* (pp. 163–170). Harrington Park Press.

DePrince, A. P., & Freyd, J. J. (2001). Memory and dissociative tendencies: The roles of attentional context and word meaning in a directed forgetting task. *Journal of Trauma & Dissociation, 2*(2), 67–82. https://doi.org/10.1300/J229v02n02_06

Deutsch, H. (1944). *The psychology of women*. Grune and Stratton.

DiAngelo, R. (2018). *White fragility: Why it's so hard for white people to talk about racism*. Beacon Press.

Duberman, M. (2002). *Cures: A gay man's odyssey*. Basic Books. Association.

Duncan, B. L., Miller, S. D., Wampold, B. E., & Hubble, M. A. (Eds.). (2010). *The heart and soul of change: Delivering what works in therapy* (2nd ed.). American Psychological Association. https://doi.org/10.1037/12075-000

Duran, E. (2007, January 24–26). *Liberation psychology: An ongoing practice in American Indian country*. Fifth National Multicultural Conference and Summit, Seattle, WA. https://bhjustice.org/wp-content/uploads/2022/02/National_Multicultural_Conference_and_Summit_2007.pdf

Duran, E., Duran, B., Brave Heart, M., & Yellow Horse-Davis, S. (1998). Healing the American Indian soul wound. In Y. Danieli (Ed.), *International handbook of multigenerational legacies of trauma* (pp. 341–354). Plenum. https://doi.org/10.1007/978-1-4757-5567-1_22

Estrich, S. (1988). *Real rape: How the legal system victimizes women who say no*. Harvard University Press.

Fals-Borda, O., & Rahman, M. A. (Eds.). (1991). *Action and knowledge: Breaking the monopoly with participatory action research*. Apex Press. https://doi.org/10.3362/9781780444239

Fanon, F. (1967). *Black skin, white masks*. Grove Press.

Fanon, F. (1972). *The wretched of the earth*. Grove Press.

Feinberg, L. (2004). *Stone butch blues*. Alyson Books.

Ford, J. D., & Courtois, C. A. (Eds.). (2020). *Treating complex traumatic stress disorders in adults: Scientific foundations and therapeutic models* (2nd ed.). Guilford Press.

Fors, M. (2018). *A grammar of power in psychotherapy: Exploring the dynamics of privilege*. American Psychological Association. https://doi.org/10.1037/0000086-000

Fox, D., & Prilleltensky, I. (Eds.). (1997). *Critical psychology: An introduction*. Sage.

Freire, P. (1972). *Pedagogy of the oppressed*. Penguin Random House.

Freire, P., & Macedo, D. (1987). *Literacy: Reading the word and the world*. Bergin & Garvey.

Freyd, J. J. (1996). *Betrayal trauma: The logic of forgetting abuse*. Harvard University Press.

Gabbard, G. (1989). *Sexual exploitation in professional relationships*. American Psychiatric Association Press.

Gay, R. (2022). *Inciting joy: Essays*. Algonquin Books.

Gaztambide, D. J. (2019). *A people's history of psychoanalysis: From Freud to liberation psychology*. Lexington Books.

Gaztambide, D. J. (2020). From Freud to Fanon to Freire: Psychoanalysis as liberation method. In L. Comas-Díaz & E. Torres-Rivera (Eds.), *Liberation psychology: Theory, method, practice, and social justice* (pp. 71–90). American Psychological Association. https://doi.org/10.1037/0000198-005

George, E. (2006). *What came before he shot her*. HarperCollins.

Gleason, J. (Creator), & Satenstein, F. (Director). (1955–1956). *The honeymooners* [Television series].

Gold, S. N. (2020). *Contextual trauma therapy: Overcoming traumatization and reaching full potential*. American Psychological Association. https://doi.org/10.1037/0000176-000

Gómez, J. M. (2023). *The cultural betrayal of Black women and girls: A Black feminist approach to healing from sexual abuse*. American Psychological Association. https://doi.org/10.1037/0000362-000

Gourevitch, P. (1998). *We wish to inform you that tomorrow we will be killed with our families: Stories from Rwanda*. Farrar, Straus and Giroux.

Greene, B. (1990). What has gone before: The legacy of racism and sexism in the lives of black mothers and daughters. In L. S. Brown & M. P. P. Root (Eds.), *Diversity and complexity in feminist therapy* (pp. 207–230). Haworth.

Greene, B. (1992). Still here: A perspective on psychotherapy with African American women. In J. C. Chrisler & D. Howard (Eds.), *New directions in feminist psychology: Practice, theory, and research* (pp. 13–25). Haworth.

Greene, B. (2000). African American lesbian and bisexual women in feminist-psychodynamic psychotherapy: Surviving and thriving between a rock and a hard place. In L. Jackson & B. Greene (Eds.), *Psychotherapy with African American women: Innovations in psychodynamic perspectives and practice* (pp. 82–125). Guilford Press.

Greene, B. (2007, January 24–26). *The complexity of diversity: Multiple identities and the denial of social privilege*. Fifth National Multicultural Conference and Summit, Seattle, WA, United States.

Guthrie, R. V. (1976). *Even the rat was White: A historical view of psychology*. Harper & Row.

Haizlip, S. T. (1995). *The sweeter the juice: A family memoir in black and white*. Simon & Schuster.

Haldeman, D. (2002). Gay rights, patient rights: The implications of sexual orientation conversion therapy. *Professional Psychology: Research and Practice, 33*(3), 260–264. https://doi.org/10.1037/0735-7028.33.3.260

Hammerstein, O., II, & Rodgers, R. (1949). You've got to be carefully taught [Song]. In *South Pacific*.

Hannah-Jones, N. (2021). *The 1619 project: A new origin story*. One World.

Harvey, M. R. (1996). An ecological view of psychological trauma and trauma recovery. *Journal of Traumatic Stress, 9*(1), 3–23. https://doi.org/10.1002/jts.2490090103

Hays, P. A. (2022). *Addressing cultural complexities in counseling and clinical practice: An intersectional approach* (4th ed.). American Psychological Association. https://doi.org/10.1037/0000277-000

Helms, J. (2019). *A race is a nice thing to have: A guide to being a white person or understanding the white persons in your life* (3rd ed.). Cognella Academic Publishing.

Herman, J. L. (1992). *Trauma and recovery: The aftermath of violence from domestic abuse to political terror*. Basic Books.

Herman, J. L. (2023). *Truth and repair: How trauma survivors envision justice*. Hachette Book Group.

Hochschild, A. (1998). *King Leopold's ghost: A story of greed, terror, and heroism in colonial Africa*. Mariner Books.

hooks, b. (1982). *Ain't I a woman? Black women and feminism*. South End Press.

Hull, G. T., Bell-Scott, P., & Smith, B. (Eds.). (1982). *All the women are White, all the Blacks are men, but some of us are brave*. Feminist Press.

Jamison, K. R. (2023). *Fires in the dark: Healing the unquiet mind*. Alfred A. Knopf/Borzoi Books.

Janoff-Bulman, R. (1992). *Shattered assumptions*. Free Press.

Jones, R. P. (2023). *The hidden roots of White Supremacy, and the path to a shared American future*. Simon & Schuster.

Josefowitz Siegel, R. (1990). Turning the things that divide us into strengths that unite us. In L. S. Brown & M. P. P. Root (Eds.), *Diversity and complexity in feminist therapy* (pp. 327–336). The Haworth Press.

Kanuha, V. K. (1990). Compounding the triple jeopardy: Battering in lesbian of color relationships. In L. S. Brown & M. P. P. Root (Eds.), *Diversity and complexity in feminist therapy* (pp. 169–184). Haworth Press.

Kaplan, H. I., & Sadock, B. J. (1985). *Comprehensive handbook of psychiatry* (6th ed.). Williams and Wilkins.

Kardiner, A., & Spiegel, H. (1947). *The traumatic neuroses of war*. Hoeber.

Kaschak, E. (1992). *Engendered lives: A new psychology of women's experience*. Basic Books.

Kaschak, E. (2015). *Sight unseen: Gender and race through blind eyes*. Columbia University Press.

Kaschak, E. (2021, December 10). Chronic traumatic terror disorder. *Meer*. https://wsimag.com/wellness/67912-chronic-traumatic-terror-disorder

Khuankaew, O., & Norsworthy, K. (2005). Crossing borders: Activist responses to globalization by women of the Global South. *Occasional Papers on Globalization, 2*(2), 1–12.

Kidder, L. H., & Fine, M. (1987). Qualitative and quantitative methods: When stories converge. *New Directions for Program Evaluation, 1987*(35), 57–75.

Klepfisz, I. (1982). Bashert. *Sinister Wisdom, 21*. https://www.sinisterwisdom.org/issues

Lahousen, T., Unterrainer, H. F., & Kapfhammer, H.-P. (2019). Psychobiology of attachment and trauma—Some general remarks from a clinical perspective. *Frontiers in Psychiatry, 10*. https://doi.org/10.3389/fpsyt.2019.00914

Lerman, H. (1996). *Pigeonholing women's misery: A history and critical analysis of the psychodiagnosis of women in the twentieth century*. Basic Books.

Lerner, G. (1986). *The creation of patriarchy*. Oxford University Press.

Lerner, G. (1994). *The creation of feminist consciousness: From the Middle Ages to 1870*. Oxford University Press.

Lerner, M. J. (1980). The belief in a just world. In *The belief in a just world: A fundamental delusion* (pp. 9–30). Springer. https://doi.org/10.1007/978-1-4899-0448-5_2

Levant, R. F. (1996). The new psychology of men. *Professional Psychology: Research and Practice, 27*(3), 259–265. https://doi.org/10.1037/0735-7028.27.3.259

Levant, R. F. (1998). Desperately seeking language: Understanding, assessing, and treating normative male alexithymia. In W. S. Pollack & R. F. Levant (Eds.), *New psychotherapy for men* (pp. 35–56). Wiley.

Lingiardi, V., & McWilliams, N. (Eds.). (2017). *Psychodynamic diagnostic manual: PDM-2* (2nd ed.). Guilford Press.

Lorde, A. (1984a). The master's tools will never dismantle the master's house. In *Sister outsider: Essays and speeches* (pp. 110–114). The Crossing Press.

Lorde, A. (1984b). *Sister outsider*. Penguin Books.

Lorde, A. (2007). An open letter to Mary Daly. In *Sister outsider: Essays and speeches by Audre Lorde*. The Crossing Press. (Original work published 1979)

Lott, B. (1995). Whoever thought I'd grow up to be a feminist foremother? In P. Chesler, E. D. Rothblum, & E. Cole (Eds.), *Feminist foremothers in women's studies, psychology, and mental health* (pp. 309–324). Harrington Park Press.

Luepnitz, D. A. (1988). *The family interpreted*. Basic Books.

Ma, Z., & Zhang, N. (2021). Brain-wide connectivity architecture. In C. R. Martin, V. R. Preedy, & R. Rajendram (Eds.), *Factors affecting neurodevelopment: Genetics, neurology, behavior and diet* (pp. 643–655). Elsevier. https://doi.org/10.1016/B978-0-12-817986-4.00022-5

Macur, J. (2021, July 24). Simone Biles and the weight of perfection. *New York Times*. https://www.nytimes.com/2021/07/24/sports/olympics/simone-biles-gymnastics.html

Maldonado-Torres, N. (2007). On the coloniality of being: Contributions to the development of a concept. *Cultural Studies, 21*(2–3), 240–270. https://doi.org/10.1080/09502380601162548

Marsella, A. J., Friedman, M. J., Gerrity, E. T., & Scurfield, R. M. (Eds.). (1996). *Ethnocultural aspects of posttraumatic stress disorder: Issues, research, and clinical applications*. American Psychological Association. https://doi.org/10.1037/10555-000

Martín-Baró, I. (1994). *Writings for a liberation psychology*. Harvard University Press.

Marx, K. (1844). *Economic and philosophical manuscripts of 1844: Estranged labor.* Marxist Internet Archive. https://www.marxists.org/archive/marx/works/1844/manuscripts/labour.htm

Masson, J. M. (1984). *The assault on truth: Freud's suppression of the seduction theory*. Pocket Books.

McFarlane, A. (2006, November 4–6). Is there a growing conservatism in the field of traumatic stress? In A. McFarlane (Chair), *Past Presidents' Symposium*. Annual Meeting of the International Society for Traumatic Stress Studies, Los Angeles, CA, United States.

McWilliams, N. (2004). *Psychoanalytic psychotherapy: A practitioner's guide*. Guilford Press.

Memmi, A. (1965). *The colonizer and the colonized*. Beacon Press.

Memmi, A. (2017). *Tunisie, an I: Journal tunisien 1955–1956 suivi de Tunisie, un pays d'opérette et Autres écrits des années tunisiennes* [Tunisia, year one: Tunisian journal 1955–1956, followed by Tunisia, a country of operetta, and other writings from the Tunisian years]. CNRS Editions.

Mitchell, J. (1971). A case of you [Song]. On *Blue*. Reprise Records.

Money, J., & Erhardt, A. (1972). *Man and woman, boy and girl: Differentiation and dimorphism of gender identity from conception to maturity*. Johns Hopkins University Press.

Montero, M., Sonn, C. C., & Burton, M. (2017). Community psychology and liberation psychology: A creative synergy for an ethical and transformative praxis. In M. A. Bond, I. Serrano-García, C. B. Keys, & M. Shinn (Eds.), *APA handbook of community psychology: Theoretical foundations, core concepts, and emerging challenges* (pp. 149–167). American Psychological Association. https://doi.org/10.1037/14953-007

Moraga, C., & Anzaldúa, G. (Eds.). (1981). *This bridge called my back: Writings by radical women of color.* Persephone Press.

Morris, J. F., & Espin, O. M. (1995). Bridging feminism and multiculturalism. In P. Chesler, E. D. Rothblum, & E. Cole (Eds.), *Feminist foremothers in women's studies, psychology, and mental health* (pp. 187–194). Harrington Park Press.

Morrow, S. L., & Hawxhurst, D. (2013). Political analysis: Cornerstone of feminist multicultural counseling and psychotherapy. In C. Z. Enns & E. N. Williams (Eds.), *The Oxford handbook of feminist multicultural counseling psychology* (pp. 339–357). Oxford University Press.

Morton, L., Cogan, N., Kolacz, J., Calderwood, C., Nikolic, M., Bacon, T., Pathe, E., Williams, D., & Porges, S. W. (2024). A new measure of feeling safe: Developing psychometric properties of the Neuroception of Psychological Safety Scale (NPSS). *Trauma Psychology: Theory, Research, Practice, Policy, 16*(4), 701–708. https://doi.org/10.1037/tra0001313

Moyers, B. (1988, November 13). *What a real president was like: To Lyndon Johnson, The Great Society meant hope and dignity* [Opinion]. The Washington

Post. https://www.washingtonpost.com/archive/opinions/1988/11/13/what-a-real-president-was-like/d483c1be-d0da-43b7-bde6-04e10106ff6c/

Nadal, K. (2018). *Microaggressions and traumatic stress: Theory, research, and clinical treatment*. American Psychological Association. https://doi.org/10.1037/0000073-000

Near, H. (1974). It could have been me [Song]. On *Holly Near: A live album*. Redwood Records.

Norcross, J. C. (2004). Tailoring the therapy relationship to the individual patient: Evidence-based practices. *Clinician's Research Digest, Supplemental Bulletin 30*(June 2004), 1–2. https://doi.org/10.1037/e375042004-001

Norcross, J. C., & Cooper, M. (2021). *Personalizing psychotherapy: Assessing and accommodating patient preferences*. American Psychological Association. https://doi.org/10.1037/0000221-000

Norcross, J. C., & Lambert, M. J. (Eds.). (2019). *Psychotherapy relationships that work: Vol. 1. Evidence-based therapist contributions* (3rd ed.). Oxford University Press.

Norcross, J. C., & Wampold, B. E. (Eds.). (2019a). *Psychotherapy relationships that work: Vol. 2. Evidence-based responsiveness* (3rd ed.). Oxford University Press.

Norcross, J. C., & Wampold, B. E. (2019b). Relationships and responsiveness in the psychological treatment of trauma: The tragedy of the APA clinical practice guideline. *Psychotherapy, 56*(3), 391–399. https://doi.org/10.1037/pst0000228

Norsworthy, K. (2007, August 17–20). Multicultural feminist collaboration and healing from gender-based violence in Burma [Paper presentation]. In E. N. Williams (Chair), *International perspectives on feminist multicultural psychotherapy—Content and connection*. Symposium presented at the annual convention of the American Psychological Association, San Francisco, CA, United States.

Norsworthy, K. L. (2017). Mindful activism: Embracing the complexities of international border crossings. *American Psychologist, 72*(9), 1035–1043. https://doi.org/10.1037/amp0000262

Norsworthy, K. L., Abrams, E. M., & Lindlau, S. (2013). Activism, advocacy, and social justice in feminist multicultural counseling psychology. In C. Z. Enns & E. N. Williams (Eds.), *The Oxford handbook of feminist multicultural counseling psychology* (pp. 465–484). Oxford University Press.

Norsworthy, K. L., & Khuankaew, O. (2004). Women of Burma speak out: Workshops to deconstruct gender-based violence and build systems of peace and justice. *Journal for Specialists in Group Work, 29*(3), 259–283. https://doi.org/10.1080/01933920490477011

Norsworthy, K. L., & Khuankaew, O. (2006). Bringing social justice to international practices of counseling psychology. In R. Toporek, L. B. Gerstein, N. A. Fouad, G. Roysircar, & T. Israel (Eds.), *Handbook for social justice in counseling psychology* (pp. 421–441). Sage. https://doi.org/10.4135/9781412976220.n29

Norsworthy, K. L., & Khuankaew, O. (2008). A new view from women of Thailand about gender, sexuality, and HIV/AIDS. *Feminism & Psychology, 18*(4), 527–536. https://doi.org/10.1177/0959353508095534

Norsworthy, K. L., & Khuankaew, O. (2020). Transnational feminist liberation psychology: Decolonizing border crossings. In L. Comas-Díaz & E. Torres Rivera (Eds.), *Liberation psychology: Theory, method, practice, and social justice* (pp. 225–243). American Psychological Association. https://doi.org/10.1037/0000198-013

Northrup, S. (1853). *Twelve years a slave.* Book in public domain, no publisher listed.

Ochberg, F. M. (1988). *Post-traumatic therapy and victims of violence.* Brunner/Mazel.

Oliver, M. (2005). *New and selected poems.* Beacon Press.

Pearlman, L. A., & Saakvitne, K. W. (1995). *Trauma and the therapist: Countertransference and vicarious traumatization in psychotherapy with incest survivors.* W. W. Norton.

Pelikan, J. (1997). *The illustrated Jesus through the centuries.* Yale University Press.

Pennebaker, J. (1997). Writing about emotional experiences as a therapeutic process. *Psychological Science, 8*(3), 162–166. https://doi.org/10.1111/j.1467-9280.1997.tb00403.x

Pope, K. S. (2016). The Hoffman Report and the American Psychological Association: Meeting the challenge of change [Appendix A]. In K. S. Pope & M. J. T. Vasquez (Eds.), *Ethics in psychotherapy and counseling* (5th ed., pp. 361–369). Wiley.

Pope, K. S., Sonne, J., & Holroyd, J. (1994). *Sexual feelings in psychotherapy: Explorations for therapists and therapists-in-training.* American Psychological Association.

Porges, S. (2011). *The polyvagal theory: Neurophysiological foundations of emotions, attachment, communication, and self-regulation.* W. W. Norton.

Porges, S., & Dana, D. (2018). *Clinical applications of the polyvagal theory: The emergence of polyvagal-informed therapies.* W. W. Norton.

Protacio Marcellino, E. (1990). Towards understanding the psychology of the Filipino. In L. S. Brown & M. P. P. Root (Eds.), *Diversity and complexity in feminist therapy* (pp. 105–128). Harrington Park Press.

Puller, L. B., Jr. (2000). *Fortunate son: The healing of a Vietnam vet.* Grove Press.

Raine, N. V. (1998). *After long silence: Rape and my journey back.* Crown.

Rippere, V., & Williams, R. (Eds.). (1987). *Wounded healers: Mental health workers' experiences of depression.* Wiley.

Rivers, W. H. R. (1918). The repression of war experience. *Proceedings of the Royal Society of Medicine, 1918*(11), 1–20. https://doi.org/10.1177/003591571801101501

Rogers, A. G. (1995). *A shining affliction: A story of harm and healing in psychotherapy.* Viking Penguin.

Rogers, C. (1961). *On becoming a person: A therapist's view of psychotherapy.* Houghton Mifflin.

Rogers, C., & Stevens, B. (Eds.). (1971). *Person to person: The problem of being human.* Pocket Books.

Root, M. P. P. (1992). Reconstructing the impact of trauma on personality. In L. S. Brown & M. Ballou (Eds.), *Personality and psychopathology: Feminist reappraisals* (pp. 229–265). Guilford Press.

Root, M. P. P. (1998). Experiences and processes affecting racial identity development: Preliminary results from the Biracial Sibling Project. *Cultural Diversity and Mental Health, 4,* 237–247. https://doi.org/10.1037/1099-9809.4.3.237

Root, M. P. P. (2000). Rethinking racial identity development: An ecological framework. In P. Spickard & J. Burroughs (Eds.), *We are a people: Narrative in the construction and deconstruction of ethnic identity* (pp. 205–220). Temple University Press.

Root, M. P. P. (2004, July 28–August 1). *Mixed race identities: Theory, research, and practice* [Continuing education workshop], 11th Annual Convention of the American Psychological Association, Honolulu, HI, United States.

Rubin, Z., & Peplau, L. A. (1975). Who believes in a just world? *Journal of Social Issues, 31*(3), 65–89. https://doi.org/10.1111/j.1540-4560.1975.tb00997.x

Russell, G. M. (1996). Internalized classism: The role of class in the development of self. *Women & Therapy, 18*(3–4), 59–71. https://doi.org/10.1300/J015v18n03_07

Saks Berman, J. (1985). Ethical feminist perspective on dual relationships with clients. In L. B. Rosewater & L. E. A. Walker (Eds.), *Handbook of feminist therapy: Women's issues in psychotherapy* (pp. 287–296). Springer Publishing.

Sanchez-Hucles, J. V. (1998). Racism: Emotional abusiveness and psychological trauma for ethnic minorities. *Journal of Emotional Abuse, 1*(2), 69–87. https://doi.org/10.1300/J135v01n02_04

Schore, A. N. (2003). *Affect regulation and disorders of the self.* W. W. Norton.

Sehgal, P. (2022, January 3 & 10). The key to me. *The New Yorker.*

Shapiro, F. (1989). Eye movement desensitization: A new treatment for post-traumatic stress disorder. *Journal of Behavior Therapy and Experimental Psychiatry, 20*(3), 211–217. https://doi.org/10.1016/0005-7916(89)90025-6

Shay, J. (1994). *Achilles in Vietnam: Combat trauma and the undoing of character.* Scribner Touchstone Editions.

Silverstein, L. B., & Auerbach, C. G. (1999). Deconstructing the essential father. *American Psychologist, 54*(6), 397–407. https://doi.org/10.1037/0003-066X.54.6.397

Smith, C. P., & Freyd, J. J. (2014). Institutional betrayal. *American Psychologist, 69*(6), 575–587. https://doi.org/10.1037/a0037564

Snell, J. E., Rosenwald, R. J., & Robey, A. (1964). The wifebeater's wife: A study of family interaction. *Archives of General Psychiatry, 11*(2), 107–112. https://doi.org/10.1001/archpsyc.1964.01720260001001

Stark, M. (1999). *Modes of psychotherapeutic action: Enhancement of knowledge, provision of experience, and engagement in relationship*. Jason Aaronson.

Sue, D. W. (2010). *Microaggressions in everyday life: Race, gender, and sexual orientation*. Wiley.

Sue, S., Zane, N., Levant, R. F., Silverstein, L. B., Brown, L. S., Olkin, R., & Taliaferro, G. (2006). How well do both evidence-based practices and treatment as usual satisfactorily address the various dimensions of diversity? In J. C. Norcross, L. E. Beutler, & R. F. Levant (Eds.), *Evidence-based practices in mental health: Debate and dialogue on the fundamental questions* (pp. 329–374). American Psychological Association. https://doi.org/10.1037/11265-008

Surrey, J. L. (1985). Self-in-relation: A theory of women's development. *Work in Progress*. Stone Center for Developmental Services and Studies at Wellesley College. https://growthinconnection.org/wp-content/uploads/2021/03/1985Self-in-Relation.pdf

Torres Rivera, E. (2020). Concepts of liberation psychology. In L. Comas-Díaz & E. Torres Rivera (Eds.), *Liberation psychology: Theory, method, practice, and social justice* (pp. 41–52). American Psychological Association. https://doi.org/10.1037/0000198-003

Townshend, P. (1971). Won't get fooled again [Song]. On *Who's Next*. Decca.

Truman, J. L., & Morgan, R. E. (2022). Violent victimization by sexual orientation and gender identity, 2017–2020. Bureau of Justice Statistics. https://bjs.ojp.gov/library/publications/violent-victimization-sexual-orientation-and-gender-identity-2017-2020

Trump, M. L. (2020). *Too much and never enough: How my family created the world's most dangerous man*. Simon and Schuster.

Tummala-Narra, P. (2016). *Psychoanalytic theory and cultural competence in psychotherapy*. American Psychological Association. https://doi.org/10.1037/14800-000

Unger, R. K. (1989). *Representations: Social constructions of gender*. Baywood.

van der Kolk, B. A. (1994). The body keeps the score: Memory and the evolving psychobiology of posttraumatic stress. *Harvard Review of Psychiatry, 1*(5), 253–265. https://doi.org/10.3109/10673229409017088

Vasquez, M. J. T. (2007). Cultural difference and the therapeutic alliance: An evidence-based analysis. *American Psychologist, 62*(8), 878–885. https://doi.org/10.1037/0003-066X.62.8.878

Walker, L. E. A. (1979). *The battered woman syndrome*. Springer Publishing.

Walker, N. (2021). *Neuroqueer heresies: Notes on the neurodiversity paradigm, autistic empowerment, and postnormal possibilities*. Autonomous Press.

Weathers, F. W., Litz, B. T., Keane, T. M., Palmieri, P. A., Marx, B. P., & Schnurr, P. P. (2013). *The PTSD checklist for DSM-5 (PCL-5)*. National Center for PTSD. https://www.ptsd.va.gov/professional/assessment/adult-sr/ptsd-checklist.asp

Weisstein, N. (1968). *Kinder, kuche, kirche as scientific law: Psychology constructs the female*. New England Free Press.

Winter, J. (2006). *Remembering war: The great war between memory and history in the 20th Century.* Yale University Press.

Zapata, K. (2020, February 27). Decolonizing mental health: The importance of an oppression-focused mental health system. *Calgary Journal.* https://calgaryjournal.ca/2020/02/27/decolonizing-mental-health-the-importance-of-an-oppression-focused-mental-health-system/

Index

About the Author

Laura S. Brown, PhD, ABPP, has practiced trauma work in Seattle, Washington, living on unceded Duwamish land, since 1976. Currently primarily a consultant, speaker, and author on decolonial, liberatory, intersectional feminist therapy theory and practice, she offers workshops and training to professionals around the world in such places as Israel, Taiwan, Australia, Ireland, and The Netherlands, as well as offering talks for the general public on such topics as trauma work, self-care for trauma workers, cultural responsivity, and the ethical challenges of this work. She is the past president of the American Psychological Association (APA) Division of Trauma Psychology (Division 56), as well as of the Society for the Psychology of Women, APA Division 35, and of the Society for the Study of Sexual Orientation and Gender Diversity, APA Division 44, and of the Washington State Psychological Association. She served as Member at Large for Diversity on the Executive Committee of the Society for the Study of Culture, Ethnicity and Race, APA Division 45, and on the Publication Board of the Society for the Advancement of Psychotherapy, APA Division 29.

She is a Fellow of eight APA divisions and the International Society for the Study of Trauma and Dissociation, and a diplomate in clinical psychology of the American Board of Professional Psychology. She was a founding member of the Feminist Therapy Institute. Throughout her career, she has received many awards, including the Lifetime Achievement Award from the Division of Trauma Psychology of the APA in 2015, the Elder Award at the National Multicultural Conference and Summit in 2019, and the Christine Blasey Ford Women of Courage Award from the Association for Women in Psychology in 2023.